Over the Influence

Over the Influence

THE HARM REDUCTION GUIDE FOR MANAGING DRUGS AND ALCOHOL

Patt Denning

Jeannie Little

Adina Glickman

THE GUILFORD PRESS

New York / London

The information in this volume is not intended as a substitute for
consultation with healthcare professionals. Each individual's health
concerns should be evaluated by a qualified professional.

Printed in the United States of America

This book is printed on acid-free paper.

Last digit is print number: 9 8 7 6 5 4 3 2 1

Library of Congress Cataloging-in-Publication Data

Denning, Patt, 1950–
    Over the influence: the harm reduction guide for managing
  drugs and alcohol / Patt Denning, Jeannie Little, Adina Glickman.
      p. cm.
    Includes bibliographical references and index.
    ISBN 1-57230-947-4 — ISBN 1-57230-800-1 (pbk.)
    1. Substance abuse—Prevention—Popular works.   2. Self-care,
Health.   I. Little, Jeannie.   II. Glickman, Adina.   III. Title.
    RC564.29.D46 2004
    613.8—dc21

                                          2003013729

To the memory of Steve, who helped me understand that the clients we see are strong and have many important lessons to teach. I learned to adopt a harm reduction approach from him as he struggled with emotional, drug, and medical problems that would have overwhelmed a lesser person and, without his guidance, would have overwhelmed me.

—P. D.

To the many members of the Sobriety Support Group at the VA's Comprehensive Homeless Center in San Francisco. Your stories and your ability to take care of yourselves and others, despite staggering obstacles, continue to inspire me. Thank you.

—J. L.

To my mom, who is a lesson in love.

—A. G.

CONTENTS

Contents

Contents

Contents

ACKNOWLEDGMENTS

A project such as this one requires great stamina not only for us, but for friends, colleagues, clients, family, and other supporters. Rather than write another book thanking all of these people, we have chosen just a few who have been most instrumental, informative, or just plain loyal!

Many people read parts or all of the manuscript and gave important feedback to us. Edith Springer returned the manuscript with pages of comments and ideas that corrected us, elaborated on our ideas, and, most important, reminded us at every turn that harm reduction is based on respect for people's strengths and love for their differences. She has enough material for a book of her own, and we look forward to reading it. Peter Goldblum (once again) helped sculpt the structure as well as the content. Fred Rotgers, who can recite every drug and alcohol treatment research study ever conducted (and did, at a moment's notice, when we needed it), keeps us scientifically honest. Michael and Michelle Aldrich, both of whom carry the entire history of drug use in the United States and the drug policy reform movement in their heads and hearts, gave us invaluable feedback about the integrity of ideas and the accuracy of our drug information. Dan Bigg, the originator of Substance Use Management as a formal intervention with drug users, kept us straight about the best ways to teach people about drugs and safer drug use. Stephanie Muro let us know how people were likely to react emotionally to both the content and the tone of the book.

Marc Kern, Dee Dee Stout, and several participants in self-help programs allowed Adina to interview them to make sure that our ideas about treatment programs and self-help options are accurate and complete.

We have two excellent, enthusiastic, and deeply involved editors: Kitty Moore and Christine Benton. Chris must have edited this book for us and with us ten times. Kitty is a major supporter of harm reduction and rallied the folks at The Guilford Press around the book. Both are extremely sophisticated about the ideas in this book, an unbelievable stroke of luck.

Our deepest thanks to the Board and the Advisory Council of the Harm Reduction Therapy Center, who work alongside us to bring our clinical work to fruition. Thanks also to Nancy Weingarten, whose support takes many delightful turns. Patt's mentor, Alan Marlatt, has opened up many opportunities for her, including her original introduction to Guilford. Jeannie's mentors, Paul Geltner and Bob Unger, understood harm reduction with no need for explanation and have contributed to the development of her skills and career for many years. Adina's team of readers, Lisa Rosenthal, Joan Corn, and Whit Fletcher, reassured often, challenged frequently, and offered up their much needed wisdom at all hours of the writing process. Lively conversations with Dr. Patience Stoddard gave Adina deeper insight into the contribution of faith to trauma recovery.

At least five organizations and their members have led the way for harm reduction: the Harm Reduction Coalition, the Chicago Recovery Alliance, the Drug Policy Alliance, Albuquerque Health Care for the Homeless, and Moderation Management have been inspirational to us over the years because of their tireless efforts to reform treatment and policy in the United States.

Finally, and most important, we offer our respect and our thanks to the hundreds of clients who have trusted us with their stories, their pain, their strengths, disappointments, and successes. Each one of them shared intimate, often humorous, details of his or her struggle with drugs and with a society that often failed to provide support. These clients gave this book its spirit and spunk.

PREFACE
Who Needs This Book?

This book is for everyone who is interested in or concerned about alcohol or other drug use—your own or that of someone you care about.

If you drink alcohol or use other drugs, and you want to be more informed . . .

If you've suffered health or relationship problems, and you think they're related to your drug or alcohol use . . .

If you've gotten into legal trouble because of your alcohol or drug use . . .

If you have emotional problems, and you've been rejected by therapists or doctors because you also drink alcohol or use other drugs . . .

If you want to quit, have tried but not succeeded, and feel discouraged . . .

If you don't buy the idea that you have a disease, or you don't feel comfortable with the spiritual program of Alcoholics Anonymous and the 12 Steps . . .

If you've been in substance abuse treatment, because there was no other option, and have failed at the only goal that's valued: abstinence . . .

If you, as the parent, child, friend, cousin, or colleague of someone who is drinking or using, are worried and want a fresh approach to understanding what's going on . . .

THIS BOOK MIGHT HELP.

If you recognize yourself among the preceding types of drinkers or drug users, you might have experienced feelings of fear, guilt, shame, or loneliness. You might have struggled with the idea that you "lose control" over yourself, once the "demon" alcohol, cocaine, speed, heroin, or some other drug is in your hands. If you have felt guilt or shame in the past, you might have gone on a binge to bury those feelings and ended up in a Catch-22 of hating your use and then using to hide from your hate. If you have felt alone, your only "friend" might have been your favorite drug.

If you are a concerned witness to someone's alcohol or other drug use, the real or imagined danger you suspect he or she is in might have caused you overwhelming fear or worry. Wondering if you contributed to his drug use might have led you to feel guilty. You might have felt helpless to stop her from sliding into ill health or legal trouble. You might have set firm limits to avoid "codependency" or "enabling" and to protect yourself from the pain of watching what seemed to be the destruction of someone you love. But now the two of you are in conflict, estranged or angry. If you are reading this book because of concern for someone else, there is a special section at the end written specifically to you. Although not necessary, you might find it easier to read if you have taken a look at what your friend or loved one is reading in the rest of the book.

If you are a drinker or drug user just starting to wonder if you have a problem, you may not see yourself in the majority of the examples in this book, because these examples come from our work as therapists and illustrate the experiences of people who are dealing with problems they already know they have. You might find it helpful, however, to learn some new ways of looking at your alcohol or drug use and to read about the process of change, should you decide at some point to try to do some things differently in your life. In the meantime, the substance use management chapter (7) and the drug information section in the middle of the book will give you tips on staying safe in your use.

For anyone using, concerned, or just curious, this book offers new ways to think about and deal with drug and alcohol use. It is an entirely new perspective in the United States, a perspective that challenges the prevailing wisdom that calls "alcoholism" or drug "addiction" a disease, while simultaneously imposing legal sanctions on the users of all but two of those drugs. This new perspective is called *harm reduction.*

We are writing to you from the perspective of therapists who have worked with hundreds of people who use drugs—both the illegal ones and the legal ones. We share the frustrations and fears of our clients who are punished for what has been accepted as a "disease" for over fifty years. We see these punishing attitudes carried over into many of the methods of alcohol and other drug treatment, where the disease model of addiction promotes the idea that "denial," considered one of the major symptoms of the disease, must be confronted before the "addict" or "alcoholic" can begin to "recover." The number of quotation marks in the preceding sentence illustrates our point of view that *the language and the methods of traditional addiction treatment are not the only way.* We are writing this book because we do not believe that drug and alcohol use should be punished. We also do not believe that addiction is a disease. We do not believe that users of alcohol or other drugs practice denial any more than anyone else. Nor, in fact, do we believe that most drug use is addiction.

What we do believe, and what this book is about, is that *people use drugs for reasons.* In our experience and observation, the most common reasons are the pursuit of pleasure and the avoidance of pain. If you use alcohol and other drugs, you are not alone. All cultures have used mind-altering substances for thousands of years in an effort to alter or expand consciousness, enhance pleasure, increase energy, or reduce pain. In the words of a prominent researcher in the biology of the brain, "The attempt to regulate affect—to minimize unpleasant feelings and maximize pleasant ones—is the driving force in human motivation."

We also believe that people develop relationships with drugs. Like all relationships—with husbands, wives, partners, parents, children, bosses, colleagues, neighbors, food, cars, clothing, or the land—some are healthy, others are not. Still others are both healthy *and* harmful. There are a few drugs that are harmful all the time. There are others that are rarely harmful. It depends on which drugs we are using, how "clean" they are, and whether they are legal. But for the most part, some drugs are harmful some of the time and not at other times. It depends on the health of our bodies and minds. It depends on our attitude and what we are looking for in the drug experience. And it depends on what's going on around us. We take a three-dimensional approach to understanding drugs and drug users: The *drug*, the *person*, and the *environment* are all important, and, at any given time, one may be more important than another.

People come to us because they, or others around them, are concerned about some aspect of their relationship with drugs. The goal of our work is to help people develop a healthy relationship with alcohol and other drugs—in essence, to help them practice harm reduction. This term—*harm reduction*—means reducing any damage caused by drug use to the user, the user's family, and the user's community. For some people, the healthiest relationship with drugs, or the best way to reduce harm, is not to use them at all. For others, it means changing the amount, the frequency, or the way they use their drug of choice.

Among the three of us, we have decades of experience working with people who come to us with alcohol and other drug problems, and many more years than that in the general mental health field. Patt developed a new way of thinking about people's relationships with drugs when she was director of a mental health clinic in the midst of the emerging HIV epidemic in San Francisco. She worked with many dying and grieving young men and came to understand that drugs were sometimes the only way to cope with overwhelming terror and loss. She went on to create an alternative approach to working with drug and alcohol users, called Addiction Treatment Alternatives.

Jeannie became familiar with harm reduction after working for two and a half years in an inpatient substance abuse program at the Veterans Administration hospital in San Francisco. She became concerned about the people whose problems were so complex that they were rejected by, or unable to attend, ongoing treatment programs. She started a harm reduction support group at what is now the VA's community-based clinic in San Francisco. This group was so popular that she, too, went on to specialize as a therapist working with drug and alcohol users.

Together Patt and Jeannie have expanded their practice into the Harm Reduction Therapy Center, a nonprofit organization that provides truly integrated mental health and substance abuse treatment in the San Francisco Bay area and that trains other therapists and treatment providers around the country to practice harm reduction.

Through her work with homeless women in New York City, and in substance abuse and outpatient psychotherapy clinics in New York and New England, Adina, too, became disturbed by the unnecessarily limited and punitive approaches of treatment programs for people with drug and alcohol problems. Given her intuition for how people best hear advice, coupled with her writing skills, she got this book started and crafted some of its more moving passages as we went along.

Through our work, and in our experience as fellow humans, we recognize that change is hard. The more we depend on something, and the more attached we are to our habits, the harder it is to change. We respect that we can't ask people to change without helping them find alternatives to whatever their drugs are doing for them. That is our job as therapists. And that is the task of this book.

In this book, we will help you understand the nature of your relationship with drugs or alcohol, the benefits you get from them compared to the harms you might be suffering. We describe a process of change that helps drug users or their loved ones develop more realistic expectations about what is involved in deciding to make changes and carrying them out. We talk about drugs and drug use in a way that reduces the stigma of drugs and the behaviors that go along with using them. We suggest strategies to help you avoid or reduce harm if you continue to use alcohol or drugs by providing accurate information about how drugs work so that you can make educated and safer choices. We also help you negotiate the complexity of quitting, if that is what you choose to do. You can do all of these things alone or with the help of this book, or you can get help from other people and places. We offer some suggestions about where and how to find the kind of help that *is* helpful to you. We offer some ways of talking about this new approach to people who might be unfamiliar with it, and therefore suspicious. And finally, we directly address the issues that might be experienced by families and friends.

The most important contribution that this book makes to the vast literature on substance use and abuse is that we offer to the general reader an insight into a movement that will forever change attitudes about drug use and treatment of drug and alcohol problems in the United States. The harm reduction movement has worked hard for twenty years to keep drug users alive and to persuade policy makers and medical, mental health, and substance abuse professionals to treat drug users with dignity and respect. We are three professionals who have been persuaded. By reading this book, you too have the opportunity to join this movement.

SOURCE

The reference to "The attempt to regulate affect ..." can be found in Allan Schore's 1999 Foreword to a reprint edition of *Attachment*, by John Bowlby. (Basic Books, 1969/1982, p. xiv).

Over the Influence

INTRODUCTION
What Is Harm Reduction, Anyway?

People use drugs. And people drink alcohol. So far, we've used drugs for about eight thousand years, and we show no signs of stopping soon. This, despite the fact that use of alcohol and other drugs sometimes causes harm—in some cases lots of harm—to the user, to his or her family, and to the community.

For much of the last eight thousand years, drugs have been used in their natural plant form as part of normal social, occupational, or religious rituals. But in the last two centuries or so we learned to extract potent active ingredients and make our own stronger drugs, including distilling alcohol (which happened much earlier). Combined with the rapid social and economic changes of the Industrial Revolution, this ability has left us with a more compelling drive to get high. It's also left us with more personal and communal harm related to drug use than our ancestors could have imagined.

This book presents a new approach to problems with alcohol and drugs. It's called *harm reduction*, and it refers to any effort to reduce the harm caused by drug or alcohol use. Harm reduction principles help us realize that when we understand our relationship with alcohol and drugs we can make decisions and choices that reduce harm in our lives and in the lives of those we care about. We no longer have to be "under the influence" of mind-altering drugs but rather we can be "over the influence"—a person with the power to learn, choose, and change.

Why a New Approach?

• Because 12-Step-based programs—which dominate the self-help landscape and account for 93 percent of all alcohol and other drug treatment programs in the United States—have a not-so-impressive success rate of somewhere between 5 and 39 percent, with hard numbers tough to come by. That's for the 20 percent or so of people who show up at those programs in the first place. And that's if success is defined as *abstinence from all intoxicating substances.*

• Because viewing drug and alcohol problems as a disease takes control and self-determination away from those who have the problems. Not everyone is comfortable with relinquishing their fate to a "higher power," and therefore many, many people avoid 12-Step programs and the potential help they may offer.

• Because the disease model says the only cure is total abstinence, which eludes up to 80 percent of alcohol and drug users who suffer harm from using these substances. Should they be left with no alternative and no hope?

• Because it's no wonder that abstinence eludes so many: demanding that "problem" drinkers or drug users give up all mind-altering substances totally, immediately, and forever leaves many people with intolerable pain, emptiness, or anxiety—a surefire recipe for relapse.

• Because insisting that everyone who has a problem with drugs or alcohol must quit right now, before they can address any of the other problems in their lives, means denying too many people the help they need to eliminate or reduce that pain, emptiness, or anxiety, and therefore leaves them alone to face it without the drugs that have helped them cope so far.

• And because the reality is that more people who have drug and alcohol problems end up moderating their use than quitting, and moderation is an excellent way to reduce harm.

Instead of the powerless state implied by the term "under the influence," people can learn to be in charge, even if not abstinent from all drugs. You can be "over the influence"—in charge of your drug use rather than having it run your life.

And Why Else?

• Because the over-twenty-year-old War on Drugs, with its efforts to control drug use through legislation, international supply control, and punishment, has left us with not less crime but more . . . with not a smaller supply but a booming black market in intoxicants . . . with not a decrease in drug use but an increase again since 1994 (after a dropoff from its 1979 peak, and except for a slight drop in teenage drug use in 2002).

- Because we have demonized certain drugs more than others. While hundreds of thousands of people are arrested for possession and distribution of illegal drugs and ten thousand die, hundreds of thousands of others die from alcohol- and tobacco-related diseases.
- Because by demonizing certain drugs over others, we disproportionately punish the people who we *perceive* use those drugs most. For example, while African Americans use drugs no more than whites (approximately 7 percent of each group), they represent 35% of those arrested, 55% of those convicted, and 74% of those sentenced to prison for drug possession.
- Because when people are locked up for drug "offenses," they are not in treatment and, despite its current limitations, treatment works better than prison when it comes to helping people with drug problems.
- All of which leads us to suspect that more damage is done by drug prohibition than by drugs themselves. And prohibition is the underlying philosophy of abstinence-based treatment.

What Does Harm Reduction Do?

Harm reduction means taking control—of your use of drugs or alcohol, of the damage that use does to you, of the harm your use causes others, and of how you live your life. It means looking closely at the role drugs or alcohol play in your survival, your ability to function, your capacity to cope with the pain you suffer, and your enjoyment of life's pleasure. It means looking at drug use in pragmatic terms—as a means to an end—rather than as a disease or as a moral weakness.

As we present it in this book, harm reduction is a means by which you can change the way you use alcohol or other drugs—including, but not limited to, quitting—to reduce the harm your use causes, whether that involves drinking less or less often, using milder drugs, or protecting yourself and others physically, financially, or legally. It is a means to make your own decisions about how much change you need or can tolerate. Harm reduction does not encourage you to hand over decision making to others. If your decisions lead you to quit, either now or later, fine. If you don't quit, that's fine too. As long as you make *any* change that reduces harm, you're practicing harm reduction, and you're moving in a positive direction. **Any Positive Change*** is the motto of harm reduction.

Harm reduction is meant to help anyone who has developed problems

*Thanks to the Chicago Recovery Alliance for promoting Any Positive Change.

with alcohol or other drugs. You don't have to define yourself (or let someone else define you) as an "addict" or an "alcoholic." You don't have to "hit bottom" before you can get better. You don't have to be living on the street, getting arrested, causing disasters, or surviving in the midst of chaos or catastrophe before you recognize the need to take better care of yourself and others. If you *do* fit any of those descriptions, harm reduction can certainly help you. But it can also help you if you've been denied therapy "until you DO something about your drug problem." Or if your life as a party animal is starting to catch up to you—if your social use of alcohol or other drugs has become more pervasive, and is affecting your work, your relationships, and your finances. Or if you feel like you're just not at your best these days, and you wonder how in the world you got to the point where you were drinking every single evening, and no longer a glass of wine or two with dinner but a couple of martinis followed by a bottle of wine. Or you've smoked just a little pot for all of your adult life and all of a sudden feel like your life hasn't changed in twenty years.

What's New about Harm Reduction?

Not much, really. Harm reduction is a holistic and humane public health approach that, in fact, is nothing new. We have practiced harm reduction for decades. Seat belt laws are harm reduction laws—driving is a somewhat risky activity, and when we buckle our seat belts we minimize the risk that we will incur serious harm if we are in an accident. When parents choose to have their children vaccinated, it is a risk–benefit decision based on the principles of harm reduction: since certain diseases can't be eradicated, the child can be immunized (protected) against the most deadly ones. On the other hand, there is increasing concern that vaccinations may not be useful, and may, in fact, be dangerous (the recent smallpox vaccine debate is one example). Where alcohol is concerned, we have enacted sane drinking and driving laws that discourage people from pairing one risky activity with another and thereby increasing the likelihood of serious harm to the drinker and others on the road.

In 1982, the same year that we in the United States launched our War on Drugs, the Dutch government responded to a campaign by intravenous drug users to expand fair access to health care. The Dutch government had banned the sale of needles in pharmacies, fearing an increase in heroin use, and drug users were concerned that many of their medical problems were caused by the resulting sharing of needles. Public health officials responded by sending medical teams out into the streets and parks to provide health care and clean needles to drug users. Several years into this public health strategy to reach out to drug users, the number of drug-related deaths in the Netherlands dropped dramatically.

In 1985, the year *before* Nancy Reagan started America's "Just Say No to Drugs" campaign, the British government opened a program in Liverpool in response to the AIDS epidemic and started using the term harm reduction. While we were pouring billions of dollars into "supply reduction" and law enforcement, the Liverpool public health department was offering medical care, clean drugs (methadone, morphine, or heroin), clean needles, and safe injection education to injection drug users. By 1989 injection drug users in New York City had an HIV infection rate of 60 percent compared to an infection rate of 0.1 percent in Liverpool.

Thus was born the international grassroots harm reduction movement. This movement has sponsored the exchange of dirty needles for clean ones to aid in the prevention of communicable diseases such as HIV and hepatitis C. It has led to overdose prevention efforts, accurate drug education, and nondiscriminatory medical care to help drug users stay alive and healthier. Methadone, a tried-and-true medical treatment for heroin and other opiate dependence, is now considered part of the harm reduction arsenal. Legal efforts to create sensible policies and laws that prevent the incarceration of nonviolent drug offenders are part of the harm reduction movement as well. And now, those of us from the mental health professions who want to offer emotional help to drug users—help based on a more realistic understanding of why people use drugs and how hard it is to change habits—have joined the harm reduction movement.

We mental health professionals who have turned to harm reduction have done so because we believe that both the moral and the disease models are inadequate to solve the problems that arise from alcohol and drug abuse. Legal approaches make them worse; the disease model is too simplistic. Harm reduction rejects the punitive moral model and moves beyond the disease model.

A Snapshot of the Disease Model of Addiction

In the United States, the standard approach to defining problem drinking and drug use since the creation of Alcoholics Anonymous in the 1930s is as follows: Addiction is a disease. It is a "primary" disease. In other words, nothing *causes* addiction—not being beaten by your mother when you were three, watching your grandfather drink himself to death, or growing up in the projects. There is now some acceptance, supported by research, that environment contributes to the development of addiction. This is the nature-versus-nurture debate. But common lore still holds that either you are an addict or you're not, and nothing else caused it. In fact, part of working the 12 Steps of Alcoholics Anonymous involves not blaming anyone else for your alcohol or drug use.

Disease model proponents assert that if you are an addict, your disease will follow a progressive course (that is, get worse over time). Furthermore, the disease is incurable: "Once an addict, always an addict." The two symptoms most characteristic of the disease are (1) loss of control over drugs and alcohol, and (2) denial of the severity and consequences of using. In other words, you are an addict because you lose control of your drinking or using. And you lose control because you are an addict. When you try to argue with someone about this, your "denial" proves his or her point.

Finally, given the inevitability that drinking or using will get worse, the only way to arrest the disease process is to stop using all psychoactive substances. You are said to be "in recovery" when the two crowning symptoms of addiction have abated—you are no longer in denial that you are powerless over alcohol or drugs, and you no longer lose control (because you don't use at all). Abstinence from all mind-altering substances, active participation in the 12-Step program of recovery (Alcoholics Anonymous, Narcotics Anonymous, etc.), and turning your life over to a higher power are your medicine. You can be in remission (or in recovery), but once diagnosed with the disease, you will always have it.

Theresa* drank a lot when she was young, got pregnant in high school, and dropped out for several years. She quit drinking during her pregnancy and went to AA but has started drinking again recently. Now that her son is in school, she has gone back to finish high school and then get a degree in education. She is in a relationship with a woman for the first time, and her family is very upset by her new identity as a lesbian. Even though Theresa drinks only a couple of beers on Friday and Saturday nights and thinks of herself as a moderate drinker, her new girlfriend doesn't like the fact that she has started drinking again. Her family thinks that the girlfriend is a bad influence on her. Her girlfriend thinks that she is an alcoholic and is relapsing. *She* thinks she's doing pretty well, finishing school, raising a son, and having a relationship. Sometimes she just gets so mad at all of them that she says, "What the hell, I might as well go out and get drunk!"

*All the cases in this book are composites based on real individuals. All identifying characteristics have been changed.

Some of the "rules" of the disease model are as follows:

• *Admit that you are an "alcoholic" or "addict" and accept that you are "powerless" over drugs and alcohol.* Research shows that many who do not define themselves as addicts stop using in problematic ways or quit completely, often without any outside help. Research also shows that better effects are achieved by helping people to *increase* self-esteem and their sense of their own effectiveness, rather than increasing their sense of powerlessness. Finally, research tells us that the worse people think they are, the worse they are. It is a self-fulfilling prophecy that when you think you are relapsing, you are more likely to relapse. The mythology is "One drink leads to a thousand." Or, as Theresa says, "What the hell!"

Daryl grew up with parents who drank a lot and used cocaine. He feels that "hard" drugs are bad, but pot is OK. He has been smoking marijuana since he was in high school. Now, at age thirty, he works part time at an auto body shop and can't decide what to do with his life. His friends tell him that he's an addict, just like his parents, and that's why he can't get himself together to find a more fulfilling career. It doesn't seem the same to him at all. He just can't figure out how to change his life.

• *Addiction is a primary disease: Take care of the drug problem before you address any other life issues.* For many people, addiction is not a primary disease. It happens because of something else. In the case of a marijuana smoker like Daryl, it is more likely that he is the survivor of a traumatic childhood with two alcohol-dependent parents, and that marijuana soothes his restlessness and inability to settle down rather than causing it.
• *Commit to lifelong abstinence from all psychoactive substances.* In the United States, abstinence from all mind-altering substances is the only way to "recover" from addiction; by definition, therefore, it is the only way to reduce harm. As is the case with Daryl, for many people, committing to the solution (abstinence) before fully exploring the problem doesn't make sense. Moreover, most people don't succeed at lifelong abstinence, even if they are committed to it.

Sylvia struggled with alcohol for quite some time. She was a part-time real estate agent, married, with two children. Her husband was a sales manager for a printing company and was out of town at least three nights a week, leaving virtually every household job to Sylvia. They had financial problems because Sylvia's father, who'd had a stroke the year before, needed daily care. She tended to collapse at the end of the day with a large vodka and tonic, which turned into three or four as the evening progressed. Sylvia's husband came from an alcoholic family, and he has strong feelings about her drinking.

After she got a DUI coming home from the kids' basketball practice, she went into a court-ordered treatment program and attended 12-step meetings for a few months. But between having her husband away so much, caring for her father, and raising two children with very little money to spare, she starting drinking again—which, of course, became a source of conflict with her husband. One time he came home early from a business trip and found her drunk and watching TV while the kids scrounged in the kitchen for dinner. He was furious. She quit altogether for about two months but was sneaking drinks in the third month and soon was drunk nearly every day. Her husband left her and took the children.

• *Be motivated for treatment: "Have you hit bottom yet?"* You have to suffer before you will accept help. It may sound convincing, but for some people the bottom is death. And a dead addict can't recover. Many other people, especially those already accustomed to social and economic deprivation, simply "adapt to the bottom," a startlingly obvious but often forgotten reality summed up by our friend and colleague Simbwala Schultz. What do you think Sylvia will do?

What's Different about Harm Reduction?

Although there is really nothing new about sane public health practices, what *is* new about harm reduction in the United States is that we embrace drug users as no different and no less deserving of compassionate care than anyone else. In this country it is a new idea not to punish people for their choice of drug. It is a new idea to give people real and balanced information about drugs. And it is a new idea to give people who use drugs equal access to medical and mental health treatment, regardless of the status of their drug use.

The harm reduction way of understanding drug use and abuse takes into account the complexity of each person's relationship with drugs. When we talk about "a relationship with drugs," we are talking about is a unique interaction of physical, emotional, social, and, some would say, spiritual aspects of an individual's inner and outer life. The relative importance of each aspect varies from individual to individual. In other words, there is no one explanation for the process of "addiction." Harm reduction values the uniqueness of each individual and helps each person define her own particular problems related to drug use.

- Harm reduction says that not all drug use is abuse—*but* all drug use does need to be safe and based on accurate information about drugs.
- Harm reduction says it is not necessary to stop all drug use to stop harm—although, for some people, that is the most efficient way, whereas for others, quitting is an unrealistic and insurmountable task.
- Harm reduction says *Just Say Know* (know what and how much you are using).
- Harm reduction means taking care of yourself, regardless of the status of your drug use.
- Harm reduction means getting nondiscriminatory care from others, especially health care professionals, regardless of the status of your drug use.
- Harm reduction means getting your mental health needs attended to, formally or informally, when you are suffering emotional pain or mental illness, regardless of the status of your drug use.
- Harm reduction means getting adequate prenatal care without fear of criminal sanctions, regardless of the status of your drug use.
- Harm reduction says you can still put business before pleasure, especially if your business is taking care of others, even if you continue to use drugs.
- Harm reduction means being free of punitive sanctions for what you choose to put into your body.
- Harm reduction means being free of the fear, the stigma, and the shame that accompany your choices.

This book aims to help people who may continue to use mind-altering substances. We want to help people to use more safely and more conscientiously if they choose to continue and to help them develop the motivation and skills to quit if that is their choice. We are, of course, aware that most of these substances are illegal. This book is based on the reality that people use drugs and always have, regardless of all efforts to legislate them out of existence.

It is clear from our experience and from the research of others that less harm is done when people make informed choices. We are not policy makers. We are not lawyers. In our work with people we do not concern ourselves with the legalization of drugs. It is not our job to address this issue. We neither condemn nor condone the use of particular drugs. We simply recognize that people use them, whether we think they should or not. We want them to stay alive and be as safe as possible. Our work, and the purpose of this book, is to provide people with information to make healthier choices, with strategies to change in a positive direction, and with help to take better care of themselves.

SOURCES AND SUGGESTED READINGS

There are many references in the Sources and Suggested Readings section at the end of the book. Here we highlight the most useful and most accessible materials.

For information about the effectiveness of the 12 Steps and treatment outcomes, in general, in the United States:

Alcoholics Anonymous: Cult or Cure? Charles Bufe. SeeSharp Press. 1991.

Hooked: Five Addicts Challenge Our Misguided Drug Rehab System. Lonny Shavelson. New Press. 2001.

Responsible Drinking. Frederick Rotgers, Marc F. Kern, and Rudy Hoetzel. New Harbinger. 2002 (pp. 6–9).

Services Outcome Research Study and other data on rates of drug use and abuse and treatment outcomes. Substance Abuse and Mental Health Services Administration Office of Applied Studies. www.samhsa.gov. 1998.

For critiques of the disease model of addiction and how this model affects people's ideas about their relationship with alcohol and drugs:

Becoming Alcoholic: Alcoholics Anonymous and the Reality of Alcoholism. Rudy David. Southern Illinois University Press. 1986.

The Diseasing of America: Drug Treatment Out of Control. Stanton Peele. Lexington Books. 1989.

Heavy Drinking: The Myth of Alcoholism as a Disease. Herbert Fingarette. University of California Press. 1988.

I'm Dysfunctional, You're Dysfunctional: The Recovery Movement and Other Self-Help Fashions. Wendy Kaminer. Vintage Books. 1993.

Relapse Prevention. G. Alan Marlatt and Judith R. Gordon, Eds. Guilford Press. 1985 (see especially the section on the Abstinence Violation Effect, or the "what the hell" effect, pp. 41–43, and the section on alcohol expectancies—the tendency to experience different effects because of expectation rather than the biological effects of alcohol, pp. 137–150).

The Truth about Addiction and Recovery. Stanton Peele. Simon & Schuster. 1991.

For critiques of the War on Drugs, drug policy, and inequitable criminal justice policies:

> *Drug Crazy: How We Got into This Mess and How We Can Get Out.* Mike Gray. Routledge. 1998.
>
> *Drug Policy and the Criminal Justice System.* Washington, DC: The Sentencing Project. 2001. All Sentencing Project publications can be obtained on their website at *www.sentencingproject.org.*

For the best library with up-to-date books and information about drug policy and the impact of the War on Drugs, and for research on the effectiveness of needle exchange, methadone, and other harm reduction interventions, see the Drug Policy Alliance website:

> *www.drugpolicy.org*

For information on the history and practice of harm reduction, and to network with the harm reduction movement, check out the Harm Reduction Coalition:

> *www.harmreduction.org*

1 ADDICTION

Is It All or Nothing?

Do you know anyone with diabetes who has ever been refused insulin by his doctor because he won't stop eating ice cream or drinking alcohol?

Or any pro ball players who are told they have to quit playing forever before they can have yet another tendon repaired?

How many heart patients are denied bypass surgery because their last meal was a hamburger and french fries, and the one before that a pizza? Or because they still haven't gotten around to getting off the couch except to let the dog out, despite their doctor's instructions to get thirty minutes of aerobic exercise at least three times a week?

How many overweight fifty-year-olds are told they must lose weight before their doctor will perform knee surgery?

How many doctors demand that you quit smoking before they will prescribe oxygen for your emphysema?

Would your doctor refuse to set your broken arm just because you don't wear elbow pads when you skateboard?

The likely answers to all of the above are "not many," "none," and "no." Doctors may ask, they may plead, they may try persuasion and education, but they generally don't refuse treatment to people who aren't ready, willing, or able to stop doing the things that are harmful to their condition.

It is not so for people who use or abuse alcohol and other drugs. People who drink too much and people who use illegal drugs—those 20 percent, or thereabouts, of Americans who often get lumped into the category of "addict"—usually hear "I can't help you until you stop drinking [quit using]." This is most often the case when people try to find help for emotional or relationship troubles or for more severe problems such as depression, anxiety, or posttraumatic stress disorder. The mythology in some circles is that getting sober will take care of all your other problems or will clear the way for you to take care of them.

The Reality of Change

Sure, sobriety's nice. So are lifelong love, unlimited wealth, and perfection. But we don't go to sleep on Sunday wanting to be wealthy and wake up on Monday with tons of money. We don't even go to sleep in February wanting to be rich and wake up in June with a stock portfolio on which we can retire. It takes time. There are obstacles. First we get some training and a good job. Then we work hard, invest well, save some money. We improve our skills, we take a few risks in the stock market.

Nor do we dream of love and wake up to find Prince(ss) Charming beside us in the morning. We talk to friends about how they found good partners, date different people, get married. We mess up, we learn, maybe we divorce—we practice until we learn to have a good love life. Eventually, we find our way.

Even then, most of us never end up rich or with the person of our dreams. But we can be happy, comfortable, even satisfied. Perfection? That, we never achieve.

The same is true with drug or alcohol problems. Most of us don't go to sleep on Sunday hoping to stop drinking, snorting coke, or shooting speed or heroin and wake up on Monday "clean and sober." (We also don't go to sleep drunk on Sunday and wake up Monday an alcoholic, but that's a different chapter.) It takes time, and there are obstacles. First you try to get control of your drinking on your own. You decide to snort coke or smoke crack only on weekends. You are determined to quit heroin completely because it has become the habit you thought would never happen. You admit to a friend that you're struggling to control your drinking and he takes you to an AA meeting. You go into a twenty-eight-day treatment program and relapse a few weeks or months after you graduate. You find a therapist to talk to about the problems you think might be causing your heavy drug use, but she confronts your "denial" so vigorously that you decide drinking is the only cure for feeling beaten up by your therapist.

Or, if you've discovered this book, you consider practicing harm reduction. In this way, you begin by first making sure you always have a ride home from the bar so you're not driving drunk. Then you quit drinking gin and stick with beer because the piercing headache that accompanies your gin hangover makes you argumentative at work. Then you drink less beer. You realize you've been depressed for a while, and you start taking antidepressant medication. Maybe find a therapist who knows about harm reduction and doesn't say you have to quit before you can talk about your problems. You begin to deal with the depression that may have started your drinking in the first place. Maybe you stop smoking pot for a while, take a "drug vacation." You exercise. You talk to a friend who also does crystal meth (speed), and together you agree to go on a run no more than once a month, to quit by noon on Sunday, and to always have condoms in your pocket. Eventually you find your way.

There Are Other Choices Besides Quitting

This book is about harm reduction. It is not about "getting clean." It is not about quitting drugs or alcohol in the hope that simply not having these things in your body will be the solution, or the beginning of the solution, to all your other problems. It is not about determining, once and for all, whether you are an addict. It is not about an all-or-nothing attitude: drink *or* be on the wagon, use *or* quit. It is about *reducing the harm* done by alcohol and other drugs in your life. Less harm *is* the solution.

Hillary works in a busy cafe. She uses speed with her coworkers to keep up with the intense pace. Usually she uses only once a day, around the middle of her shift. Sometimes, though, it feels good to do a hit later because she's *so* tired. But then she has trouble sleeping. Which means she needs a hit the next day even more. She knows she can't go on like this forever. She has a child who needs attention, she's exhausted, and she'll burn out at this rate. She thinks about quitting speed or maybe getting a different job. She's already beginning to practice harm reduction just by worrying about the problem and thinking about solutions. She will have many options for taking better care of herself and her child.

If, for you, reducing harm means abstaining entirely, that's fine. But if it means beginning with tiny changes that move you in a positive direction, that's fine, too. If it means drinking, but for the first time in your life not driving drunk, that's wonderful—lives are no longer in such danger when you get in your car. If it means limiting your marijuana use to whatever is supplied by your most reliable drug dealer so that you know you're not getting a joint laced with PCP, that's wonderful—you're reducing your risk of a potentially violent, psychotic, or lethal drug experience. If it means getting more sleep on Sunday so you don't get so tired at work on Monday and can avoid that first hit of speed to get through the day, you're on your way. Even if it doesn't work out so well from Tuesday through Saturday. That's the reality of change for most of us. We do as much as we can the best way we can. And that's harm reduction.

Moreover, *you* are the expert. You know better than anyone what works and doesn't work. You are the only one with the power to choose what's best for you. Whether consciously or not, you always balance the risks and the benefits of using drugs versus quitting. Harm reduction merely helps you find more options between keeping on as you are and quitting altogether. And the most radical idea from harm reduction is that *drugs work*. The speed you use does, in fact, get you through the day; alcohol helps you *enjoy* your wife's office Christmas party; pot makes the music so much more beautiful; cocaine was around before Viagra; and heroin takes away *all* the pain. Drugs work; otherwise you wouldn't be using them.

The Reality of Harm Reduction

Since this book is about reducing harm, there will be times when you'll be invited to identify the harm you experience in your life, whether it's harm that has caused or is caused by your alcohol or other drug use. We appreciate the magnitude of such an invitation. If most of us had to strip down and look at our lives with brutal honesty, we'd climb into the nearest dark hole with as much of our drug of choice as money could buy and stay there till hell froze over. To some degree, we all avoid looking closely at the damage, pain, anger, sadness, loneliness, or depression in our lives. And we do this for an understandable reason: it hurts to live it, and it hurts to think about it.

We understand that you may begin reading this book feeling like you've failed at the only step usually accepted—total abstinence from all psychoactive substances. So when it comes time to look again at the harm incurred by your drug or alcohol use, go at the pace that's right for you. And if you do get into that hole, drink lots of water and get plenty of rest. This book is waiting patiently for your return.

We offer the plainest and most difficult advice: **Be patient with yourself**. Being patient with yourself means going at your own pace, no matter whose agenda is pressing you to DO SOMETHING NOW, OR ELSE!

Practicing harm reduction means taking an active interest in your own welfare and the welfare of those around you. It means being curious about why you drink or use. It means reviewing how you got here, why you started using in the first place, and how you got to the point of needing this book. It means examining, *without harsh judgments*, the risks of your drinking and the trouble you've gotten into because of it. It means accepting, *without guilt*, that you like things about your drugs, that they are helpful or pleasurable, even if they cause problems.

Harm reduction is not the easy way out. It's not an "excuse" to keep using. It is, in fact, very hard work. Harm reduction is based on the reality that most of us don't quit doing something unhealthy or start doing something healthy just because someone says so or just because it's the "right" thing to do. But that doesn't mean we do nothing at all.

When facing a problem, our first job is to think, not to do. Of course, if you have to quit immediately because you're a doctor and you've been threatened with suspension from your job . . . or you're on parole and you'll be locked up for a violation . . . or your wife has said she'll leave you and that's the last thing you want, then fine, quit. But it's hard to do and hard to maintain. Change is difficult, and it's stressful. If you can't or don't want to quit, even thinking is hard, too. Because so often what we have to think about is painful. On the other hand, you've already shown that you can tolerate pain, stress, or frustration. In everyday life, you have probably (at least once)

- Gone without food, new clothing, or other pleasures when those around you were indulging.
- Broken up with a partner when you were still in love.
- Withstood humiliating lectures from teachers or bosses.
- Endured a broken ankle and taken three months away from your favorite sport.

Having done any of those things tells you that you have the *ability* to do something painful, difficult, uncomfortable, or boring, even when you don't want to. You also have the ability to exercise control. If you've gotten into trouble drinking and using drugs, it could almost certainly be worse. You've already set limits on your use, or you wouldn't be reading this book right now. You'd be in the hospital struggling to live, living in the streets struggling to survive, or, worst of all, dead.

But What If People Say I Have to Quit?

So you wake up Monday morning. Whatever pleasures the weekend provided for you, you find yourself in pain now. Your head hurts, you're nauseous, anxious, and tremulous. You're late for work and your pockets are empty. This morning, the options are laid out, crystal clear and so depressing you can barely bring yourself to think of them. There's an NA meeting that starts at noon. Or an AA meeting at the church in half an hour. Insurance would probably cover a detox, maybe even rehab. The possibilities all jumble together in your head, and the only clear feeling you have is that nothing has ever worked. Either you go whole hog, quit, "join the program," suffer another detox, or keep on going the way you are. Either way, you're doomed.

The people around you believe you're suffering because of your use of alcohol or other drugs. The term they know for this is *addiction*—if you drink too much or use drugs, you must be an addict. The only solution they know is for you to quit—quit using all "mind-altering" drugs. It's the only way. That's what they've been told, and that's what they believe is best for you.

Kendra got laid off from her job at a large law firm and can't find another job. She's very worried. For the past five months she's been hanging out with other unemployed friends, watching TV, smoking pot, and occasionally snorting heroin. Some of her friends also drink a lot. But her brother had a big problem with alcohol, lost jobs and family, finally quit, and is much better off now. So she stays away from drinking. He says he was an alcoholic and that she's an addict. He tells her that the only way she'll ever get back on her feet and find work is to quit.

Addiction is a strong word, and we use it very freely in this country. It's a casual term that sometimes just means you're using a drug regularly and don't want to give it up. It's often used to peg a user with negative images. Because we have such a strong tendency in the United States to be puritanical about pleasure (pleasure is indulgent; being indulgent is bad), the word *addiction* denotes stigma. People who are addicted are seen as being weak and out of control. The word *addiction* really has no official meaning. Someone in your life who uses this term may not know whether you are "addicted" or not. He is just communicating to you that he's worried. Using an illegal drug doesn't make you an addict. Nor does drinking more than most other people around you.

The actual terms used by substance abuse treatment professionals are *substance abuse* and *substance dependence*. Substance *abuse* refers to continuing drug use even after it has begun causing problems such as legal, financial, or family trouble. Substance *dependence* refers to a number of things related to use, including possible physical dependence (see the special drug section in the middle of the book for more information about this aspect), craving, or seeking and using drugs to the exclusion of other activities. The term *addiction* generally refers to chaotic, compulsive use that can no longer be understood or controlled by the user. But this by no means describes most drug use.

Since addiction has become such a common term, it's likely that your friends and family use it freely. They see that you use drugs or alcohol, they see problems in your life, they experience problems in their relationship with you, and despite their requests, demands, or pleas for you to stop, you continue to use. Therefore, you must be an addict. As we explained in the Introduction, these ideas about addiction come from the disease model of addiction, known elsewhere in the world as the *American disease model.*

In reality, there are many types of problematic use patterns that are not described easily as "abuse" or "dependence" or "addiction." There are also many ways to use drugs more safely. The continuum of drug use is much more complicated than the disease model allows. To get an idea of the difference between the approaches of the disease model and harm reduction, consider this:

According to the Disease Model ...	Harm Reduction Says ...
IF DRUGS AND ALCOHOL CAUSE PERSISTENT PROBLEMS IN YOUR LIFE, YOU'RE AN ADDICT.	Your *use* of alcohol may be related to some trouble in your life, but you are not necessarily *addicted* to alcohol.
ADDICTED TO ONE THING MEANS ADDICTED TO ALL THINGS.	You may be addicted to the *heroin* you use every day but not to the *marijuana* you smoke on weekends.
ONCE AN ADDICT, ALWAYS AN ADDICT.	You can stop drinking and later learn to drink moderately. Or you can stop drinking and just be over it. You are no longer an alcoholic.
THE ONLY ANSWER IS TO QUIT ALL MIND-ALTERING SUBSTANCES.	Most people don't quit, or not forever. They end up moderating their use. And most people who quit one substance—like heroin, crack, or alcohol—don't quit everything, especially alcohol or pot.

So What Do You Do?

You picked up this book because you or someone in your life is worried about your drinking or drug use. If you haven't been living under a rock, you've heard of, or even been to, Alcoholics Anonymous or drug treatment. The fact that you're reading this book suggests that they haven't been helpful enough so far. You are in the majority. Although, many people find extraordinary help through AA and its 12-Step cousins, most don't. That doesn't mean there is something wrong with these programs. Nor is there anything wrong with you. It just means that AA, or NA, or any other 12-Step program, with its disease approach to understanding and dealing with drug and alcohol use, is not a good match for you. But you're still worried and looking for help.

For the moment, you're willing to coast on the hope that this book might have a few new ideas for you. In spite of your searing headache, the unexplained bruises on your leg, or the zero balance in your bank account, you're willing to entertain the possibility that there's a way to make life better. It's a delicate thing, that hope you cling to, daring to try one more thing before you decide your life is going to suck from today until you die. Thus you invite harm reduction into your life.

Harm reduction does not intend to take over or boss you around. Harm reduction is not an expert on you or your personal relationship with drugs or alcohol. Harm reduction does not insist that you are like every other drinker or drug user out there. Harm reduction does not require that you be "clean and sober" to read this book.

You have a number of options if you disagree with other people's opinion of you:

1. *Reject their opinion outright.* The upside to this is that it exercises your ability and your right to think for yourself. You remain the expert. The downside is that other people, especially those close to you, might see something you don't. If you're like most people, you have at least some difficulty looking inward. You might have spinach in your teeth, have forgotten to turn off the coffee machine, or be using cocaine problematically, and when someone else points it out to you, rejecting that observation could be anything from embarrassing to fatal.

2. *Accept their opinion completely.* The upside to this is that you can probably avoid a fair amount of conflict with the people who say you're an addict by simply agreeing with them. Also, if you are, in fact, addicted to drugs or alcohol, agreeing with your friends or family might enable you to get some help from them in working on the problems. The downside is that it may not be true, and it may not help you understand your relationship with drugs or alcohol realistically—and a *realistic* understanding of your relationship with drugs or alcohol is the strongest ally you have in reducing any harm done by your use of them.

3. *Accept some, reject some.* The upside to this is that you can keep a flexible balance between your own perceptions and those of the people around you. Where there is flexibility, there is understanding. Where there is understanding, there can be harm reduction.

Harm reduction is not an either/or proposition. It's not get help *or* keep using. You can do both. We just suggest that harm reduction be invited to sit next to your weed, your booze, your dope, as you make the very important changes that will help you reduce the harm in your life caused by your drug use. And for now, harm reduction and your drug of choice are just going to hang out and introduce themselves to each other.

The conversation might go something like this:

"Hello, I'm Harm Reduction."
"What the hell's that?"
"It's a way of making life better."
"My life is fine."
"OK, then can I just hang around for a while?"
"Suit yourself. Just stay out of my way."

Have this conversation as many times as you want. A minute, three months, whatever. Put down the book. Pick up the book. Put down the book. Have mixed feelings about the whole thing. Take a break. That's fine. The right way to do this, to make things happen, is to pay attention to whatever feels the most manageable. Bombard yourself with too much too soon, and you'll have every reason to stock up and climb into that hole.

Yes, sobriety's nice, but harm reduction could save your life.

SOURCES AND SUGGESTED READINGS

For data about the efficacy of 12-step programs and traditional treatment and the varieties of treatment actually used or needed by people:

Alcoholics Anonymous: Cult or Cure? Charles Bufe. SeeSharp Press. 1991.
Hooked: Five Addicts Challenge Our Misguided Drug Rehab System. Lonny Shavelson. New Press. 2001.
Recovery Options: The Complete Guide. Joseph Volpicelli and Maia Szalavitz. Wiley. 2000.
The Truth about Addiction and Recovery. Stanton Peele and Archie Brodsky. Simon & Schuster. 1991.

2 SO IF WE'RE NOT ADDICTS, WHAT'S THE HARM?

Now that you know you're not suffering from an incurable disease, you can begin to look at harm without the hooded face of death looming over you and threatening you to stop using all mind-altering drugs right now. (Lest we throw out the baby with the bathwater, *addiction* is a perfectly fine word, *as long as it is used carefully and accurately*. Later in this chapter, we define the various levels of drug use and put addiction in its proper place.) *Harm* is, simply, anything that happens, no matter what causes it, that damages any part of you, your life, or those around you. Harm can be physical, emotional, social, or, some would say, spiritual.

Harm is relative. In other words, different people are damaged in different ways and at different rates, even by the same event, crisis, or drug. If you drink a glass of wine every night with dinner, you're generally not considered an alcoholic. But if you have hepatitis C and your liver is already damaged, one glass of wine could speed your death. On the other hand, we all know of people who drink large amounts of alcohol for decades and remain "as healthy as a horse" until they die of "natural causes."

Marijuana, generally considered one of the least harmful recreational drugs, still has harm associated with it, depending on your health and situation in life. For example, a young person might find learning interrupted by daily use, since marijuana impairs short-term memory. If you don't know what to do with your life, marijuana will help you avoid hard decisions and hard work. (This effect could be harmful or beneficial, depending on your point of view.) But for someone with schizophrenia or other psychotic disorder, marijuana is one of the drugs most likely to trigger a psychotic episode. The effects of a hallucinogen like LSD depend enormously on your circumstances. Because hallucinogens are perception-altering drugs, you're more likely to have a bad trip in unfamiliar surroundings than in a comfortable place with people you know. A little-known fact is that the same is true for heroin: you're more likely to overdose in an unfamiliar environment. **Harm can occur regardless of the frequency or intensity of your use.**

Then again, maybe no harm is done by your drug use. Most people who drink don't have a problem. Most people who use illegal drugs work and function fine in the world. There's a whole generation of casual marijuana smokers and purposeful and intelligent users of hallucinogenic plants and LSD. Entire cultures use such drugs in careful and ritualized ways. In fact, most drugs that are used in their original plant form, including the coca leaf, are not abused. The vast majority of people who use opiate drugs prescribed by their physicians for pain do not abuse them. And certainly most people who try drugs do not get addicted. Finally, many people use drugs for pleasure—and what's the harm in that?

In other words, it depends. The harm you experience with drugs is based on the unique combination of the condition of your body, your psyche, and your environment. The presence of harm and the degree of its intensity are a result of you and your life circumstances *as well as* specific to the drug or drugs you're using. If you are going to continue using mind-altering substances in any way, you can begin to reduce their harmful effects by getting to know more about your body, your mind, your environment, and your drugs.

What are all of these drugs—recreational, abused, whatever? In Chapters 3 and 4 we list the harmful as well as beneficial effects of all of the drugs of pleasure and abuse. And in the special section in the middle of this book we detail each drug or class of drugs and give a few ideas for avoiding harm. If you choose to use drugs, both of these sections will help you figure out how to minimize potential harm.

Please note that most of the drugs we talk about in this book are illegal in the United States. There is nothing more dangerous or harmful about the drugs that are illegal than those that are legal. Alcohol damages more organ systems than any of the illegal drugs. Cigarettes cause three times more deaths than all the other drugs, including alcohol, combined. Four hundred thousand people die each year from smoking-related illnesses (a full 20 percent of all deaths in the United States; see Schmitz, Schneider, and Jarvik). And solvents (glue, gasoline, lighter fluid, etc.), which are inhaled by more children in the world than any other mind-altering substances, may not only be legally obtained but are found on any street corner or under any household sink and are absolutely the most dangerous drugs known to humankind. In fact, unlike many other recreational drugs, solvents were absolutely *never meant* for human consumption.

Despite there being no chemical rhyme or reason to a drug's illegal status, engaging in illegal behavior automatically puts the user at risk of harm. For now, unfortunately, getting caught using illegal drugs can result in your suffering more harm at the hands of society than the drugs themselves are causing. Going to jail is a serious problem; smoking pot or using may not be. The stigma and shame associated with illegal drug use are harmful to one's relationship with others and damaging to one's own psyche. Finally, a drug's illegal status means there is no quality control. Thus it can be cut with dangerous substances or infected with potentially lethal bacteria.

The legal status of certain drugs is a given, and we won't belabor it throughout the book in the interest of addressing the other aspects of drugs and people's relationship with them.

A Word about Hidden Harm

While there are harms that hit you over the head, and harms that become obvious once you start learning more—wine for someone with hepatitis C or marijuana for a person with schizophrenia—there is a special type of harm that is usually not obvious. We call this "hidden harm" because the person who suffers from the harm is not aware that it is occurring. The painful hangover headache, the despair after your spouse leaves you, the fact that your children have stopped speaking to you or your parents have kicked you out—these are easy to see. But you may be incurring harms that are not so visible.

Say you're a teenager who feels awkward in social situations (and what teen doesn't?). You may experiment with alcohol and discover that drinking increases your confidence, makes you witty and fun to be around. Or you use ecstasy so you can dance and connect with your peers, even though you think you're a horrible dancer. Seems to work. What's the harm in it? You don't drive after you've been drinking, so it's okay. The hidden harm, however, might be that you don't ever really get to practice being yourself around other people, to learn how to tolerate *not* being totally cool in public. This missed experience can keep you tied to drinking long after you want to be.

Maybe you're a musician or an artist who finds that smoking marijuana enhances your creativity. Ideas flow more smoothly, the music dances off your fingertips. And so you use it, and you produce art. The hidden harm may show up a few years down the road, when you discover that your creations are good but you haven't really produced anything marketable. Or you've produced a finished piece but just can't quite get yourself an agent, so no one gets to see it. You've tolerated the obvious harms of smoking marijuana—your girlfriend's nagging, the way your physique has lost its edge, occasional lapses of memory—but this hidden harm to your career takes you by surprise.

You might have been molested as a child. You learned to dissociate—the ability that some people have to mentally leave their bodies to get away from the horrible thing that's happening to them. Dissociating is a more extreme version of "spacing out." The problem is, you don't always have control over when it happens, so you've missed important things, like what your teacher was saying back then or what your boss is saying right now. You discover that heroin or alcohol allows you to check out too. It quiets the demons that haunt you. The dangers of heroin and alcohol are no mystery. The advantages of these drugs to victims of abuse, however, are not given nearly enough credit. They make many people feel protected from going insane. What is less obvious, however, is the lack of emotional development you experienced during the years that you were "spacing out." We've heard thousands of people say, once they started examining their relationship with drugs, "I feel like I'm still fifteen years old, like I missed growing up with regular emotions."

You may be vulnerable to harm beyond what you're aware of, particularly if you've stayed under the radar of addiction detection and your drug use has been considered "normal" or benign, as we considered cigarette smoking for so long, for example! Our lack of accurate and detailed information about drugs, in the interest of pushing abstinence, is appalling. The D.A.R.E. program, our "Just Say No" approach to drug education in schools, which has received much media attention lately for having failed, has left young people with warnings against drug use that are too general to be useful when they inevitably experiment. Yet we learned from the RAND Corporation's Drug Research Policy Center in the 1980s that young people who experiment with drugs and use them moderately are more psychologically healthy than those who use heavily *and than those who abstain.*

Do You Have to Be an Addict to Be Harmed?

Harm can occur with *any* use of drugs or alcohol. The (primarily) young men who have died during fraternity drinking bouts at colleges were probably not alcoholic. Although they were certainly drinking way too heavily on those occasions, they may not have been chronic or heavy drinkers in general. In fact, if they *had* been regular heavy drinkers, they might *not* have died: their ability to tolerate large amounts of alcohol, to "handle their liquor," would have been stronger. They died because they drank more than their central nervous system could tolerate. (See a definition of *tolerance* in the section on drugs in the middle of this book.) For exactly the same reason, your first experiment with heroin could result in a fatal overdose. Again, we're talking about *tolerance*—your body's ability to handle the effects of drugs improves with more exposure to the drugs. Most people know by now that a single dose of heroin or speed, if injected with a shared needle, can result in your getting HIV or hepatitis C. Experimenting just that one time therefore means risking one of the most seriously harmful consequences known to all drug users. Ecstasy is usually used on an occasional social basis, which is generally not thought of as an addictive pattern. But it may still be harmful to brain chemistry and cause depression during withdrawal. Ecstasy is most dangerous if you mix it with alcohol or don't drink enough water when you're dancing; it can cause fatal kidney failure due to dramatically high body temperature.

So, no, you don't have to be an addict to be harmed.

A New Way of Thinking

Mike is an attorney who has been married for fifteen years. He has two teenage kids and a new baby. Mike has been drinking since college, heavily at times. Occasionally he goes on the wagon when he thinks he's drinking too heavily. No one else in his family had alcohol problems, so he never thought about alcoholism. But then he was arrested for DUI on his way home from a conference. He's under a great deal of stress at work right now. The economy has caused some layoffs, increasing his workload and causing him to feel uneasy and edgy. He is also adjusting to the unplanned new baby. Over the past few months, he has been drinking heavily, a cocktail or two and several glasses of wine, and arguing about child care, housework, money. For a while Mike's wife increased her drinking along with him, as they unwound together after the kids went to bed, until she realized she couldn't stay up late and drink, manage the kids, and work. She has now quit. The older kids notice when Mike gets drunk and are upset. His wife thinks he's an alcoholic and must quit drinking altogether.

Is Mike an alcoholic who can't control his drinking? Is he just suffering from stress? Is he "allergic" to alcohol? Should he quit altogether? And what does Mike think about all of these questions?

If Mike has stumbled on to one of the disease model's myths mentioned in the Introduction, he has probably not gotten much help in understanding his true relationship with alcohol. If you're using alcohol or other drugs, getting to know this relationship is very important, because it will help you understand how to reduce harm in your life, and it will show you if your efforts to reduce harm have been effective. For example, if cocaine is your favorite drug but you also drink heavily on occasion, and the arguments with your wife occur only when you drink, this connection suggests a causal relationship between *alcohol* and *arguing*. It will be easier for you to stop drinking if you don't also have to stop using cocaine. If indeed the arguments with your wife stop, you might then check in on your relationship with cocaine. If the arguments don't stop, you might consider checking in on your relationship with your wife. In other words, you evaluate each relationship on its own merits and then look for what might be causing which problem, if there is any causality at all. Mike needs to study his emotional life, job stress, home life, and the chemistry of alcohol, then study the *interactions* between them, to change his relationship to alcohol.

Harm reduction offers a new way of looking at your drug and alcohol use. From our perspective, you don't have a disease; you have a *relationship* with the drugs or alcohol you use. The relationship is probably complicated. Like all relationships, some are healthy, some unhealthy. Some are both.

According to harm reduction, drug use is a three-dimensional phenomenon. It is based on your biology, your psychology, and your environment. *Biopsychosocial* is the term used by the social work profession and more recently adopted by many drug treatment professionals. More simply, your use of drugs or alcohol is a complex combination of what is happening in your body, your psyche, and your environment.

For each person, the importance of body, psyche, and environment varies. Each person's relationship with drugs is different. To begin reducing the harm in your life caused by drugs, *your* relationship with drugs deserves careful and unique attention.

What Is a "Relationship with Drugs," Anyway?

There are two ways of looking at this question. The first is to understand drugs the way we understand people or things. We have relationships with people. Whether they are permanent or fleeting, satisfying or unhappy, passionate or dull, hostile or indifferent, they are relationships. We long for a new girlfriend the first weekend she goes out of town on business. We argue with our rebellious teenager. We plead with a defiant toddler to *please* eat her oatmeal. By now, our partner of thirty years knows whether we like mushrooms, tuna fish, or green peppers better than we do.

We have relationships with things. Favorite couch, so comfy. The car I love that costs too much to repair. I'd be lost without my cell phone.

We relate to drugs as we do to people and things. That first shot of vodka is the lover who holds all of your most intimate secrets. The eighth hour of a crack binge feels like a nagging parent. The pipe is even more comfy than your favorite chair. The needle full of heroin is the couch at the end of a bad day.

Relationships with people differ. You can love your husband and loathe his father. You can have fun with your eight-year-old but find your fourteen-year-old totally stressful. And, of course, sometimes you want to divorce your husband and move in with your father-in-law or put your eight-year-old in a blender and relax into an intelligible conversation with your fourteen-year-old.

Likewise, you may have different relationships with different drugs. Can't start the day without a large coffee but can do fine without vodka till the weekend. Love smoking marijuana with your boyfriend, but cocaine makes you paranoid these days. Can get through the day without a cigarette, but not without at least three sodas.

Finally, *relationships change.* Nothing is static. Our relationships with drugs also change. The drinking you did in college would put you in bed for a week now that you're fifty. You were a light social drinker until your partner died. Now the only thing that gets you to sleep at night is a half a fifth of whiskey. You smoked pot every day in your twenties. These days, the stronger pot and the fact that your memory isn't so great anymore means you save it for parties. On the other hand, the cocaine you snorted at parties in the eighties became the crack you started smoking five days a week in the nineties, a habit you still haven't gotten rid of.

In other words, a relationship with drugs is complex. We have found it useful to base our understanding of drug use and abuse on a set of five principles. These principles form the basis for the rest of this book.

Harm Reduction Principles

Not All Drug Use Is Abuse

In fact, drug use occurs on a *continuum* that ranges from no use at all to chaotic, out-of-control use, the kind of use that is often thought of as addiction. On the next page is a very simple spiral showing snapshot points along this continuum.

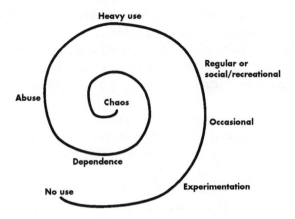

The general meaning of these levels of use is probably obvious enough. In Chapter 3 we go over these different levels of use in detail. For now, here are a few points to consider:

- It is possible to be *physiologically dependent* at any point after occasional use without any *psychological* dependence. In other words, when you take opiates like Vicodin or Percoset for pain, or when you take Paxil for depression, once you build up tolerance to the drug, you will feel bad when you stop. You will get "sick" and have other symptoms such as headaches. This is not addiction, it's *physical* dependence. It is just what happens when your body adjusts to certain medications or drugs and needs time to readjust when you quit. *Psychological* dependence is when you have to have it—you crave the drug, perhaps use more and more, and feel lost without it.
- *Regular use* can be for any *reason*—recreation, medical need, communal or personal ritual, perception or performance enhancement, etc.
- *Heavy* is a relative term—what is heavy alcohol use in one culture (Asian or Jewish) may be moderate in another (Irish or Italian). What is moderate to a healthy body may be heavy to one that is coping with diabetes, hepatitis C, or major depression.
- *Substance abuse,* the continued use of drugs despite negative consequences, is an official diagnostic category in the drug treatment profession and is generally the point at which people start to think *addiction.* This is an oversimplification that is misleading.
- *Substance dependence* is the most serious of the two official diagnostic categories. It can, but does not necessarily, include out-of-control drug-using behavior that supersedes all other life activities. People can be sub-

stance dependent, however, and still function quite well in many areas of life, with their drug use remaining hidden.

• *Chaotic* is the term used by the harm reduction movement to set apart drug use that is out of control and causes chaos in the life of the user and those around him or her. Chaotic use is most accurately described as addiction.

• Most people do not progress to the point of chaotic use, or to heavy use, abuse, or dependence, for that matter. They can, nevertheless, incur harm if they are uninformed about their drugs or themselves.

Many people (estimates vary) who *do* progress to one of the more serious levels of use back off on their own, without any help. Many people, as you probably well know, go back and forth between heavy and not heavy use, just like Mike.

People Use Drugs for Reasons

Gloria and her husband were in a car accident and got a large financial settlement. This money allowed them to retire, so they've been traveling a lot. Gloria's neck keeps bothering her. The muscle relaxant, Soma, that her doctor gave her works OK, but only if she takes more than prescribed. Her doctor wouldn't give her more, and she ran out once and got very anxious and shaky. Now she goes to a few different doctors to make sure she doesn't run out. Is she a drug addict? Does she have a disease, or is she managing in the best way she knows how to control her pain?

Gloria's story shows us that it is natural to look for comfort in an uncomfortable world and that indeed drugs help. Looking at drug use through the eyes of harm reduction allows us to see it as a function of normal life. While AA and traditional treatment tell us addiction is a disease and alcohol and other drugs are the things that cause all the trouble, harm reduction understands that trouble usually comes before drug use. Even though using drugs or alcohol can create a whole set of other troubles and harms, for many of us things could be a whole lot worse without them. Heavy alcohol use destroys liver tissue and creates depression in some people, but its ability to numb painful feelings has stopped more than a few people from soberly jumping off the Golden Gate Bridge. Marijuana and alcohol, when used in large quantities, impair the storage of new memory—a very useful function for survivors of trauma who have problems with flashbacks and intrusive memories. In other words, even though they cause harm, drugs often serve as a warm blanket on a shivering psyche.

Think about getting dressed in the morning. In most parts of American culture, you were shown, ever since you were little, that the right way to leave the house is fully clothed. It may be in ripped jeans, or it may be in a silk suit, but the nonnegotiable way to feel OK out there in the world is to wear clothes. It feels odd and embarrassing just to consider being around strangers, colleagues, even friends or family, without our clothes. We would feel exposed and vulnerable. So we wear clothes.

But let's say you have a big scar on your elbow. You fell through a window when you were six and don't like people looking at the scar or asking about it—it reminds you of the dog that was chasing you when you fell and of the cold hospital room where you got stitched up. So you always wear long-sleeved shirts to hide your scar. Without sleeves you feel exposed, naked.

For some of you, this is how drugs and alcohol work. You suffered abuse or neglect in childhood. Or your heart was broken by losing someone important. Most drug and alcohol abusers have experienced some type of trauma earlier in life—abuse or neglect. Trauma often leaves the survivor feeling not only scarred but unworthy and vulnerable. Drugs or alcohol now clothe these scars like long sleeves over a vulnerable elbow. They help you deal with the emotional or physical pain you have weathered. Just as you want to wear clothes to feel protected, you might want to walk around high to feel insulated. There is actually a chemical basis to this desire—early trauma impairs the development of certain brain systems, particularly in the emotional and judgment centers of the brain. So your feeling of unworthiness or vulnerability is actually "wired" into you. These same brain systems are heavily affected by alcohol and other drugs. In other words, drugs often fix—temporarily—what's broken! Take away the drugs and you feel unsafe, unprotected, naked.

No one would dream of stripping the shirt off your elbow to get a closer look at that scar. It would be unthinkable to demand that you walk around in a T-shirt while you go through psychotherapy to deal with the dog, the stitches, the hospital room. And no one should ask you to strip yourself of what may be the only thing that helps you survive your pain, *even though your methods may also cause you trouble.*

There is a growing belief among some drug treatment professionals (a belief that we subscribe to) that heavy alcohol and other drug use or abuse is linked to some common difficulties—trouble with relationships, trouble with taking good care of oneself, trouble with handling strong emotions, and most of all, struggles with self-esteem. And the drugs are not the cause of these troubles; the troubles came first, and the drugs help to soften the pain.

31

In other words, people use drugs and alcohol for reasons, and those reasons may be quite good, even if some of the effects aren't what we had in mind. It is not a requirement that you be without adequate "protection" to reduce harm in your life. **And so it is *not* a requirement that you must be clean and sober in order to reduce harm in your life.**

Problems Don't Just Come from Drugs Themselves but from a Combination of Factors and Circumstances

Yolanda has always been a good student, even though life at home with her parents was a constant battle. She finally moved out and is working and going to school. It's a hard life. She and her friends started smoking heroin on the weekends, and it really helped her relax. This guy she met talked her into letting him inject her with heroin, and it was heaven! They talked and made love, and she feels better than she has in years. He says that as long as she shoots only with him, she'll be safe and won't get addicted. Yolanda is caught between her desire to succeed in life and the emotional scars from a difficult childhood. And now she's in a relationship with a man who makes her feel wonderful but is introducing her to a whole new, more dangerous level of drug use. Her drug use might be driven by her need to relax, but starting to use intravenously seems to be driven by her relationship with her boyfriend.

Have you ever wondered why some people get into trouble with drugs and others don't? How can some people put down their wine glass when it's half full? Who are those people who just smoke other people's cigarettes every now and again? How come there is such a high correlation between substance abuse treatment and a history of childhood trauma, but there are still so many people with traumatic childhoods who *don't* abuse alcohol or other drugs? Why, if heroin is such an addicting drug, do most people who try heroin not become addicted? Why, if addiction is a disease with no cure, do the majority of people who act like addicts as young people "mature out" somewhere between their late twenties and early thirties without ever thinking about an AA meeting and without ever returning to heavy drinking or using?

Problems with drugs develop out of a unique interaction between the drug and its compelling properties, the person and his or her unique needs and characteristics, and the environment with its combination of stressors and sources of supports—in other words, what the drug is and what it does, who you are and what you are looking for, and the circumstances surrounding you and your use. This model is called Drug, Set, Setting, and it is described in more detail in Chapter 6. The drug, set, setting model influences how we understand and evaluate the many people with whom we have worked. It is a little different from the traditional addiction model. The combination of drug, set, and setting means that no one has the same relationship with drugs. In other words, *everyone is unique.*

You Are Your Own Expert

Many people will tell you that there is only one program of recovery, the 12 Steps of Alcoholics Anonymous or one of its many sister programs. If you follow your own wisdom about your body and mind, you're trying to do it "your way." We can't resist saying "That's the point!" In fact, your wisdom is best. Only you know your pain. Only you know that you cannot tolerate the anxiety you feel when faced with the prospect of a relationship. Only you know whether you can quit heroin, pot, *and* cigarettes. You are the best person to evaluate what you need and why you use drugs to fill that need.

When you are given advice or feedback, or when someone in your life gets mad at you and insists you DO something, make sure the message you absorb is kind. When your husband insists that you come home after work without stopping for several drinks, is it because he doesn't want you to die in a DUI accident, or because his business meetings at night require that you be with the kids? Try to distinguish which part of the message is for the other person's benefit—which is surely his or her right to consider and perhaps your responsibility to honor—and which is for your benefit. Avoid getting overwhelmed by others' opinions and look to what you know to be true. You still might have to negotiate, but you won't take care of yourself for long by bending to others' will. If you aren't sure, check it out with someone you trust to understand you. If you don't know such a person, look for one. In Chapter 9, we give suggestions for how to go about finding the right therapist.

Change Is Slow

In the past half-century, the United States has been witness to phenomenal inventions of all types. We have watched LPs shrink into CDs. We have watched communications melt pounds off desk phones into lighter-than-a-credit-card cell phones. And while some of us were still struggling to program our VCRs, sound bites became the essence of communication. One of the most famous sound bites of recent years has been Nike's "Just do it!" We watch Michael Jordan practicing his art, the result of a lifetime of skill building on top of raw talent. If we have seen the commercials, we have been encouraged by Nike to go out and do it ourselves. So we rush out there and then halt, courtside, peer down at our sneakers, and ask ourselves, "Who, me? Do what?" Even if we *had* some idea of how to replicate Michael's magic, we would flounder hopelessly, wondering "How *does* he do it?" But Nike doesn't include instructions.

The field of addiction has been no different. Nancy Reagan's "Just Say No to Drugs" campaign preceded Nike's 1988 ad slogan by years. Commonly considered to be the out-of-control use of intoxicating substances, addiction is an extraordinarily complex phenomenon involving thought, emotion, biology, environment, and behavior. Success rates at "treatment" are notoriously low, and the consequences of failure can be everything from disappointing to life threatening. Yet we give in to the impulse to embrace simplistic explanations as the *truths* about addiction. We watch the world change with dizzying speed and think that we, too, should be able to change quickly.

Our love of sound bites results in such slogans as "Keep it simple," "Let go, let God," "One day at a time," "Keep coming back," or "Once an addict, always an addict," and, of course, "Just say no." While catchy and even persuasive at times, these quick-fix phrases don't always reflect the reality or the complexity of our feelings and behavior. The most famous from AA, adopted into the popular culture to refer to all manner of things, is "One step at a time." That's all very well, and we couldn't agree more, but the steps they're referring to are taken only after the user is "clean and sober." There is no program of steps for the active user to *get* "clean and sober," just a slippery slope to the "bottom." Sobriety—or *abstinence*, as we prefer to call it— is supposed to happen when the user "hits bottom," "surrenders to a higher power," and "gets with the program."

The many words and phrases in quotation marks indicate our lack of belief in the ideas expressed, despite the respect we have for their usefulness to a dedicated group of people who have found help in the program of AA. Unfortunately, it is a small group, possibly as low as 5 percent of the people who get into trouble with alcohol and other drugs.

In contrast, harm reduction, the newest model for understanding drug use and abuse, involves embracing the full complexity of each individual's relationship with his or her drug of choice. This approach is about reducing drug-related harm in individual and small ways. The steps start before the drug user even thinks about the nature of his or her drug use. They start as soon as *anyone* begins to worry. They progress through a series of stages that is both predictable and human, called (not surprisingly) the Stages of Change. In real people with real lives, change, although constant, is most often slow.

What if you don't want to acknowledge harm? George has been playing music lately with some other guys. They sometimes go to clubs to hear other bands. Everyone seems to be doing ecstasy. He's tried it a few times, and it's great. It makes everyone seem friendly and makes him feel close to his friends. Someone at the club got really sick the other night, though, and ended up in the hospital. They said he almost died from heat exhaustion. George doesn't know whether or not to take ecstasy again. No one else he knows ever had any trouble with the drug. Maybe it was just a fluke and won't happen to him. He won't worry about it for now.

Perhaps by now you've probably been told that your unwillingness to look at the harmful consequences of your habit or make substantial changes in your using, means you're in denial. In our experience, it's unlikely that you're in denial. It's more likely that you're either uneducated about the drugs you're using or ambivalent about what to do. In other words, you're actually unaware of the relevant information, or you are of two minds, have mixed feelings, are stuck on the fence. George is most likely a little of both. All that means is that he is at an early stage of the change process, the stage where he feels little pressure to worry about what's happening with his drug use.

A problem in our "just do it" society is that once we acknowledge a problem, we are supposed to DO something about it. However, the slogan is a trap that keeps us from looking. *Doing* means *changing*. And when it comes to drugs, *changing* means *quitting*. How on earth do we know, when we take the first peek, what we want to change, never mind whether we want to quit?

Feeling ambivalent about changing your relationship with your drugs is normal, especially if changing that relationship means leaving it forever. No one would suggest that you leave your husband or wife of ten, twenty, or thirty years as soon as you got that "Oh, no, what have I been doing?" feeling. That sudden thud of reality that your relationship is a mess, even if the two of you have been fighting since the day you married, doesn't mean you're packing your bags tonight. You talk, you fight some more, you wonder how the kids would handle a divorce, you try to imagine yourself single again, and you just can't see it. Of course, your drugs don't have feelings like your wife does. And you probably don't have children with your drugs. But you *have* had a close relationship with them for a long time. And if they are help-ing you cope with something else equally or more serious, you may not want to just throw them out.

It's actually healthy to be able to have conflicting feelings. It means you're able to see the upside, the downside, and the gray areas in between. But, normal as it is, ambivalence can be paralyzing if you're not aware that you're being pulled in two or more directions. You may not realize that the weight gain to which drinking contributes is in conflict with alcohol's ability to make you the life of the party. Take heart. Being stuck on the fence is sim-ply a reasonable reaction to the sinking feeling that you're going to be pres-sured to DO something. Who on earth would want to launch an exploration of his drug use, knowing it would only lead to pressure to make difficult de-cisions or changes? Staying unconscious simply means you're trying to tee-ter comfortably on that fence. Teetering on the fence is the legitimate begin-ning of the process of change. You don't have to *do* anything. Just try not to fall off.

Looking at harm is sometimes the very thing that *drives* drinking and us-ing.

> "I feel guilty about how much money I've blown on crack, so I use more to erase the guilt."
> "I'm already a junkie with AIDS, so why bother using clean needles or even *trying* to quit?"
> "My wife left because I drink, so what the hell? Might as well keep drink-ing."

This reaction is normal. Looking at harm is a big step, and a very painful one if the damage is serious. Take your time. Give this book to your cousin who *really* needs it. Or just leave it on the shelf and head for the bar.

When you are ready, when you become curious or more relaxed, when some other crisis in your life has calmed down, when you feel it's safe to move forward, or when you can't stand the pain anymore, you can start to look at where the harm in your life is occurring and where you might begin considering some changes. Any time this step starts to overwhelm you, just stop.

How do you know if you're feeling overwhelmed? Some signs are: Your head hurts. Your stomach churns. Distractions come fast and furious. You want to use. You want to drink. You feel hopeless. You hate yourself or your life. The dark hole looks awfully tempting. Stop reading and wait until your curiosity returns. Wait until the safety comes back.

You Can Make Positive Changes While Still Using

Up until now, it has not felt manageable to quit drugs and alcohol completely. It has not felt OK to surrender or feel powerless. And it has not felt okay to look out on your future and see yourself sentenced to a life of permanent recovery, always defined by an identity as an addict you may wish to shed. Harm reduction believes you are entitled to look in the mirror and see a person with problems, not a problem person with an incurable disease.

Is abstinence the only way to start taking better care of yourself? The disease model says you should quit all mind-altering drugs before you can begin to deal with other problems. Harm reduction says otherwise—you can pick any problem on which to start. So what if drinking is contributing to weight gain? You might also not be exercising much these days. You don't have to quit drinking to go back to the gym or take a walk every other day. If you're having marital problems, you could go ahead and start couples counseling as long as you find a therapist who won't make you quit cocaine before letting you talk about your relationship. If you use speed and have unsafe sex when you're high, you could devise tricks to increase the likelihood that you will use protection when you're having sex. Put condoms in every pocket and in your wallet. Go out with a buddy who's safer than you. Go to clubs where the management pushes condoms. Try nonpenetrative sex. You don't have to quit shooting dope to start eating better. You can *always* drink more water and, if you can control your using schedule even a little, get more sleep. People do manage all of these things and more. It helps to find a using buddy, a friend, a therapist, someone who will help you think of these things and remind you to practice them.

Just Say Know: Substance Use Management

If you take only one thing from this book, take this: **You don't have to label yourself an alcoholic or addict to examine and make sensible decisions about your use of drugs and alcohol. You do, however, have to *know* something about the drugs you use.** The practice of using alcohol and other drugs sensibly is called *substance use management.*

Even if you or your family, employer, or probation officer decide that quitting is the only choice, it will probably take more than a day to get there if you're like most of us. On the road to abstinence are many ways that you can take better care of yourself and those around you. If abstinence is not your destination, rest assured that there is almost no drug in the world that can't be used safely by at least some people.

You don't have to quit smoking crack altogether to get more sleep. You might have to quit smoking earlier in the evening, however. You don't have to quit ecstasy to avoid having heatstroke, but you might have to drink plenty of water, avoid alcohol, and wear lightweight clothing and no headgear. You don't have to quit drinking to avoid trouble at work. But you do have to know how long it takes for all the alcohol to get out of your system and quit drinking in time to be sober, with no smell of alcohol on you, when you show up.

There is a lot to know to use drugs safely. There is a lot to know about your relationship with alcohol and drugs. It's not all hard work, though. If you use drugs or alcohol, you're probably already pretty motivated to get real, unbiased, nonjudgmental information. And you already know a lot just by using. What might be new is that we're asking you to *pay attention*. Harm reduction assumes that you already know a lot about drugs, your reasons for using, and the problems you might be experiencing. You already have a lot of wisdom. We want to draw it out and perhaps offer something you haven't thought of yet.

SOURCES AND SUGGESTED READINGS

This chapter introduces ideas that are developed in the rest of the book. Therefore, the entire reading list is applicable. Here are just a few references to supplement what we have talked about:

On "Maturing Out"—how people's drug use changes over time without help:

> *The Truth about Addiction and Recovery.* Stanton Peele and Archie Brodsky. Simon & Schuster. 1991.
> "A Life-Span Perspective on Natural Recovery (Self-Change) from Alcohol Problems." Linda Sobell, John Cunningham, Mark Sobell, and Tony Toneatto. In John Baer, G. Alan Marlatt, and Robert McMahon, Eds. *Addictive Behaviors across the Life Span: Prevention, Treatment and Policy Issues.* Sage. 1993.

For the most useful explanation of the Stages of Change model and help to work the stages:

> *Changing for Good.* James Prochaska, Carlo DiClemente, and John Norcross. Avon. 1994.

Drug, Set, Setting. This book is out of print, but probably at some libraries:

> *Drug, Set, and Setting: The Basis for Controlled Intoxicant Use.* Norman E. Zinberg. Yale University Press. 1984.

For the most accessible description of the biology of the brain and how drugs work (there are many others in the Sources and Suggested Readings appendix. Allan Schore and Bessel van der Kolk, in particular, address the damage to brain systems caused by trauma. They're technical but not impossible and worth a look for those of you who want to pursue this topic):

> *Buzzed: The Straight Facts about the Most Used and Abused Drugs from Alcohol to Ecstasy.* Cynthia Kuhn, Scott Swartzwelder, and Wilkie Wilson. Norton. 1998.

For the self-medication hypothesis:

> "The self-medication hypothesis of substance use disorders: A reconsideration and recent applications." Edward Khantzian. *Harvard Review of Psychiatry,* 4, 231–244, 1997.

For the study on the psychological health of teens who use drugs versus those who do not. This is a good source for publications on many different aspects of drug use, abuse, and policy, including another excellent study from the early eighties on the different patterns of resolving alcohol problems:

> RAND Corporation Drug Research Policy Center. *www.rand.org/centers/dprc/DPRCpubindex.html*

For the yearly National Household Survey of drug use and abuse:

> Substance Abuse and Mental Health Services Administration. Office of Applied Studies. *www.samhsa.gov*

For data on the impact of nicotine:

> "Nicotine." Joy Schmitz, Murray Jarvik, and Nina Schneider. In Joyce Lowinson, Pedro Ruiz, Robert Millman, and John Langrod, Eds. *Substance Abuse: A Comprehensive Textbook* (3rd ed.). Williams & Wilkins. 1997.

3 HOW MUCH IS TOO MUCH?

You've probably heard these questions before:

How much do you drink? How many grams of coke in a week? How many doses of E in a night? Do you smoke pot before work or just in the evenings? How often do you shoot up—are you on a maintenance or a recreational schedule? Do you drink every night, or do you confine it to weekends?

And these:

How many times have you been in trouble—DUIs, fights with your spouse, arrests, job losses? How many people are being hurt by your drug use?

It's traditional to identify a problem with drugs and alcohol by *measuring*—the amount of alcohol consumed, the frequency of drug use, the number and severity of personal consequences, the people hurt. There's some validity to that approach, to be sure. But there are problems with it as well.

First, most such measuring has been two-dimensional. One of the most widely used tools, the Michigan Alcohol Screening Test, asks two-dimensional questions about dynamic, three-dimensional areas, such as "Have you ever lost friends because of your drinking?" If you answer yes, you chalk up a point on the "you are an alcoholic" side. But what if the answer is not a simple yes? What if your answer is "I lose friends all the time, but it's because I borrow money from them for rent." *Yes* does not reveal the complex relationship among you, alcohol, money, and friends. And a simple *no* would not surface these issues either.

Take another question: "Have you ever gone to a doctor, social worker, clergyman, or mental health clinic for help with any emotional problem in which drinking was part of the problem?" Although a simple *yes* adds another point toward understanding yourself as an alcoholic, it does not reveal more subtle, but important, information about emotional problems or how alcohol has effectively muffled your grief since your spouse died or your anxiety since September 11, 2001. Nor does a simple *no* reveal that you often have the *desire* to seek help but have not mustered the courage to walk through the door.

Second, measuring in the traditional way can be overwhelming if you're not ready for the information it can yield. Consider a brief questionnaire intended to get at key elements of a drug problem that goes by its acronym, CAGE:

Cut down: Has anyone ever recommended that you cut down or stop drinking?

Annoyed: Have you ever felt annoyed or angry if someone comments on your using?

Guilty: Have there been times when you've felt guilty or regretted things that occurred because of drinking or using?

Eye-opener: Have you ever used alcohol or other drugs (don't forget coffee!) to get started in the morning or to steady your nerves?

By all means, if you find these questions useful, answer them and use the answers to learn more about your relationship with your drugs. But also pay close attention to your internal signs of distress. Questions like these are often designed to hit you square in the face with the hard truth. The trouble is, the truth *does* hurt, especially when it's condensed to the point of oversimplification. Questions of this sort also assume the perspective of the person judging your use, and that person may have ideas about what is "too much" that do not match your own. This mismatch in views can make you feel even more overwhelmed, and feeling overwhelmed pushes some people to use. If you find even *thinking* about measuring your drug or alcohol use exhausting, overwhelming, irrelevant, or just plain useless, DON'T DO IT. Put down the book, take a deep breath, and go do something else.

(P.S. You have just practiced harm reduction! You have reduced the harm caused by reading this book, and that will probably help you come back to it without feeling beaten up.)

Finally, measuring doesn't tell the whole story. We are three-dimensional creatures. Any drugs we use affect all dimensions of our being—physical, emotional, spiritual, cultural, social, environmental—and are, in turn, affected by these dimensions.

41

Consider a different issue—weight. A man weighs 240 pounds. If he is 5'8", we would probably agree he is on the heavy side, and his doctor would recommend that he lose eighty or so pounds. If he is 6'2", those among us who are football fans would see him as robust and healthy, maybe a little heavy for a quarterback and too light for a center, but just about right for a cornerback. Now imagine that this man lives in Afghanistan, the Sudan, or Somalia and is facing famine and starvation. Or he lives anywhere and has cancer or AIDS. Two hundred and forty pounds become a blessing. In Africa it may be an indication of wealth or former wealth; in the case of cancer or AIDS, a boon to withstanding the rigors of treatment. In any case, the more the better. Depending on culture, environment, and personal circumstances, there will be varying levels of concern or celebration, not to mention differing goals, for weight management.

So it is with drugs and alcohol. Measuring is—and should be— a complex process, and how much of this or that is a *problem* depends on many factors. But as in everything, the more one strays from "moderation," the more likely one is to encounter problems.

Measuring substance use within a harm reduction framework asks you to entertain far more than traditional measures or evaluation tools ask you to do. Harm reduction asks you to measure in an interactive format. For example, a man who drinks a glass or two of wine a night with dinner is considered to be a moderate drinker in most Western cultures. He is practicing what is called *normative behavior.* However, if he has diabetes or hepatitis C and has been instructed by his doctor not to drink any alcohol, his drinking pattern immediately falls into the category of heavy, if not potentially lethal.

Measuring your use within a harm reduction framework is complex and shifts according to many personal and environmental factors. Next we will introduce you to another tool for measuring your drug use, a tool that will help you understand your relationship with drugs or alcohol in a more complex, and therefore useful, way.

In Chapter 2 we introduced you to the continuum of drug use. The continuum is an interactive measure of the amount consumed, the frequency of use, and the harm done by your use. As in the preceding example, one glass of wine with dinner each evening can fall into the category of typical social use until we discover that the drinker has diabetes or hepatitis C. That moves the quantity and frequency of use into the category of heavy use, because any alcohol at all has the potential to negatively impact a medical problem. On the following page is a review and a more detailed explanation of each level of use.

THE CONTINUUM OF ALCOHOL AND DRUG USE	
No Use	You abstain from all psychoactive substances. Depending on your culture or your health, you may or may not count coffee, tea, or chocolate among these. You may have never used, or you may have quit.
Experimentation	You are curious about the effects of a drug. You use once or a few times. You don't maintain a supply.
Occasional	There may or may not be a particular pattern of use. You use occasionally at parties, events, or holidays, maybe because a particular drug is being used by others. You drink cocktails after work or beer watching a football game. You use "poppers" (amyl nitrite) to enhance sex. You use ecstasy at a dance club to feel close to friends and dance all night. Or you smoke other people's cigarettes when you're around smokers. You are able to attend events where people are using and abstain yourself because you don't feel like using at that time. You use alone for a particular effect, such as smoking pot to make reading science fiction more interesting.
Regular	Using becomes predictable. A pattern has been established. You might drink beer only on weekends, but it is every weekend. You smoke weed whenever you're stressed, and that's about every other day. Or maybe it's once a month. Otherwise, you smoke when you're with friends at a party. You shoot speed when you go to clubs and meet a guy to have sex with, about every weekend. You shoot heroin every day. You may use recreationally or as an emotional "crutch" (*coping mechanism* is the term we prefer).

(cont.)

THE CONTINUUM OF ALCOHOL AND DRUG USE *(cont.)*

Heavy	The fuzziest level of use, "heavy" depends on your health and on the norms of your group or culture. You use more than you "should." This evaluation is often a confusing and very subjective one. If you have hepatitis C, two beers is probably more than you "should" drink. If no one else in your social group smokes pot every day, you might be considered a heavy user, but not if they do. Daily heroin use could be considered "regular" or "heavy" depending on whether it interferes with the other activities in your life.
Abuse	A formal designation in addiction medicine and the drug treatment profession. You continue using despite having incurred negative consequences: angry family, warnings at work, DUIs, medical problems, legal consequences, running through your bank account like wildfire.
Dependence	The other formal designation in addiction medicine and drug treatment. Your life becomes organized around using. You might be physically dependent. In other words, you have developed tolerance and you go into withdrawal without the drug. You crave your drug and go out of your way to get it. You try to quit and can't.
Chaos	Out-of-control use that best corresponds to what people mean when they use the term *addiction*. Your life and activities become organized around drug use (getting it, getting money to get it, finding a place to use, using, coming down, enduring withdrawal symptoms). You do not take care of other aspects of life—work, family, friends, your health. You feel lost in your drug use. You keep making promises about quitting. You can no longer identify your motivation for using— you use because you use or to avoid getting sick from withdrawal.

If you remember from Chapter 2, drug abuse and drug dependence refer to particular *kinds* of relationships to drugs. Not all use is abuse. The alcohol user who calls in to work sick once a week because of a hangover and
receives a verbal warning, then continues drinking in the same way, has en-
tered the realm of alcohol abuse. The cocaine user who drains his bank account, loses his job, and endangers his children's livelihood has probably en-
tered the realm of dependence. If he continues in this way and leaves his
family, switches from powder to crack cocaine because it is cheaper and
more compelling, becomes homeless, stops eating regularly, and keeps
smoking crack, he has become a chaotic user.

On the other hand, the drinker who doesn't drink on Sunday before the
start of the work week and waits until Friday to start again, *even if she drinks
heavily*, may not be abusing alcohol. And the cocaine user who maintains a
balance between getting high, working, paying the bills, and relating to family and other important people is not a drug abuser, *even though the drug is
illegal*, provided she makes sensible decisions about when, where, how,
and how much to use and can avoid arrest and incarceration for illegal drug
use.

Hopefully by now we have persuaded you that you don't have to
worry about whether or not you are an addict. Without the diagnosis of
addiction nipping at your heels, perhaps you can make realistic and can-
did statements to yourself about the level of your use. Here are three special considerations to bear in mind when placing your drug use on the
continuum.

1. Consider the continuum drug by drug. Each drug may have a different
place in your life. It is common for people to become heavy or abusive users
of speed, cocaine, or heroin but remain moderate or social users of alcohol
or marijuana. People who become abusers of marijuana may occasionally
party with cocaine or drink socially.

2. Your use of each drug will not remain the same over time. How many
people have been heavy drinkers, marijuana smokers, or party drug users as
teenagers, in college, into their early twenties, only to slow down as they approach thirty and have more financial or work responsibilities or can't stay
up so late anymore? At least 50 percent of heavy drug or alcohol users. This
is sometimes called "maturing out." What about someone who has lost a
child or a lover or a spouse and who then begins drinking or smoking
heavily? It seems like the world has stopped and the pain is interminable,

but in reality it doesn't last forever. The same can happen with drugs and alcohol.

3. Finally, your use does not automatically progress to abuse and dependence, even if you get into trouble. Moreover, even people who reach the chaotic stage of drug use can back off to a less destructive level of use. Many people's use waxes and wanes in response to both internal (emotional and mental) and external pressures and situations.

So now you may be able to guess where each drug falls on the continuum, based on the amount and frequency of your use. However, you still may not know how much *harm* is done by the drugs you use. You may not know about the drugs themselves, their medical and psychological effects. You also may not know everything about your own medical and psychological conditions. You certainly know if you've gotten one or more DUIs. You know if your partner has left you because you're stoned all the time. You know if you were arrested for growing pot. You know you can't concentrate at work because you've started partying during the week. You know you disappear for a day or two after every payday. You know you got HIV by sharing needles. But did you know that you can contract hepatitis C by sharing straws when you snort cocaine? Did you know that alcohol and marijuana both impair the storage of memory, so if you're a student who has to take a lot of exams, they may not be the greatest drugs to use? Did you know that alcohol and cocaine together produce another chemical, cocaethylene, a more toxic substance in the liver than either drug alone?

How Drugs Harm

On the next page is a chart that gives you some information about the medical, psychological, and social harms of each major class of drugs. By no means is this list comprehensive. For that we would need to write a textbook. We offer some good and readable resources, both print and online ones, at the back of this book, if you want to know more about how specific drugs work. In the middle of this book is a comprehensive description of each class of drugs.

THE HARMS OF THE MAJOR CLASSES OF DRUGS

Drug	Psychological risks	Medical risks	Social risks
Stimulants Amphetamines Cocaine	Increase anxiety, sometimes to the point of paranoia. Can cause what is called "stimulant psychosis," with paranoia and hallucinations, which almost always resolves with discontinued use.	Raise blood pressure and heart rate—risk of stroke, heart attack. Constrict blood vessels. Poor nutrition can accompany use. Risk of blood-borne diseases such as HIV and hepatitis with IV use.	Illegal, except for some amphetamines or amphetamine-like drugs prescribed for weight control, attention-deficit disorder, or narcolepsy (and by the militaries of the United States and other countries). Chronic use is expensive. Isolation can result from paranoia. Use during sex can lead to unsafe sex.
Stimulants Nicotine	Very habit-forming. Difficulty concentrating or irritability in situations where you can't light up. Embarrassment or guilt at being a smoker in the midst of others' disapproval.	Well-known risks to the heart and lungs, most famously, cancer and emphysema. Less known effects on health of skin due to oxygen deprivation.	Social isolation due to stigma about smoking; more prominent in some environments than others.
Stimulants Caffeine	Dependence to "get going" in the morning. Anxiety at high doses (4–5 cups of coffee a day for some people). Increase in panic attacks.	Irritant to the gastrointestinal system. At very high doses (8 cups of coffee or more) can be toxic, causing vomiting. Headaches in withdrawal. Sleep problems.	None, in our society. It is the most accepted drug. It is rather expensive, however, if you don't brew your own.

(cont.)

47

THE HARMS OF THE MAJOR CLASSES OF DRUGS *(cont.)*

Drug	Psychological risks	Medical risks	Social risks
Hallucinogens LSD Peyote Mushrooms DMT, as in ayahuasca Salvia divinorum	Difficulty functioning while using. Can trigger psychosis in vulnerable people.	None known. Some cause nausea and purging, which can be uncomfortable.	Illegal. Using at the wrong time, in the wrong place, or with the wrong people can lead to a bad trip.
Ecstasy	Depression hangovers the day after using. Damage to serotonin neurons, the brain cells that help control our mood, observed in studies on rats that were given enormous doses, giving rise to concerns about long-term mood problems. (So far, not proven in human research.)	Increases heart rate, blood pressure, body temperature. Risk of death from kidney failure due to high body temperature. Can be cut with more dangerous substances or ones that react badly with it, such as dextromethorphan (the drug that is in over-the-counter cough medicine).	Illegal. Becoming bonded to a group because of the drug might limit connections to other people or encourage overuse.
Alcohol	May increase depression or cause sleep disturbances. Anxiety in withdrawal. Interferes with memory and learning.	Disrupts body's ability to absorb nutrients. Damages liver over time. May cause brain damage with long-term use. Delirium tremens (DTs) in withdrawal. Accidents. Alcohol poisoning at large doses—depends on each individual's tolerance level.	Disinhibition can lead to inappropriate behavior, saying things you regret, having unwanted or unsafe sex, or becoming aggressive. Being a victim of violence the highest risk for women. Driving while intoxicated.

Barbiturates, benzodiazepines, including Rohypnol ("roofies") GHB	Anxiety in withdrawal. Cognitive problems while intoxicated and with long-term heavy use (barbiturates). Interfere with learning new things.	Withdrawal can be dangerous—risk of seizures. High risk of overdose with barbiturates or GHB. Dose is often uncertain with GHB. High rate of accidents.	Disinhibition can lead to inappropriate behavior, saying things you regret. Unsafe sex or date rape with GHB and roofies, which are sometimes slipped into drinks without a person's knowledge.
Opiates and opioids Opium Morphine, codeine Heroin Oxycontin MS Contin Vicodin Percoset Percodan Demerol Darvon Fentanyl	Dependence is psychologically compelling, making quitting or controlling hard. The lifestyle associated with illegal opiate use can cause depression, anxiety, guilt, and low self-esteem due to the stigma of being a "junkie." Heavy use may lead to difficulty tolerating stress, anxiety, and pain after quitting. Opiates do not cause, but are heavily associated with, depression and history of trauma.	All cause physiological tolerance and dependence, with risk of very uncomfortable withdrawal for those who are dependent. Risk of HIV, hepatitis, and infections with needle use. Heroin's purity is often unknown, increasing the risk of overdose. It also can be cut with unknown substances or contain bacteria, causing abscesses or serious infection. Poor nutrition and self-care may accompany abuse, as may constipation.	Heroin illegal. Others are prescribed medications. Strong social stigma, except for community-accepted painkillers or if you belong to a drug-using subculture. Very expensive to maintain a regular habit, leading to illegal or antisocial behavior.

(cont.)

49

THE HARMS OF THE MAJOR CLASSES OF DRUGS (cont.)

Drug	Psychological risks	Medical risks	Social risks
Inhalants Poppers (amyl nitrite) House-hold solvents (glue, gasoline, aerosols)	Dissociation, poor judgment, impulsive and risk-taking behavior. Possible paranoia and aggression.	High risk of traumatic injury and overdose with inhaling solvents (brain deprived of oxygen in many cases). High risk of brain damage.	Aggressive behavior. Unsafe sex.
Dissociative anesthetics PCP Ketamine Nitrous oxide Dextromethorphan	Dissociation, anxiety, possible aggression (usually only PCP).	Accidents (falls). Death from lack of oxygen.	Unsafe sex. Illegal.
Cannabis	Paranoia for some people. Motivational problems observed but not proven to be caused by marijuana. Memory impairment.	Minimal—possible increased risk of lung disease if smoked.	Illegal unless used by physician recommendation in states where this is allowed.

Special Considerations

Harm is relative to how much vulnerability you bring with you and to your life circumstances and goals. For example . . .

If you are an older adult, you need to be aware that your metabolism will have slowed with age. It's a bummer, but the amount of alcohol, speed, or Valium we can absorb without getting too high is likely to be less when we're sixty-five than when we're twenty. It's hard to be precise, since we're all individuals with many other differences, but it's worth bearing in mind before you take your drugs—or medications, for that matter—although your doctor will likely have been aware of that issue when prescribing your medicine.

Gender and race can have an impact on how high we get on which drugs. Again, it's hard to be specific, since there are many differences within groups of people. One easy example is the fact that women have half the enzyme that metabolizes alcohol than men do, so they tend to get more intoxicated. The same is true for some proportion of Asians who lack the ability to metabolize alcohol. Bear in mind that racial groups are vulnerable to different diseases as well, and those diseases or vulnerabilities might impact one's ability to use certain drugs.

If you are pregnant or have infants or young children, a few things are worth considering. Recreational drugs cross the blood–placenta barrier as well as get into breast milk. What this means is that your fetus is getting the same drugs you are. Before you panic, research has not substantiated what this means, except in the case of Fetal Alcohol Syndrome, which affects both physical and intellectual characteristics of a child. We also know that some infants are born physically dependent and in need of detoxification from drugs. However, these drugs are probably not uniformly damaging, and there is much to learn. For example, the "crack baby" syndrome has been debunked. It is more likely that learning and emotional difficulties of children born to women who use crack are related to environment (poverty, poor nutrition, neglect, and abuse) rather than to drug effects. Which brings us to the issue of caring for infants and young children. You might ask yourself whether using drugs impedes your ability to be attentive to your child. This question gets more complicated when you consider that you might be using to avoid paying attention to all kinds of hard things about life, with the unintended consequence that you are also less attentive to your baby.

If you are trying to get pregnant but are having difficulty conceiving, you will, no doubt, have asked the question about the effects of all those years of smoking, drinking, coffee, or pot. You might even be blaming yourself for your inability to conceive. There is certainly research that pairs different drugs with male and female infertility, but the data is inconsistent across studies. We can only suggest that you try to weed out the well-researched from the circumstantial evidence. Then weigh your attachment to your drugs against what you learn about their possible impact on your fertility in figuring out what to do. And also bear in mind, before you decide to punish yourself, that people use drugs for reasons.

Certain diseases are closely associated with alcohol and other drug use. HIV, hepatitis, and diabetes are three of those diseases. Some have been contracted as a result of use, some are negatively impacted by use. For example, some drugs interfere with one's ability to absorb HIV medications; alcohol is a sugar, and alcohol interferes with one's ability to absorb nutrients. Again, before getting down on yourself, use the decision-making process we talk about in Chapter 5 and the more detailed information about drugs in this book to figure out what to do.

Now you may be thinking that it's time to crawl back into that hole with your favorite drug, dangerous or not. This is the time that most other books want you to be motivated by what you just read to quit immediately. Go ahead and quit if you want to. But for many of you, it's not that simple. How much of which drug you use is not the whole picture. People use drugs for reasons, and those reasons are often the benefits you get from the drugs you use. In the next two chapters we talk about how drugs help and about the complex interactions among you, your drugs, and your life circumstances. In the meantime, you might read these four stories about some other people and their relationship with drugs.

Is My Drug Use *Really* a Problem?: Four Stories

Cheryl wonders if she will ever get married. Thirty-six years old, established as a successful attorney in Atlanta, she has good friends and a close relationship with her parents, who still live in the small Georgia town in which she was raised. She is on the board of a couple of local arts organizations; is a well-known member of her church, through which she does volunteer work; and is quite respected in the community. Her private grief is that she cannot seem to maintain long-term relationships with men. She dates, her relationships become intimate, but a few months after the sexual relationship has begun, the fighting starts. Conflicts seem to rage over everything, large and small. After six such relationships, it is clear to her that *she* is the common denominator.

As an African American woman raised in the small-town South in the not-so-enlightened 1970s, the respect Cheryl has earned is a point of pride. She is ashamed that she has not completed her success by having a marriage and children. Her friends and acquaintances shake their heads, mystified at her relationship failures, and regularly introduce her to new men. Those who know her well, however, point to her drinking as the source of her problem. Indeed, she drinks regularly—wine with meals or when at home alone watching a movie. Once a sexual relationship starts, her drinking goes from being a regular part of her routine to a necessary ingredient for sex. That is all very well, and common enough for many women and men, but it also loosens her tongue. Once she starts noticing things about her partner that irritate her, she does not hold back her criticisms and picks fights.

Cheryl doesn't argue that alcohol plays a part in escalating the conflicts in which she finds herself embroiled. Her dilemma is that she is too uptight to have sex without it. She craves sexual intimacy, but she is also afraid of it. What no one but her best friend and her therapist know is that her oldest brother, who is seven years older than she, sexually molested her for three years beginning when she was eight years old. As is often the case, he told her he would kill her if she told anyone. The abuse stopped when he left home at eighteen. He has always been difficult and is in and out of trouble now as an adult. Her parents have suffered so much over their oldest child that she could never bear to tell them about what he did to her. So it remained a secret, until she sought therapy to try to resolve her relationship problems.

Despite her part in starting fights with boyfriends, she also notices that she has been in a lot of relationships with men who do not respect her needs once they become intimate. They pay her a lot of attention when they first start dating. But after a while, they become arrogant and demanding. She gets angry at their coldness—she feels that once they have gotten her into bed, they no longer need to woo her or care for her. So she feels she is fighting for more fairness and consideration. A couple of times she dated men who were sweet and gentle. After a while, she lost interest. Unfortunately, their sweet natures went along with their not being particularly ambitious. She sees herself more suited to a man who is high-powered professionally. The others were, in her words, "just too much like my father, who is a nice man and worked hard all his life, but didn't have much to show for it."

Cheryl's shame and frustration have caused her to drink more heavily, up to a bottle of wine some nights, whether with a partner or not. She is feeling less healthy, not eating well or exercising regularly, and not spending as much time with friends. Like most people's, her job is hard and she is feeling more tired and irritable. Everyone is focusing on the damage she is doing to her health, her relationships, and her psyche. But more and more, having a drink or two or three is the most effective way for her to unwind at the end of the day. It also prevents her from having to notice her loneliness. Her friends have suggested that she go to Alcoholics Anonymous, but she gets mad at that advice. After all, she's not an alcoholic. She works and has friends, and besides, she doesn't always drink too much. But she knows that sounds defensive. She knows her life is not quite right and that she is drinking too much and too often. She just can't imagine giving it up.

Masa's life has been hectic for quite a while. He was named *Masahiro* twenty-one years ago by his first-generation Japanese American parents but nicknamed *Masa* recently by his friends, a partying bunch of gay men and lesbians and other cool people living in San Francisco. He is a student and doing well, although his social schedule leaves little time for study. Born and raised in the Midwest, Masa "came out" to his parents when he was fifteen, and the resulting storms at home about his being gay left him very depressed. During his senior year in high school, he spent a month in bed followed by another month just wandering around the house, unable to do anything and unable to talk to anyone about his suicidal feelings. He didn't even have any friends to talk to or hang out with—he didn't know any other gay kids. But by spring he was over it—felt great, in fact—and graduated with no difficulty.

The summer before he left for college he started going to dance clubs and discovered ecstasy, which seemed like the perfect companion for his good mood. Away at college over the next two years, Masa made friends more easily and continued going to clubs, doing ecstasy on the weekends and drinking a little as well. During that time Masa had his first sexual relationship. The man had some speed, and together they discovered the pleasure of sex with speed. Then he discovered dancing with speed. When he's high, his friends joke with him and call him a "dance demon" because he gets wild and loose. He gets up with speed and finishes the night with intense sex.

One day recently, Masa was trying to study but was so agitated that he had to go out for a while to get some air. He thought he heard footsteps following him and so began to run, but then the voices started: "You aren't running fast enough, speed demon, you can do better." He started running through town and couldn't stop. When he ran down the center of a busy street, laughing and yelling, the police tried to stop him. It took several of them to catch him, and even then, in the back of the police car, he sang songs and tried to dance despite the restraints. The doctor at the emergency hospital gave him some medicine to calm him down, then released him the next day with a warning to stay away from drugs.

Finally Masa ran out of steam and slowed down—but went too far and couldn't get out of bed. He was scared. "I haven't been doing any drugs lately, so why am I feeling so bad?" It seemed that only drugs could take him out of this depression, so he went back to the clubs and began partying all over again. But he knew deep down that something was not right. His other friends didn't seem to have the dark moods that he did. He saw an ad in the campus newsletter for a lecture on college students and depression. It was a first step for him that eventually led him to the student counseling center, where he could talk with someone about his life, his depression, and his drug use.

Stella has been out of it for two years. Pills (Xanax) and alcohol are the culprits. She lost her husband, Victor, two years ago. They had been married for thirty-four years, since she was nineteen and he was twenty-one. He died of pancreatic cancer. Their four children, ages twenty-two to thirty-two, are all off on their own, except the youngest.

Stella and Victor were close. They had been constant companions since she was fifteen. She has been beside herself with grief and loneliness since he died. She is nervous and restless, cries a lot, can't sleep, and often has the feeling that he is with her or trying to talk to her. This only makes her feel lonelier. The only way she gets any relief is by drinking. A few years ago her doctor prescribed Xanax for her occasional panic attacks. They didn't happen very often, so she didn't need the pills much. But they've been around the house, and she remembered how relaxed they made her feel. Since she obviously can't drink at work, she started taking Xanax when she gets so anxious she can't think. Her kids are worried about her. She's lost a lot of weight, and she looks terrible.

Her boss is worried, too. Stella is the most competent of all of the bank managers. She suggested that Stella see the EAP (Employee Assistance Program) counselor. It was comforting to talk to someone. The woman asked lots of questions and was sympathetic about Stella's loss. When Stella said that she was drinking and using Xanax to calm down, the counselor got concerned. She said that Stella had developed a substance abuse problem, and she would never get over her husband's death if she kept using drugs. She said that Stella had to feel her feelings to get better, and drugs were keeping her from her feelings. Stella couldn't argue, but the idea of feeling the feelings she was having made her panic. She thought she might die. In fact, many times she had felt such a pain in her chest that she thought she was having a heart attack.

The counselor said Stella should first go to a women's alcohol support group and to AA to stop using pills and drinking. Only then, she was told, could she benefit from grief counseling. So Stella went to a group twice a week at a substance abuse treatment program, which in turn required three AA meetings a week. Some of the people were very nice but told her that all of her problems came from her drinking. This was confusing. It just didn't feel right, especially the idea that she was out of control. And when she said that she had never had control problems with alcohol or drugs in the past, that she was only drinking and taking pills to stop the feeling that the earth had caved in, she was told she was "in denial." She knew she shouldn't be relying so heavily on pills and alcohol to keep calm, and she was trying to talk to people about how she felt, so how was she in denial? It seemed no one wanted to talk about anything but alcohol, never about her.

People told her that drinking and pills were a slow way to suicide. She wasn't so sure about that. They seemed to be *saving* her from suicide. Or at least from the feeling that she didn't want to live anymore. So it was all very confusing. In the meantime, her boss was telling her, in the kindest way she could, that Stella had to pull herself together or she would be suspended from work because she was dragging down the whole team. Not only was she panicking at the thought of not being able to drink, but she was panicking at the thought of the trouble she was in at work. Without Victor, her job was her only friend left. What was she to do?

She thought of taking some time off work, going on disability for a while before she got fired. But she can't live on that little money, and besides, she doesn't want to let people down. Maybe she could go into a program, but she doesn't want people at work to think she has a drug problem. Sometimes she just gets mad at herself for being so weak—she should just quit the pills and drinking and get on with life. But she can't. Not yet, anyway.

Danny is twenty-eight years old. Right now he lives in a halfway house for people with mental illness. He has schizophrenia. He has been in and out of this particular halfway house, as well as several others, because he doesn't always take his medication. Eventually he gets paranoid. Then he becomes delusional and starts hearing voices. His delusions are generally focused on his counselors and peers having intentions to get rid of him. He gets belligerent and threatening. Then he does get kicked out.

Danny also uses drugs, pretty much whatever he can get, but he particularly likes cocaine, speed, and alcohol. Marijuana is relaxing for a few minutes, but then he gets paranoid. Cocaine and speed help him have fun—he feels more energetic and can forget his mental illness. He especially prefers these two drugs when he is on his medication. He complains that his meds make him feel "dull." He feels sleepy and isn't as sharp or observant. Even the new medications like Risperdal and Zyprexa, though they aren't anything like Haldol or Thorazine, change his usually sharp thinking. So every now and again he stops taking his meds. He feels better, but then the voices start. That's when alcohol really helps. Danny doesn't use opiates like heroin because it's too hard to get the money and the equipment, but he's heard that lots of people who hear voices like it better than alcohol. They're the lucky ones, because if they can get on methadone, they feel a lot better, the voices aren't so bad, and they don't have to chase their drugs all the time.

In between halfway houses, Danny is usually homeless. He receives money from Social Security but spends a lot of it on drugs. He thinks, "You can't get a place to live on Social Security anyway. You can't get a place if you're mentally ill, either, unless you're in a program. But then you have to take your meds. And you can *never* use any other drugs. What's with that— you can take the drugs your doctor prescribes, but not the ones you like? Who made these rules anyway? You can't win. So why bother?"

Danny occasionally ends up in drug treatment when he gets really sick and can't get back into his psychiatric halfway house. He'll tell you, though, "the problem is that the people who run drug treatment don't know much about mental illness. And they don't usually have psychiatrists who can prescribe medications. Everything is 'drugs' to them. You're supposed to 'do it on your own.' They don't even know the difference between crack, Prozac, and Thorazine. Mostly, they don't even take people who are 'mental' because they don't understand us." So Danny can get into drug treatment only if he is "clean," meaning no street drugs or psychiatric meds. But then if he gets paranoid and can't stay in the groups, he is accused of "working the program his way." Enough rule infractions and he's out. Back to the streets.

The other place he goes is home to his parents. They are middle-class folks who live in a middle-class neighborhood. His parents are used to him. Their neighbors get a little nervous when he's around, though, because they know how much heartache he has caused his family. Danny was the good kid. His brothers and sisters were all in trouble at some point or other—tru-

ancy, fights, drugs, car wrecks, a teenage pregnancy or two. He was obedi-
ent, quiet, supportive of his parents, a good student. He was "the sensitive
one." His siblings even liked him, too. He gave their parents a much-needed
break. When he went away to college, he was okay for a while. Then he got
anxious. Then more anxious. He started worrying about everything. Then
the voices started. Then doctors, medications, and the roller coaster that is
his life now.

For nine years now, Danny has lived with schizophrenia. Everyone tells
him he could make something of himself if he'd just take his medication and
never use drugs. They tell him coke and speed make the voices worse. They
tell him alcohol makes *everything* worse, that it will rot his brain. But he
can't live without them.

Cheryl, Masa, Danny, and Stella show us how complicated a relationship
with drugs is. You can be suffering harms and getting benefits at the same
time. In Chapter 4 we talk about the specific ways drugs help, and in Chapter 5 we explain how complicated it really is and give you a model for laying
out your entire relationship with drugs so you can more easily examine it.

Before you move on, you might want to try measuring the level of your
use of each of your drugs.

SOURCES AND SUGGESTED READINGS

For a good professional book on assessment:

> *Handbook of Alcoholism Treatment Approaches: Effective Alternatives.* Reid
> Hester and William Miller, Eds. Pergamon Press. 1989.

*How alcohol affects women differently from men, and other information about alcohol
can be found in:*

> *Responsible Drinking: A Moderation Management Approach for Problem Drink-
> ers.* Frederick Rotgers, Marc F. Kern, and Rudy Hoeltzel. New Harbinger.
> 2002.

How people naturally change their drug use over time:

> "The Natural History of Drug Use from Adolescence to the Mid-Thirties in a Gen-
> eral Population Sample." L. Chen and D. Kandal. *American Journal of Public
> Health, 85,* 41–47, 1995.
> *The Truth about Addiction and Recovery.* Stanton Peele. Simon & Schuster. 1991.

THE CONTINUUM OF DRUG AND ALCOHOL USE WORKSHEET

Here is an example:

Drug	Amount	Frequency	Harms (your own observations)	Level of use (guess)
Speed	About 1 gram	Every weekend	Too speedy when I first shoot up (so I drink). Bad crash—horrible day on Monday. Losing a lot of weight. Teeth and skin looking bad.	Heavy? Abuse?

Use the worksheet on the next page to measure the level of your own use.

This worksheet is intended to help you figure out the level of your use for each drug you use.

THE CONTINUUM OF DRUG AND ALCOHOL USE WORKSHEET *(cont.)*

Drug	Amount	Frequency	Harms (your own observations)	Level of use (guess)

There are many, many books to help you understand how drugs work. These are the most accessible. Others can be found in the Sources and Suggested Readings appendix:

> *Buzzed: The Straight Facts about the Most Used and Abused Drugs from Alcohol to Ecstasy.* Cynthia Kuhn, Scott Swartzwelder, and Wilkie Wilson. Norton. 1998.
>
> *Drugs, Behavior, and Modern Society.* Charles Levinthal. Allyn & Bacon. 2002.
>
> *Drugs and the Brain.* Solomon Snyder. Scientific American Library. 1996.
>
> *From Chocolate to Morphine.* Andrew Weil and Winifred Rosen. Houghton Mifflin. 1993.
>
> *A Primer of Drug Action: A Concise, Nontechnical Guide to the Actions, Uses, and Side Effects of Psychoactive Drugs.* Robert Julien. Holt. 2001.

4 SO WHY DO I KEEP USING?

Because it works. People use drugs for reasons.

The good that drugs and alcohol do is the dirty little secret whispered among those who use—unless the stigma of being a user keeps you from speaking at all. Why so hush-hush? Because asserting any positive impact from drugs or alcohol usually brings the response "You're in denial (and, since denial is a symptom of addiction, you're an addict)." Buckling under social pressure, with its induced guilt or shame, drinkers and users of illegal drugs themselves may deny any benefits. Ironically, though, we Americans are famous for our faith in and use of pills—the prescribed ones for depression, anxiety, sleep disorders, sexual dysfunction; the over-the-counter ones for coughs, fevers, allergies; and the health-food-store ones for mind or body performance enhancement. Despite our love of medicines, we separate out alcohol and street drugs, even though they differ little from those prescribed. It is when we self-prescribe that we become suspect.

People don't gravitate to certain drugs randomly. Alcohol gives people a certain type of experience, PCP another. Even though availability, cost, and social/cultural environments have some impact on what type of drug someone decides to use, the choice is also made by the body's internal voice calling for a particular kind of experience. With the understanding that drug use is an effort to relieve or "medicate" distress, to enhance pleasure, or to expand consciousness, let's look at what attracts us to different drugs.

For Cheryl, alcohol plays an important role in allowing her to have intimate relationships with men by reducing her inhibitions. It also helps her destroy these relationships. Danny bounces between drugs and medications in an attempt to balance a life of mental illness and loneliness with a life where he feels more alive. Masa was able to manage the depression that followed coming out as a gay teenager only with drugs, the drugs that help him party and have great sex, but these are the same drugs that now make him para-noid. Stella will have to feel the loneliness of a life without her husband if she quits alcohol and pills. Which is worse?

Often people assign a moral value to how, or whether, we choose to deal with hard feelings or difficult situations. We hear that we should face our problems, not run away from them. This is not necessarily bad advice. It just might be unrealistic. We all must be careful about these moral values—who should judge whether someone should go out to a movie when he doesn't want to face his deteriorating marriage, or eat chocolate chip cook-ies when he can't balance his checkbook? We don't usually think of those avoidance tactics as morally bad. We laugh with them. We reserve our harshest judgments for people who use drugs to deal with hard things. But once we start judging how people cope, it's a slippery slope.

For many people, it seems crazy to place "drugs," "alcohol," and "help" in the same sentence. The moralistic judgments that stem from Puritan-based prohibition remain in the minds of Americans today. When people hear the phrase *using drugs,* there is an automatic association with crime, antisocial behavior, dirt, skid row, the downfall of society, prostitution, pov-erty, laziness, and other "bad" things. But drugs and alcohol do more than just damage. In reality, drugs and alcohol are more closely associated with relief, fun, relaxation, and pleasure than they are with crime, antisocial behavior, and the like. Of course, the Puritan ethic also decries too much pleasure, so drugs just can't win. Nevertheless, in order to use a harm reduc-tion model to address substance use, appreciating how drugs help is as vital as seeing the harm they produce.

Read these three paragraphs:

*Every weekend, my brother and I go downtown and **use drugs**. It is something we do together. It helps us feel like part of the group in our neighborhood. Our friends all **use drugs,** too. It makes us strong. It makes us feel good.*

And now:

*Every weekend, my brother and I go downtown and **eat a good dinner**. It is something we do together. It helps us feel like part of the group in our neighborhood. Our friends all **eat good food,** too. It makes us strong. It makes us feel good.*

Try again:

*Every weekend, my brother and I go downtown and **use drugs**. It is something we do together. It helps us feel like part of the group in our neighborhood. Our friends all **use drugs,** too. It makes us strong. It makes us feel good.*

Our leap from using drugs to eating well may be a challenge. But perhaps you will allow that there are, in fact, benefits of drug and alcohol use. People who use drugs use them for reasons, just like we eat good meals for reasons. Drugs help us cope—with painful emotions, with unbearable social situations, or with the embarrassment of just being in our own body. We should not take away what helps, even if it also causes harm, without understanding the help it provides.

Each class of drugs has certain effects, many of which are of great benefit to us. Generally people search for and find a particular drug that meets their needs for pleasure, relief from pain, or altered reality. Some drugs have accepted medical uses: most commonly, stimulants for attention deficit disorder, opiates for pain, and marijuana for symptoms of cancer, HIV, multiple sclerosis, or glaucoma (in some states). Many drugs are used to enhance social relationships, creating a sense of community among people who use. The ritual uses of drugs like peyote, ayahuasca, or alcohol are excellent examples of communal use of drugs. The chart in this chapter is just a snapshot. The special section on drugs in the center of the book gives a more comprehensive description.

Richard has a serious drinking problem. Now thirty-six, he has been drinking most days since he was twelve. At the insistence of a friend, he came into treatment when he began experiencing blackouts soon after he got married; his friends were furious with him for the things he did during his blackouts. As Richard revealed the origins of his relationship with alcohol, it became clear that he had started drinking the liquor in his parents' cupboard to muffle the noise of his father beating his older sister and mother. He had tried to intervene to protect them, but his attempts just enraged his father more. Richard found that drinking allowed him not to react and to be able to sleep so that he could concentrate in school and get good grades. He moved away from home and earned a college degree that allowed him to find a good job. He cut back on his drinking for a while. He feels very lucky to have found someone with whom to build a new family. But he's drinking a lot again, and this is very upsetting to his wife. Sometimes it scares her that he seems so angry when he drinks.

Why would Richard start drinking more when his life is going so well? It doesn't make sense to him or to his wife and friends. It would be easy to say that he is an alcoholic and his disease is just progressing. But we think it's more complicated than that. Richard may have a lot of anger that he has never dealt with and is terrified to repeat the family relationships of his childhood. Staying drunk helps him avoid his feelings now, just as it did then.

How Drugs Help

The chart on the following pages provides some detail about the benefits of specific classes of drugs.

Alcohol, Richard's drug of choice, has two major effects that are important to him: suppression of pain and memory and disinhibition. The former may allow him to shut out memories that are being stimulated by his new marriage. The latter may allow him to express anger that has remained repressed.

So Why Do *You* Use? What's Outside . . .

Why you use drugs or alcohol is not simple. You could probably list several reasons, including "just because." If you're coming to the conclusion that you should *do* something about your drug use—get a grip on it, control it, or quit altogether—it's important to begin noticing your adaptive use of your drugs. *Adaptive* is another way of talking about how you bring drugs into your life to help you cope with or manage difficult things, enjoy pleasurable things, or escape the unbearable. If you are usually too busy shielding yourself from moral condemnation—your own or that of others—please take a break for a while and take a nonjudgmental look at your relationship with drugs. Generally speaking, reasons for using drugs arise from two factors: what's outside of you and what's inside of you.

What's outside is the environment: where you live, where you work, who you deal with every day, the weather, the bus schedule. All of these environmental factors can contribute to stress that you must then figure out how to manage. Some people eat hot oatmeal on a cold morning. Some people drink brandy. Eating oatmeal before you encounter bad weather may seem like a better idea to some, but if you're homeless and don't have a way of getting hot food, the booze will serve as a welcome substitute (even though it doesn't really warm you).

What's outside also includes other people and their attitudes. Danny

Drug	Psychological benefits	Medical benefits	Social benefits
Stimulants (amphetamines, cocaine, caffeine)	Perk up your mood, create a sense of euphoria and power. Improve focus and concentration.	Improve alertness and physical stamina. Reduce appetite, help weight loss.	Increase stamina for late-night parties, driving or flying, studying. Improve sexual stimulation and performance (speed especially, but not caffeine). This effect can wear off after chronic and heavy use.
Nicotine	Creates relaxation. Reduces anxiety. Good way to take a break. Enhances focus and concentration. Reduces psychotic symptoms.	None known.	Used to be, and still is among some people, a group social activity.
Hallucinogens (LSD, psilocybin, peyote, DMT, etc.)	Interesting, often spiritual, "journeys" and experiences. Distort or expand reality. Enhance insights. Various hallucinogens, most recently ibogaine, are researched for their help in curbing addictive use of other drugs.	None known.	Powerful experience of shared, expanded consciousness.

Ecstasy	Improves mood and sense of well-being. Increases sense of closeness to other people. Has been used to enhance communication in individual and couples' therapy.	None known.	Creates feelings of openness and warmth toward others. Used in religious rituals.
Alcohol	Disinhibition, mental relaxation, reduces stress. Inhibits memory (useful for victims or survivors of trauma).	Muscle relaxation. Dulls pain. Cardiovascular health in small-to-moderate doses—cuts LDL cholesterol.	Social "lubricant"—reduces shyness or anxiety.
Benzodiaze-pines, barbiturates, GHB	Disinhibition. Very effective antianxiety medications.	Slow heart rate. Some (especially Valium) are good muscle relaxants. Sleep aids.	Help you feel part of things—eases social anxiety and diminishes social isolation.
Opiates (heroin, morphine, codeine, Dilaudid, Oxycontin, etc.)	Reduce stress and emotional pain. Enhance pleasure. Create feelings of well-being.	Pain relief. Cough suppression. Control diarrhea.	Create sense of warmth in social situations. Strong rituals of sharing drug-using experience.

(cont.)

Drug	Psychological benefits	Medical benefits	Social benefits
Inhalants (amyl nitrite, butyl nitrite, household solvents)	Disinhibition. Stimulation. Get "out of one's mind."	A type of nitrite is used in cardiac medicine. Nitrous oxide used in dental work.	Enhance sexual experience (nitrites). Decrease social anxiety. Common peer activity.
Dissociative anesthetics (PCP, Ketamine, nitrous oxide, dextromethorphan)	Pleasant, dreamy, or hallucinatory experiences. Reduce self-consciousness.	Surgical anesthetics (ketamine and nitrous oxide; PCP no longer used, as it is too unpredictable in its effects). Cough suppressant (dextromethorphan).	Risk-taking experiences. Party drugs. Some enhance sexual experience.
Cannabis	Enhances perceptual experiences for some people. Decreases depression, decreases anxiety. Can impair memory (useful for trauma survivors).	Stimulates appetite. Suppresses nausea (useful for people with HIV, cancer). Controls pain. Relaxes muscle tissue (useful for multiple sclerosis). Reduces intraocular pressure of glaucoma.	Helps you feel relaxed, connected to peers. Have great conversations.

knows that other people think he's crazy and don't want to be around him. He doesn't act so crazy when he first starts using—he looks more like everybody else for a while, and he has a group to hang around with who have nothing to do with mental illness. Other people with drug or alcohol problems have suffered from racism. Being a person of color in the United States can be full of trauma, insult, and massive disappointment. Poverty is another physically damaging and emotionally terrifying circumstance. If you're a person of color *and* you're poor, it's sometimes hard to tell whether people are treating you the way they are because of your race or your poverty. Cheryl grew up poor and black and is fiercely proud of her climb out of poverty. As an attorney in a large Southern city, she has earned the respect of her white peers as well as of other people of color. But it would be naive to think that Cheryl doesn't carry some scars, not only from her childhood in the rural South but also from day-to-day interactions with the people who still disrespect her and her race. If she feels secretive about her drinking and relationship problems, her hesitancy makes sense. She's come a long way and doesn't want to lose ground at this point in her life by being pigeonholed as an alcoholic.

A disproportionate number of gay, lesbian, bisexual, and transgendered people use or abuse alcohol and other drugs. The assumption is that being a part of a hated and ridiculed group causes so much fear and shame that the only way to cope sometimes is to get high.

But you don't have to be part of a stigmatized group to feel pressure from outside. Am I smart enough, thin enough, beautiful or handsome enough, buff enough, rich enough, powerful enough? Do I live in the right neighborhood, in the right house? Am I hip enough? Do I listen to the right music, see the right films, wear the right clothes? Inadequacy in the face of pressure to conform to externally imposed standards is something we all face and is a demon that some have finally conquered—through a spiritual quest, enough therapy, or just plain age and maturity.

It is also true that the use of intoxicating drugs has been part of social interactions for thousands of years. Sometimes these culturally approved uses, such as the ritual use of tobacco or peyote by Native Americans, have been what we might call "moderate." Other rituals may be quite extreme, however. For example, bachelor parties, weddings, and New Year's Eve celebrations typically involve large amounts of alcohol consumption. Social bonding and celebration bring people together in communities and decrease a sense of alienation and isolation. The use of mind-altering substances to deepen and expand those celebrations is almost as old as our oldest major civilizations.

. . . and What's Inside

What's inside of you is even more complicated. What makes sense about your drug use? What benefits does it bring you that nothing else does? One way of recognizing these benefits is to imagine how you'd feel without the drug or to remember how you felt during times that you didn't use. Irritable? Impatient? Depressed? Tense? Bored? While it is also true that your alcohol or other drug use may cause or intensify those feelings, right now it's important to see how you have helped yourself deal with difficult emotions, not how you might have harmed yourself.

Masa started using ecstasy to help overcome depression and shyness. Cheryl drinks to deal with sexual inhibition. Stella uses pills and alcohol to protect herself from the intense grief that she feels at being left alone in the world. And Danny's reasons for using change depending on the phase he is in—first he wants to feel normal, then he wants to quiet the voices of his psychosis, and finally he gets into a state where he uses "just because."

For you it could be simpler or more complicated. Maybe you don't like the way you feel the next morning, but the previous night many things could have driven you to finish that bottle of wine, smoke an extra pipe, snort the whole gram, or shake up a triple martini: The humiliation over that run-in you had at work with an arrogant employee? The fact that you and your husband simply get along better when you're drinking together? The fact that you were more tired than usual? Whatever it is that's on your schedule for the next day that you don't want to think about? Sheer boredom? All of these and more could send you to the liquor cabinet or drug stash; it's just something you do. The external pressures listed in the preceding section—stigma of mental illness, racism, panic at being identified as gay, and the myriad ways that success is judged in America—all have internal consequences. In other words, being found wanting leads to feelings of distress: low self-esteem, shame, guilt, anxiety, self-pity, self-loathing—you name it.

Then there are the emotional or psychological problems *not* created by the attitudes of those around us now, *not* caused by whatever external events or circumstances bring us pain or discomfort. These are problems we were born with or developed early in life. Schizophrenia, bipolar disorder, and some depressive and anxiety disorders are lying in wait in some of our genes. Other depressions and anxieties come from experiences in childhood that, even if not clearly abusive or neglectful, caused us sufficient distress that we had to look for ways to cope. Some of us found defenses such as lying, manipulation, arrogance, passivity, avoidance, rationalization, or aggression. Others of us found the church choir, rock music, sports teams, the school newspaper, mystery novels, or physics. Some of us found drugs.

Psychological Theories of Drug Use

There are a few psychological theories of drug use and abuse that many people find interesting or comforting. We have already referred to Edward Khantzian's concept of "self-medication." This is a theory that has gained widespread acceptance among drug treatment professionals, despite the tendency for some people to mock "excuses" for drug use. We have also mentioned drugs as tools to help people cope with, or adapt to, difficult circumstances or emotions. Another useful idea is that drug users do not *lack* control so much as need drugs to *release* the control of overly critical internal voices. Alcohol, for example, does a great job of shutting up the internal critic. Another theory is that people who can't express intense emotions in words learn to express them with their bodies. To do this, you might get sick a lot, fight, sing, play football—or use drugs.

Finally, a very interesting idea is that we use drugs because we don't have good attachments to people. Karen Walant goes so far as to say that our society values autonomy at the expense of attachment needs. When we encourage young children to be independent, whether it is because we are proud of their achievements or because we are just too busy or too tired to be with them as much as they need, we practice something that Walant calls "normative abuse." Normative abuse is behavior that people do not consider unusual but that is, in fact, damaging to children. An example of this type of abuse would be the days when we thought that spanking children was good for them, something we now consider potentially harmful. Walant's point is that drugs help to soothe the trauma that most of us experienced as children in this country.

The Interacting Nature of Emotions, Biology, and Drugs

There are biological reasons why drugs help us manage difficult feelings. To understand these reasons, however, we have to start with emotions. There is one factor that we believe to be common to all people who chronically abuse alcohol and other drugs: if you have a problem with drugs, you have a problem with emotions. You might be highly sensitive to criticism. You might get angry over small things. You might find sadness unbearable. You don't, however, have to figure out whether emotional sensitivity or drug use came first. You just have both. Your drinking and your depression, your smoking and your anxiety, your shooting up and your psychosis coexist, side

71

by side, in the eyes of harm reduction. Figuring out which is the dominant "primary diagnosis" (sort of like asking, "Which came first, the chicken or the egg?") might make your therapist, your drug counselor, or your psychiatrist more comfortable, but it won't help you understand how to reduce harm in your life. To do that you will have to give your relationship with drugs *and* your emotional life equal treatment and attention. You *might* have to do some work on your emotional reactions. You *might* have to learn how to notice, express, and manage your feelings. You *might* have to control when, where, with whom, and how much you use. But who doesn't?

Research in the United States suggests that over 50 percent of people with the major psychiatric disorders mentioned above—schizophrenia, bipolar disorder, major depression, reactive depression (to loss or trauma), anxiety or panic disorder, and posttraumatic stress disorder—abuse drugs at some point in their life. All of these disorders have a chemical basis in the brain—and, of course, so do drug effects. The official term for coexisting psychiatric and drug problems is *dual diagnosis*. If you have one or more of these mental disorders, drugs and alcohol can have powerful effects, both positive and negative, on how well you feel and on how much you suffer. You don't have to have one of these conditions, though, to experience serious emotional and biological interactions when using drugs.

One of the crucial aspects of practicing harm reduction is to gain some understanding of what is at work in your choice of which drugs to use. As we said before, alcohol gives people a certain type of experience, PCP another. People don't gravitate to particular substances arbitrarily. Although cost, availability, and peer culture influence what we use, the drug we *fall in love with* is the one that speaks most clearly to our search for pleasure and/ or our need for comfort. This is what is referred to as your "drug of choice."

With the understanding that drug use can be an effort to self-medicate distress, you can look at how different substances may soothe, or *medicate*, different kinds of distress. We'll start by looking at how these drugs act in your brain and why you might choose to use one or more of them as a way to change your brain chemistry and thus your experiences.

And Now for Some Science: This Is Your Brain On and Off Drugs

We keep stressing that drug use is the product of a complex interaction of biological, psychological, and social factors. Some people also like to acknowledge spiritual aspects as a factor. There is an enormous amount of research on each of these areas and a growing amount of information on the interactions between them. This combination is referred to as a *biopsycho-social* (and sometimes spiritual) model of addiction. Here we focus on the chemistry of the psychological part of the equation: the chemistry of the brain.

The brain takes in, transmits, evaluates, and gives orders based on all sorts of information from both the external and internal domains. While some people worry that focusing on the function of the brain reduces the complexity of being human to "just chemistry," we believe—and research indicates—that the physical workings of the brain are an important part of the drive to use drugs.

The brain is filled with nerve cells and the fibers that connect them. Nerve cells are the information centers, or the messengers, in the brain. They contain our genetic coding, the blueprint that makes our bodies and minds operational. They also carry information from one cell to another, using their fibers, via electrical charges. There are gaps or *synapses* between these fibers. The electrical charges don't simply jump across the synapse—they "float." Nerve cells manufacture chemicals, and when an electrical impulse travels through a cell, the chemicals in the cell are released and float

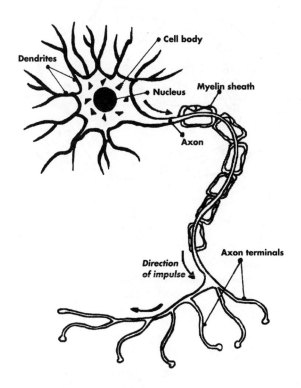

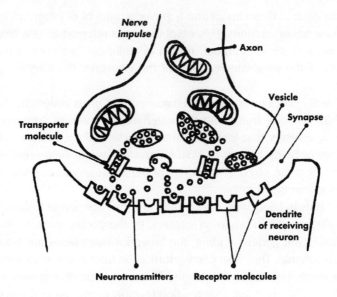

Nerve impulse

Axon

Vesicle

Synapse

Transporter molecule

Dendrite of receiving neuron

Neurotransmitters   Receptor molecules

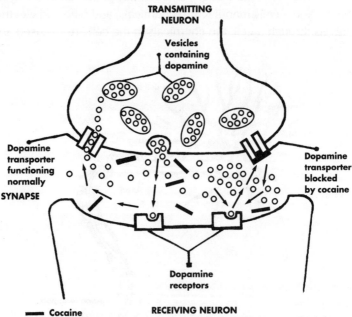

TRANSMITTING NEURON

Vesicles containing dopamine

Dopamine transporter functioning normally

SYNAPSE

Dopamine transporter blocked by cocaine

Dopamine receptors

▬ Cocaine

RECEIVING NEURON

When cocaine enters the brain, it blocks the dopamine transporter from pumping dopamine back into the transmitting neuron, thereby flooding the synapse with dopamine. This large amount of dopamine intensifies and prolongs the stimulation of receiving neurons in the brain's pleasure circuits, causing a cocaine "high." Drawings courtesy the National Institute on Drug Abuse, from its website, *www.nida.nih.gov/MOM/TG/ momtg-introbg.html.*

across the synapse, where they attach for a short time to the next cell and transmit the message from the last cell.

For example, when you burn your hand on the stove, the nerve fibers in your hand send a signal up through your spinal cord to your brain, where the signal gets translated into "OUCH." This information is then transmitted by more fibers to the cells that manufacture the brain's natural pain relievers—endorphins—which are commanded to wake up and DO something. They obey the command and release enough endorphins to relieve the pain enough so that you can think to run your hand under cold water to stop the inflammation. Once the endorphins (or any other messenger chemicals) have transmitted their information to the next nerve cell, they are reabsorbed by their cell of origin by a process called *reuptake*. Now back in the "home" cell, they wait until another electrical impulse sends them back out into the synapse.

The chemicals that transmit information from cell to cell are called *neurotransmitters*, and there are many dozens of them in the brain. Some of the most important ones are the very chemicals that drugs such as alcohol or marijuana affect. These neurotransmitters are related to, and often control, feelings and moods and are involved in many mental disorders and emotional problems. You might have heard of some of them—such as dopamine, serotonin, and the endorphins.

Drugs that affect the brain directly are called *psychoactive*. When you take a psychoactive drug into your body, it gets into the brain and affects which neurotransmitters are released into the synapses. Psychoactive drugs mimic, stimulate, or replace neurotransmitters. In other words, some drugs stimulate the release of neurotransmitters, some block their reabsorption, and yet others, such as marijuana and sometimes morphine, act *instead* of neurotransmitters. Blocking reabsorption has the effect of leaving more of the chemical in the synapse to continue to activate the next cell, so it's similar to the effect of releasing more. The effects, depending on the particular neurotransmitter itself, either stimulate or depress the brain's activity.

Chronic use of a psychoactive drug may alter not only the process (physiology) of chemical release but also the actual brain structures (anatomy) themselves. It's unclear whether these changes are permanent. We also don't actually know whether the brain is made worse by chronic drug use, or if the brain of the user wasn't quite right to begin with and the drug is a temporary solution. The chart below helps explain this idea. But first, we offer brief definitions of the most important neurotransmitters for understanding how drugs work in the brain.

Dopamine is present in several different parts of the brain and is most well known as the neurotransmitter responsible for feelings of pleasure. It is also related to coordination of movement and logical thinking. *Recreational* psychoactive drugs have their first effect on dopamine. (Psychoactive *medications* such as Prozac or antipsychotics tend *not* to stimulate dopamine in noticeable quantities.) By dumping large amounts of dopamine into synapses (or preventing its reuptake, depending on the drug), we experience "the rush"—that first pleasurable feeling of euphoria, relief, or excitement—that is so intensely satisfying and rewarding. Dopamine links directly to survival areas in the brain. Anything that stimulates these areas creates a response of "Aaaahhh. That feels good. Do it again." Dopamine explains why most people repeat experiences that are pleasurable or reduce suffering. It's why some of us use drugs more than once!

Norepinephrine is one of the brain's natural stimulants, increasing alertness and mental focus. It is also responsible for a complex "fight or flight" response termed the *human stress response*. This series of chemical reactions gets us ready to deal with danger by pumping adrenaline into our bodies to allow us to think fast and move even faster. (Adrenaline, by the way, is also called *epinephrine*, and, it is just about the same chemical as the norepinephrine in the brain.) This output of energy releases stress hormones, which, over time, can weaken our immune system and cause us to be more susceptible to illnesses.

Serotonin plays several complicated roles in the brain. It affects or controls mood and is well known to be related to depression. Low levels of it also seem to be associated with aggression, irritability, and premenstrual syndrome (PMS). It helps regulate sleep, appetite, and sexual functioning. Some serotonin cells are responsible for hallucinations. Serotonin also may regulate the actions of other neurotransmitters. If we don't have enough serotonin, it could result in the dysregulation of neurotransmitters that affect other conditions (anxiety, panic, and pain sensitivity, to name a few).

GABA (gamma-aminobutyric acid) relaxes the brain. Sometimes called "the brain's Valium," it suppresses certain kinds of brain activity, hyperactivity, or overexcitement, while allowing higher cognitive processes to remain unaffected. With the release of GABA, we can feel calm but still alert. Without a healthy supply, we feel anxious and worried. We are also at risk of seizures, which are the result of excessive electrical activity in the brain. GABA calms electrical activity.

Endorphins are several different types of chemicals that are all related to pain perception and pain control. There are many different types of pain, physical and emotional, and relief from emotional pain may be part of this neurotransmitter's job. Perhaps this is why a release of endorphins not only decreases pain but also gives us a sense of well-being and happiness.

We have yet to learn a lot about **anandamide** (from the word *ananda*, which means "bliss" in Sanskrit), but it is found in an area of the brain called the *hippocampus*, which coordinates memory formation and retrieval. Forgetfulness, whether related to age, disease, or psychological conditions, may be related to this chemical.

Glutamate is widely distributed in the brain and stimulates different activities. Its role as a mind- or mood-altering chemical is not well understood.

Acetylcholine works in several different areas of the brain and the body. Its main functions in the brain are to transmit orders to the muscular system (such as telling your hand to get away from the hot stove) and to help with memory formation.

These are the most prominent neurotransmitters related to emotions, moods, and behavior. It is important to remember that, as far as we know, all drugs of "recreation" or "abuse" act on these normal brain chemicals and either increase, decrease, or somehow affect their release or reuptake. Practically speaking, what this means is that the brain is wired to receive these chemicals, recognize them, and accept their messages as a part of its "normal" functioning. The difference between the release of neurotransmitters as a part of the brain's "normal" daily functioning and their release in response to the ingestion of recreational drugs is that drugs do it better, faster, and much, much bigger.

We keep putting the word *normal* in quotation marks. As we have discussed, life experiences, especially in childhood, affect how our brains develop, how we feel, and how we cope emotionally. It is now understood that early experiences affect the development of our brain structures, including the manufacture of neurotransmitters. People who have suffered childhood trauma have been found to have low levels of dopamine, serotonin, and endorphins, leading to a suppressed ability to feel pleasure, to soothe pain, or to regulate mood and aggression. Norepinephrine, as the neurotransmitter most directly activated by stress, has been overworked and tends to cause hypervigilance or overreaction to stress. So the "normal" brain of someone who has experienced trauma may, in fact, be a brain that needs externally supplied drugs to balance its neurotransmitter levels.

Each drug has its own profile of which neurotransmitters it affects. The relationship between particular neurotransmitters and emotional or mental disorders is not necessarily a causal one. The jury is still out. Nor do we know precisely what each recreational drug does in the brain. Some drugs are better understood than others. The section on drugs in the center of this book gives a more detailed description of how each class of drugs works. We also include a list of references that do an excellent job of talking about the chemistry of the brain and how drugs work. In the meantime, here are some examples of what you could be trying to achieve by using different drugs.

People often search for the drug that fits best with their underlying problems. If you're feeling depressed, sluggish, bored, or plagued by low self-esteem, you might gravitate toward stimulants like amphetamines or cocaine. They give you a big rush of dopamine and a dose of norepinephrine, which boost feelings of pleasure, energy, and focus. You feel euphoric for a while. (*Euphoric* is the opposite of *dysphoric*, which means feeling low or depressed.) Focus, of course, is the sought-after effect for people with attention-deficit disorder.

If you feel irritable, moody, or stressed, you might be drawn to opiates or marijuana, which act on endorphin and anandamide receptors, respectively. We know that endorphins are soothing and relieve both physical and emotional pain. We know less about anandamide, but we think it may have something to do with forgetting. It certainly blocks the storage of new memories. If memories are painful, what better resource to have than a drug that helps us forget? People who have experienced trauma might therefore also find relief from opiates and marijuana. Or they might turn to dissociative anesthetics, which can give you an out-of-body experience and reduce self-consciousness. (Dissociation—when your mind separates itself from painful reality—just happens to be one of the main protective symptoms of posttraumatic stress.)

Alcohol both soothes and disinhibits (makes you feel loose and carefree), so it's also the drug of choice for people who have been traumatized and feel inhibited from expressing themselves, and for people who are anxious, especially socially anxious. Some people with schizophrenia have found that alcohol quiets their auditory hallucinations (voices). The same effect has been found with opiates: people with schizophrenia who are on methadone often have an easier time managing the symptoms of their mental illness. Although stimulants like cocaine and speed can *cause* psychosis, people with schizophrenia are also drawn to them for the same reasons as other people, as well as to counteract the emotional flatness that comes with the illness or from antipsychotic medications. Nicotine, used by 95 percent of people with schizophrenia, increases activity in the areas of the brain responsible for concentration and focus—a useful effect when you feel your brain is out of control. A useful effect, too, for people with attention-deficit disorder.

Although alcohol does make us feel looser and we often use it to ease social interaction and sexual encounters, it is not the greatest drug for sex, especially large amounts of alcohol. Speed and cocaine are great for sex, however, especially speed. But after a few years of cocaine use, it stops being effective and starts interfering with sexual performance. We are supposed to be focusing on benefits in this chapter, but since we're on the topic of sex . . . one of the downsides of getting to like sex with speed is it's a struggle for a lot of people to return to "normal" sex—it's just not as exciting. Since speed can be a physically harmful drug, continuous use can be a big problem.

Remember, everyone is unique. You might have a different experience from anyone else. Then again, all of these drugs release dopamine to a greater or lesser degree, which makes you feel good. Since these drugs literally work on the same systems as prescription drugs, you might consider speaking with a pharmacologist or a psychiatrist about whether an antidepressant or antianxiety medication would be helpful in assisting you to control your use of illegal drugs and thus avoid some of the downsides of using.

The four people we have been following may have chosen their drugs for particular reasons related to the interactions just described. Cheryl drinks alcohol, which releases GABA, a natural relaxant. Her experience of being sexually abused left her with fear and anxiety about sex. Alcohol helps her calm down and get in the mood. It also makes her less inhibited in other ways, as when she gets critical of her boyfriends and picks fights.

Danny has a lot of complicated things going on in his brain. Many researchers think that schizophrenia is related to having too much dopamine. Indeed, if you take dopamine, which is in some medicines for Parkinson's disease, you may experience psychosis and perhaps hear voices or have hallucinations. Likewise, speed and cocaine, which strongly stimulate dopamine, eventually cause psychotic symptoms, such as paranoia and hallucinations, in many people. So Danny, when he uses street drugs, might be getting too much dopamine released in his brain. But, at the same time, some antipsychotic medicines rob his brain of dopamine, so he feels slowed down and dull. By using, he is trying to balance things out. He can stop taking his medicine, but then he hears voices. He can use speed, and he won't feel dull anymore, but it might make him hear voices, too. But if he drinks alcohol, he has discovered, he can keep the voices down to a whisper instead of a shout. Danny may or may not be totally aware of how he is playing with his moods and symptoms, but from our perspective, it sure looks like he's trying to accomplish a complicated task—to feel as normal as he can.

Masa also has a lot going on inside his brain. He may have a condition called *bipolar disorder* (it used to be called *manic–depression*). This condition could be the cause of his mood swings between feeling great and being depressed. When he's feeling good, ecstasy and speed make him feel even better. But the brain chemicals that are being released when he uses these drugs can easily throw him over the edge into mania (feeling on top of the world, reckless, able to dance all night, and eventually, maybe hearing voices or becoming paranoid). On the other hand, Masa may not have bipolar disorder—the drugs might be causing psychosis and depression. Both ecstasy and speed cause depression in withdrawal, and speed can cause psychosis. It's easy to say to someone like Masa, "Well, you better not do drugs, because they might be making you sick." But that's not the whole story. Masa started out depressed, and the drugs helped him get out of bed. Just like Danny, you can see how Masa is trying to balance things out. Sometimes it works, but sometimes it just makes things worse—if not in the short term, then in the long term.

Stella is using pills and alcohol that release some dopamine, the pleasure neurotransmitter, which makes her feel better in general, and GABA, the brain's natural Xanax (similar to Valium). She feels better able to cope with her life and her grief. She wants to stay functional, keep her job, get on with her life. Grief is robbing her brain of vital chemicals she needs to help her cope with the everyday trials of life. Stella is getting the chemicals she needs with the help of external drugs.

Richard's story is complicated as well. Just prior to entering treatment, he had fallen in love for the first time. The amount of alcohol he drank when he was away from his girlfriend nearly doubled within a few months of their meeting. The increase in alcohol accounted for his blackouts. Even after they were married, his drinking didn't slow down, as he thought it might. His new wife asked him not to drink as much, and he was trying. He had no idea why falling in love would result in his increased need to drink. His friends told him that he was an alcoholic trying to destroy the first good relationship he has ever had. Richard wasn't convinced that this was the explanation, but he could offer no other. He felt bad about himself and helpless to control his drinking. He had not yet realized that it might be serving a useful purpose, as it had in his past. It took therapy to help him unravel this complicated pattern of why he was drinking so much. As we examined his experience, it became clear that his use of alcohol in his childhood muffled the violence in his house.

For Richard, as for many of us, these experiences and our ways of coping with them don't just go away once we become adults and leave the scene of our pain. In fact, starting a new family can bring up old feelings from our original family. Try as we might to make things different, sometimes we get stuck in patterns. Richard realized that, while he was very happy with his wife and looking forward to having children, it also felt like a huge step, a big responsibility that made him feel weak, not up to the job. He remembered how panicked his father always was, trying to make ends meet. He realized he was afraid he'd turn out like his father, anxious and abusive. Alcohol made him feel relaxed, made him forget about his fears, made him less likely (he thought) to become abusive. It had worked when he was a kid, so why should he think that alcohol might now cause a problem?

The people around you, frustrated by your choice to use drugs as part of your effort to live your life and concerned about the harm they witness, have an ideal vision of you "clean and sober." Their vision is based on their misunderstanding that it is only the presence of drugs or alcohol that makes you sick, irritable, impatient, or depressed. Although it's true that withdrawal from heroin, alcohol, ecstasy, or speed, among others, can make you sick, irritable, or depressed, these troubles may have been there before you took your first hit or your first sip. It is difficult to help your friends and family understand that their vision is not where you begin to practice harm reduction. It may not even be where you end up. For now, it's most important to understand what's driving your use and to respect your creativity for having found some solutions.

If you would like to plot the reasons you use different drugs, here is a worksheet to help you:

THE BENEFITS OF DRUG AND ALCOHOL USE WORKSHEET

Here is an example:

Drug	Amount	Frequency	Benefits
Speed	1 gram	Every weekend	Great sex. Get lots done, too. Can't think of any better way to get out of the funk I'm in since I lost my job and can't find another one.

THE BENEFITS OF DRUG AND ALCOHOL USE WORKSHEET *(cont.)*			
Drug	**Amount**	**Frequency**	**Benefits**

SOURCES AND SUGGESTED READINGS

For some history of why and how people use drugs, and more about drugs and their cultural and medical uses:

> *Buzzed: The Straight Facts About the Most Used and Abused Drugs from Alcohol to Ecstasy.* Cynthia Kuhn, Scott Swartzwelder, and Wilkie Wilson. Norton. 1998.
>
> *From Chocolate to Morphine.* Andrew Weil and Winifred Rosen. Houghton Mifflin. 1993.
>
> *The Pursuit of Oblivion: A Global History of Narcotics.* Richard Davenport-Hines. Norton. 2002.

For information about drug use among different groups of people:

> *Substance Abuse: A Comprehensive Textbook.* Joyce Lowinson, Pedro Ruiz, Robert Millman, and John Langrod, Eds. Williams & Wilkins. 1997. (See especially chapters 62, 66–73)

For psychological theories of addiction (these are on the technical side, written for therapists):

> *Creating the Capacity for Attachment: Treating Addictions and the Alienated Self.* Karen Walant. Aronson. 1995.
>
> "Contemporary Psychoanalytic Theories of Substance Abuse: A Disorder in Search of a Paradigm. Jon Morgenstern and Jeremy Leeds. *Psychotherapy, 30*, 194–206. 1993.

If you're a drinker, this is a great way to begin your assessment—it's an interactive software program.

> Hester, Reid. *Drinker's Check-Up.* Order from *rhester@behaviortherapy.com*

5 TO CHANGE
OR NOT TO CHANGE

If you woke up tomorrow morning to find all your problems had disappeared, what would your life look like? How many things would be different? How many obstacles to happiness would be gone? Which people would have disappeared? And who would have taken their place? What kind of car would you drive? How old would your children be? What would you do for work, and how much money would you be earning? Or perhaps you'd be retired. What would your partner be like? What would your body and mind feel like? And would you, or would you not, have alcohol or drugs in your life?

You will probably wake up tomorrow with everything looking much the same as it does today—your room, your house, the car outside, your partner and children, your internal life, and the drugs in your system, beside your bed, or waiting in your liquor cabinet. What would it take, then, to achieve some of the fantasies we've invited you to call up? And how long would it take to achieve them? The process of getting from here to there, of course, involves change.

The Dilemma of Change

On a good day, most of us can appreciate that changing has both good and bad aspects. On a bad day, the prospect of having to change any part of our routine, surroundings, or outlook is simply overwhelming. If this chapter has caught you on a bad day, feel free to stop reading. Come back on a better day. Contemplating change in an atmosphere of fear, hopelessness, or exhaustion is a self-defeating exercise. Self-defeating efforts are harmful. Reduce the harm in your life by coming back when you feel better.

An irony of life is that change is actually inevitable. We and our world are changing all the time, for better or worse. It happens whether we are looking or not. It's when we deliberately go about making a change that things get trickier. Actually *trying* to change creates a dilemma.

The dilemma of change is that it means loss. Getting thin means losing weight, perhaps weight we have had around since childhood, weight that is part of our identity. Our children's growing up means losing them from our day-to-day lives. Moving to a new place means leaving the last one, with all the experiences we had there. Getting a new job means leaving the one where we felt so at home and so competent, even if we hated the boss or the politics. And where drugs or alcohol are concerned, we have always thought change meant quitting—losing the medicine that has gotten us through so many hard times, or losing the magic potion that has given us our most intense highs.

The word that best describes how most of us feel about the dilemma of change is *ambivalence*. Ambivalence means having mixed feelings about something. Mixed feelings are normal: I'm proud that my children made it to adulthood, but I'll miss them when they go. I'm glad to get a new place to live, but it'll never be the same as the one where I spent my first ten years out of school. I need to stop drinking, smoking crack, shooting dope, or smoking cigarettes because I know how much trouble my using is causing but I'm not sure I can leave it behind—after all, it helped me reach my forties.

Harm reduction invites you to embrace both sides of the dilemma of change. It is the only way to make decisions about what and how much to change. Both sides are real and will influence what you actually do. The more conscious you are of your ambivalence, the more realistic you will be in the promises you make and keep. As you come to accept how drugs are harming you and yours, also appreciate that you love them—the drugs, that is. Denying that love will have you sneaking around behind your own back to keep stoking the embers of a relationship you promised to extinguish forever.

The Choices: To Change . . .

If you find yourself faced with the dilemma of doing something about your relationship with drugs, you have choices about how to proceed. In all simplicity, listed in no particular order, and with absolutely no sarcasm, they are:

1. Change.
2. Don't change.

Within each of these choices is enormous variety. *Change* can mean changing everything, like discontinuing all use of all drugs. Or it can mean changing only some things, like limiting when you use or how much. It can mean changing how you use, like switching from needles to snorting. Various ways of changing your drug use might look like the following:

• **Change everything**. Totally abstain from using all drugs. Do this all at once ("cold turkey"), with the help of others—a program or a therapist or friends—or on your own. Do it slowly—cut down on one drug at a time, until you've eliminated it from your life—or cut down on all of them simultaneously by tapering at a pace that you choose. Try periods of abstinence just to see what it feels like. You'll also lower your tolerance to most drugs, so you don't have to use as much to get a buzz when you start again–it's a tapering device. Again, do this on your own or with professional help.

• **Eliminate one drug and keep the others.** Eliminate the most harmful one all at once, and don't do a thing about the others. The most common example of this option is people who detox from heroin and stop using it altogether but continue to drink or smoke pot. Another common change is to quit smoking crack but keep using alcohol. You can also eliminate the most harmful drug slowly while leaving the others alone. The easiest way to stop heroin is to use methadone, although methadone is hard to get, especially outside of major cities. We know many people who have gradually cut down on their crack smoking, despite its reputation for being very difficult to use moderately.

• **A variation on the theme: eliminate more than one of the most harmful drugs and keep the rest.** You might stop snorting cocaine because it's draining your bank account *and* quit drinking because you have hepatitis C, but keep your pot and enjoy ecstasy or mushrooms from time to time.

• **Another variation: switch from more harmful to less harmful drugs.** If you're clear that you aren't ready for, or interested in, a drug-free life, consider pot instead of heroin or pills. Or, if your drug use is driven by anxiety, see if you can find a doctor who understands that drugs like Valium (but preferably longer-acting ones like Klonopin) are valuable antianxiety medications and are not used addictively by most people, including those who have a history of addiction. Or, try an SSRI like Prozac or Celexa.

• **Change how you use.** Change the route of administration–snort instead of shoot so you eliminate the harm of needle use. Mix your scotch with water and ice so the first drink doesn't hit you so hard and cloud your judgment about whether to have another. Stop using alone, so you won't die if you overdose—have someone there to call 911 or do rescue breathing.

• **Change how often or when you use.** Stop using before work. Don't drink during the week, or at least not every night. Give your body a break. Snort after the kids are in bed or only when they're with a babysitter and you're out of the house.

In short, changing means taking control of *whatever* you can *whenever* you can. It's all progress, and progress breeds progress. It doesn't have to be all or nothing to be better. Remember, any positive change is harm reduction.

. . . or Not to Change

Although we've specifically mentioned this point earlier, it deserves to be repeated. No change, in traditional substance use circles, is a deal breaker. It's usually seen as the one option that puts you outside of any treatment or support network. The traditional thinking is that once you have decided not to make any changes, you're "resistant" to getting better. Therefore, you will not get better.

But not changing your drug use doesn't mean you're doing nothing. It can mean doing more research. It can mean talking to some people about your problems. It can mean sitting with your fears and your mixed feelings and getting to know them better as you continue to use. It can mean doing absolutely nothing except noticing you've made a choice to do nothing. Changing can also mean returning to a previous pattern or activity that was positive for you. Maybe you've stopped reading books lately. Change might mean going back to the library. It doesn't always have to be something new or scary. And it doesn't have to be about drugs.

You could do many things while not changing your drug use:

• **Accept yourself as a drug user and embrace your ambivalence about your use.**

• **Find people who accept you as a drug user.** Avoid judgmental people. Or work on them to stop ragging you about your relationship with drugs.

• **Educate yourself about safer use of drugs.** Learn overdose prevention and proper injection techniques. Don't let others shoot you up. Use clean syringes. Don't share crack pipes or coke straws. Make sure your ecstasy is really pure E. Use hallucinogens in a planned way and in the right setting for you. Don't let anyone else give you a drug you don't know about. Have a guide around, a "designated driver."

- **Pay attention to yourself on drugs.** This is hard, especially if your goal is to get out of it, to not be conscious, and if obliterating feelings of shame is one of your driving motives for using. But notice what you can. How impulsive are you when you're high on speed, and what tricks can you develop to have safer sex? What are you like when you drink, or what do people tell you about your behavior if you drink yourself into a blackout? Do you fall down a lot when you use ketamine? Just notice these things, or try to accept others' observations, to build an accurate picture of yourself on drugs.

- **Ponder what you use drugs for.** You might already know a lot about why you use drugs, about your history of abuse, your social anxiety, your discomfort with your body. But as you use, get specific about what precise experience you are looking for with each drug and wonder why you use the amounts you do. What do you feel after two drinks, and is it what you wanted to feel before you started? Then how do you feel after four, five, or six? What does pot do for you, and how many hits does it take to do it? Observe how you feel at different levels of use. You might even jot some of these observations down in a journal *while you're using* and read them later.

- **Do other things to be a healthy and balanced person.** Eat. Drink water. Stay warm. Exercise. Just a little. Go look at something pretty every day. Talk to somebody nice. If you don't know anyone nice, go to a friendly store and buy a soda, just to talk to the cashier for a minute.

- **Use within your means, both financial and emotional.** You don't have to quit alcohol or other drugs to keep some money in your pocket, your house, your job, your family, your friends, or your spirit.

Since intentional change is a process that involves making conscious choices, the choice *not* to change is an equal option in the process. If you find yourself weighing all the options, exploring your resources, feeling the burden of your ambivalence, and you decide to quit working on it, *you have still been engaged in a positive process that has already changed you*. Despite the fact that no apparent change has been made, you are still on the right road. It may not result in an obvious reduction of harm, but it is a start, and a start is more than you had yesterday. That's harm reduction.

How to Weigh the Choices:
The Decisional Balance

The decisional balance is just a fancy way of describing the discussion we often have with ourselves that begins "On the one hand . . . " and is followed closely by "but on the other hand. . . . " Comparing the pros and cons, finding the delicate balance between the upside and the downside of change, or the upside to staying exactly the same and its downside, is what constitutes a decisional balance. Doing a decisional balance means mulling over the possibilities, the pros and the cons, the possible impact of making a change. No action is required at this juncture. There is nothing to be "done" in the run-out-and-change-your-hair-color-right-now kind of way.

The key to using this tool for change is to *go at your own pace*. Remember, your own pace is indicated by how tight or relaxed your belly feels, how sweaty or dry your palms are, and how calm or choppy your breathing is when you think about the pros and cons of your drugs. If you are hyperventilating while you massage your tight belly with clammy palms when you think about quitting, now would be a good time to step back and take a break. But if you feel yourself relax—or you even feel proud of yourself— when you contemplate adding ice to your Scotch, then the decisional balance is tipping in favor of the latter. The decisional balance is a process of looking at the benefits and costs of change versus staying the same. It is not usually hard to untangle the information about costs and benefits, but uncovering things about yourself and your drugs can bring up a lot of strong feelings. Remember to be tender with yourself. Uncover enough to enlighten but not bombard. The chart on the following page can help you get a clear picture of the benefits and costs of your alcohol or drug use.

Once you've put together your lists of benefits and costs, you can compare them. On one hand, you have the **benefits** of changing. On the other hand, you have the **costs** of changing. Then you have another list, which might not be a mirror image of the first one—the **benefits** of not changing and the **costs** of not changing. Your goal in the decisional balance is to bring both sides into focus. The easy part is creating the list. The hard part is figuring out how much each item *weighs* to determine which side "wins." This could take months or years of pondering. Following the laws of both physics and human experience, the **benefits** of changing will eventually have to outweigh the **costs** before you're persuaded to do anything.

In the following story, Jorge is doing a decisional balance, even though he might not be writing it down.

	Short-term benefits/gains (positive)	Short-term losses/costs (negative)	Long-term benefits/gains (positive)	Long-term losses/costs (negative)
To Change If I change my use of _____ [insert drug], I expect to experience these results or consequences.*				
Not to Change If I do not change my use of _____, I expect to experience these results or consequences.*				

*Physical health, emotional well-being, self-esteem, relationships, family (including everyone else's attitude about your use that you haven't managed to ignore), life goals, community.

It's awful. Whenever I'm at my parents' house for Sunday dinner, it always turns into a total nightmare. Everyone's drinking, my parents get into some stupid argument, and the only way to survive is if I start drinking as soon as I step in the door. My two brothers usually join me, and we hang together and try to ignore our parents. Sometimes we watch TV. My one brother is pretty heavy; technically, I think, he's obese. My other brother is okay, but he yells at his wife as nasty as my parents yell at each other. I don't date much. I'm not really heavy, but my gut hangs over my belt, and I don't think the girls I go for are too attracted to that. It might be my meds [Jorge has a seizure disorder], but I don't know for sure. Besides, why would I want to date when it's so clear that relationships end up in yelling matches?

I probably smoke more pot than I should, but I drink too much only at my parents' house. I think about maybe drinking less when I'm there, maybe leaving when the yelling starts. Or maybe just not going at all. But then I'd never see my brothers. Of course, it's not like the three of us have such a great time at my folks' house. And after we've been drinking, nobody really has much fun. I wouldn't mind tossing a ball every now and then, but who can move that fast when you're plastered? I hate it even after I get back to my apartment. I usually get into trouble on Monday because I'm so hung over, I'm really disorganized. My boss, who is pretty cool, has started asking me those "everything okay with the family?" questions, so I pretty much know he knows I'm drinking a little too much on the weekend. If only I was drinking at a great party, it would be worth it. But like I said, I don't date much. If I could get buff, I might. I guess I better get a handle on it before I get into trouble and lose another job. Next time, maybe I'll leave my folks' a little early before the worst starts.

As a part of the process of change for Jorge, his decisional balance does not begin with action. It begins with thought, or contemplation. All of Jorge's thoughts about his drinking, his family, his job, his future take place before he ever makes a solid promise. Becoming active in his decisional balance will lead him to a decision. Becoming more active means focusing on each decision, one at a time. For example, Jorge could focus on whether he will drink less when he is at his parents' house. He thinks about the advantages of *drinking* and the disadvantages. Then he thinks of the advantages of *drinking less* and the disadvantages. An advantage of drinking is being able to tune out the yelling. A disadvantage of drinking is his hangover the next day. An advantage of drinking less would be losing weight. A disadvantage would be not being able to handle the yelling, so more stress. Then he goes through the same process to think about not showing up for Sunday dinner. He goes through the pros and cons of not seeing his brothers, how his parents would feel. Maybe they'd stop helping him with his car payments. And so on.

Eventually he makes a decision about what to try. His decision will lead him into a planning process, and the planning will eventually become action. If he decides to take a break from going over one Sunday to see if that helps, then he has to plan for what he's going to say when they call him up and are upset. Does he lie and say he was sick? Does he tell the truth and say he can't stand the fighting anymore? If he decides to go but drink less, he has to think through what he'll do if he starts to get stressed at the fighting. Does he go to another room, take earplugs, pretend he has a stomachache and leave early? Once he feels prepared to try one of these actions, he'll see what works best, causes the least trouble, and that's what he'll try to maintain.

We will describe a well-researched set of stages that are the basis for understanding change in the harm reduction model. But first, a little more about the difficulties of change.

Normal Difficulties of Changing: Resistance and Ambivalence

Being opposed to change supports the notion that you're just fine as you are. And why wouldn't you feel this? After all, you've gotten this far, and you're still alive. Change is disruptive, implies a rejection of what *is* for what *might be*. It requires a judgment against the present situation and a judgment in favor of something possibly better. But then again, it could be worse. Even though there are problems with a current situation, it is sometimes simply easier and less painful than the benefits change *might* bring. The current situation is the devil we know. Change invites in the devil we don't know.

Resistance

Someone has said to you "Do something about your drinking," or "Spend more time with me," or "If you don't quit soon, you're going to ruin your life." Your reaction to these commands and predictions is to cancel the next dinner with the person, forget to call her back, miss the next appointment, use more drugs. This is called *resistance*. You are reacting to other people's scolding and warnings, because they mean you have to change. And you're not ready to do that.

Even when there's no outside pressure, most people are allergic to change. When faced even with our own impulse to do something different, we break out in a rash of resistance and fear. Maybe it's because being stuck is easier than creating momentum of any sort (the law of inertia!). Or maybe it's because change always suggests going from the known to the unknown and having to lose something in the process.

Despite our tendency to resist new things, most people would, in fact, like to change *something*. If you could get rid of the hangover after a night at the bar, life would be great—no problems concentrating at work and no suspicious glances from your boss or colleagues. Or if you could afford a babysitter so you *and* your partner could be out late, then no more ragging. If you could control your crack smoking so you could maximize the euphoria and avoid the paranoia that follows, you'd be happy. These situations illuminate the hidden wishes to change *at least something*. Notice that all of these changes would be valuable and that none of them require that you quit.

Ambivalence

Imagine you're at sea in a lifeboat. It's flimsy, but it will keep you out of the shark-infested water until you drift toward land. There is one oar, sitting at the far end the boat. If you get up and reach for the oar, you might capsize the boat and get eaten by sharks. If you don't reach for the oar, you might starve before you drift to shore. Deciding what to do constitutes the central dilemma of change.

If you're comfortable with change, you reach for the oar. If you are not comfortable with change, you sit very still and avoid eye contact with the sharks. Changing involves unknown risks. Not changing involves known ones. If you're like most people, the decision to change or stay the same is an agonizing one. The dilemma of change is knowing we should reach for the oar, yet clinging to the instinct not to rock the boat. This dilemma is the stuff of ambivalence.

Sure, change is a good thing that has cured cancers and put twenty-eight varieties of breakfast cereal on the grocery store shelf. Change has helped difficult marriages become easier ones and sad children become happy ones. Change, although often difficult and risky, is a good thing. But our "just do it" society makes very little room in the human experience for ambivalence. "Just do it" means we are expected to go from thinking to action in a nanosecond. "Just do it" suggests that even if there are obstacles to action, we should "just get over it" and move on. If you're not able to "just do it," you're out of the game. In traditional addiction models, "just doing it" means quitting drugs.

Harm reduction puts the human experience of ambivalence ("I'm not sure if I want or *can* just do it") at the center of its philosophy. Ambivalence is the single most important feeling to pay attention to in practicing harm reduction. It means giving equal weight to "on the one hand, maybe yes, but on the other hand, maybe no." This "yes, but" is often seen as making excuses when really what's happening is that you're considering the complexity of your relationship with drugs and with anything else about which you're ambivalent. Making room for your ambivalence about drugs, alcohol, love, work, family will shape your best efforts to reduce harm.

Using drugs in a way that produces harm in your life is like being adrift in a lifeboat. The choice to reach for the oar exists all the time. Not rocking the boat, continuing to use without making any changes, may not lead to inevitable death by starvation, but you will get pretty parched and sunburned. In other words, sitting very still in your substance use will continue to yield the same or more harm, even while it yields some benefits of which, by now, you are aware.

The ambivalence that comes with considering a change in your life is simply the feeling produced by your attempts to balance the harms and benefits of using. Honesty is needed to admit to yourself that change might be needed, but tremendous honesty is required to think of all the reasons why *not* to change. It's virtually impossible to move through the process of change without struggling with ambivalence. The stronger the pull in either direction, the deeper the ambivalence. Being ambivalent is a useful part of the change process. It doesn't mean you're stuck. It doesn't mean you're in denial. It means you're waking up to the different directions in which you're feeling pulled.

The Stages of Change

Change is not a threshold that you just step over. It is an ongoing, living process. An excellent description of this process has been developed by James Prochaska and his colleagues, who use the term "Stage Model of Change." The idea is that we change in stages, not all at once. They identify seven stages: precontemplation, contemplation, preparation, action, maintenance, relapse, and termination. Notice that *action* is not the first stage, and *relapse* does not end the process.

Precontemplation

The **precontemplation** stage is the **"Who, me?"** stage. You wonder who they're talking about when they say you have a drinking problem. People give you a ton of information that you might accept or reject. Either way, you don't know what to do with these suggestions, warnings, ultimatums—except feel pangs of irritation or resentment before you pick up the glass or the pipe again. This is the stage at which many people think you are "in denial." But you are not denying anything; you just don't see what the people around you see. You haven't made the connection yet between your drug use and the problems in your life. You feel hassled, and you don't get what all the fuss is about.

Contemplation

Eventually, you get a DUI, you get diagnosed with hepatitis C, you get a bad dose of ecstasy, and you start to believe what people say about the harms of drug use. Or people give you information in a respectful enough manner that you listen. Then you start thinking about your using. The **contemplation** stage is the **"Yes, but"** stage. This is when you become torn between the "on the one hand" and "on the other hand" conflicts. "On the one hand, nothing takes me out of my boredom like a few hits of crack. On the other, I am really not doing well at work, and my boss is noticing." You're attracted to books that educate you, maybe even read a few that make you think about your use. Maybe you start talking to someone or check out a self-help meeting. You begin considering what making changes might look like. You begin to consider what choices you have. At some point, after weeks or months or years, you make a decision to *do* something.

Preparation

At this point, action is still not your next move, although there's nothing wrong with just going ahead and doing something, as long as you don't fail at what you do and get frustrated at yourself. Generally, people move into the **preparation** or the **"Uh-oh"** stage. The rubber begins to hit the road as you zero in on what to do. You might have decided not to smoke pot when you're taking care of your kids or not to share needles. But *how* to follow through on this decision? If pot's in the house, you could roll a joint even in your sleep. And you haven't a clue where to get a large supply of needles. You explore ways to make your decision happen. Still, you're scared it won't help or you're just not up to it. If that happens, you should consider any other areas you should take care of first—perhaps getting treatment for depression, moving to a different neighborhood, hanging out with different friends. In addition you might begin to visualize a life that's different from the one you've lived up to now. This fantasy makes you feel jazzed about taking action, and you map out realistic plans for the action stage. You find out where the needle exchange program is in your community. You plan to store your pot at someone else's house and just get a limited supply every day.

Action

Finally, the **action** stage is the **"Do it"** stage. You've made a plan that includes a series of steps that are just the right size, and now you're taking those "right-sized steps," continually evaluating how it's going. Sometimes you feel like you can conquer anything. For example, you may quit drinking altogether. Or you stop injecting heroin and snort it instead. Whatever action you take, you try to take steps that won't be so big you trip on them. Despite your exhilaration at times, every day you might feel like you're having your teeth extracted, and every minute the world feels like a scary place.

Maintenance

The **maintenance** stage is **"The grind."** You're solidifying your progress, using support to work through underlying psychological troubles, and getting used to your new routines. Your sense of unfamiliarity and risk begins to fade. The world is not such a scary place, but it can be pretty tedious. There are times when you're bored out of your brain and pissed off that so much work is involved. This is a time when you might decide that you need therapy to deal with the loneliness, anxiety, or depression that has plagued you for years. You make some new friends who will support your efforts to stick with your changes. You change your environment to support your new behavior—a new job, a new friend. This might be when you realize that you may need some antidepressant medication to help you stay on course. It might be that you take up playing the guitar to keep your hands busy or go back to your neighborhood church for a sense of community.

Relapse

Relapse is not actually a stage. It simply means taking a step or two back, and you can do this at any point. In **relapse** you head **"Back to the**

drawing board." Relapse simply means breaking a promise you made to yourself or to someone else. It may be just a momentary lapse. It does not necessarily mean a return to using or using in the way you did before. It means looking at how the promise you made to yourself was unrealistic because you didn't take something into account.

You promised yourself that you wouldn't drink during the week, and it has worked pretty well for months. But your cousin's wedding was on a Wednesday evening, and they had an open bar, and you just hadn't planned on that. Or you had promised yourself you would use only clean needles but found yourself with a group of people who hadn't brought their own, and you ended up sharing. You smoked crack the day you learned your wife had a miscarriage. Relapse often happens when you find yourself in a "high-risk" situation, without a specific plan. Many of the harms that led you to action have been forgotten, but you can clearly remember the benefits of your favorite drug.

You might also develop an "Oh, to hell with it" feeling after breaking your promise and be tempted just to trash the whole thing. Then you beat yourself up for your failure. But relapsing doesn't mean you didn't work hard enough. It means the plan was flawed or not complete enough to take into account all possible pitfalls—given the complexity of human life, what plan could possibly anticipate everything? You're allowed to go back to work on it. In doing so, you explore what worked and what didn't work. Congratulate yourself for your success. Feel as little shame as possible. Take it for what it was—a bump in the road. Move on and reevaluate your plan so that the next bump won't trip you up.

Termination

Termination is when you say **"I'm over it."** The work is done, you've ceased doing the harm you originally sought to reduce. It's at this point that you begin to recognize that your harmful relationship with drugs and/or alcohol is resolved. The difference between this stage and precontemplation is that true awareness, or consciousness, has taken the place of your lack of knowledge and understanding of your experiences. You're harm-free, but not necessarily drug-free.

These stages don't always progress smoothly, as we're sure you can imagine from your prior efforts to change things in your life. However, when you *actively* participate in your own process of change, and when you have new tools to work with, things often go much easier, if not faster. Some people spend years in **precontemplation**. There are many factors that might get you stuck in that stage of "Who, me?" The most serious factor is mental ill-ness. Some forms of serious mental illness make it almost impossible to think about yourself rationally. If you or a family member suffers from para-noia, from schizophrenia, or from debilitating depression, for example, there will be many times when you can't see cause and effect very clearly. At other times, even people with serious mental illness can observe them-selves and move out of precontemplation, only to suffer setbacks when their emotional problems become worse again.

There are other people whose personalities don't allow them to blame themselves or take responsibility for much in their lives. Often these people have been humiliated and abused as children, and they've learned not to accept any feedback from the world, especially if it makes them look bad.

In general, though, the majority of people who have trouble at this stage have simply not had the opportunity to consider all the facts, all the connec-tions between their alcohol or drug use and the problems they are suffering or causing. They are ignorant, in a sense, of cause and effect. Rational, re-spectful information is the best approach for you or for a friend, if this is the stage of change where you get stuck. With this type of intervention, you can expect to get moving much more quickly than if someone browbeats you.

While many people think the stage of **contemplation** is something to get over quickly, it's actually the time when you will be doing the richest, hardest, and most important work. This is the stage in which you're encour-aged to be honest about *your true thoughts and feelings*, not about what oth-ers say or think. Although this type of honesty may be painful, at least it's of your own doing. It's a time for you to respect how complicated you are. Some people go through this stage relatively easily: "Gee, I really like to smoke pot, but it's true that I'm not as sharp at work as I need to be" or "The last time my kid got sick, I'd had too many beers to safely drive her to the hospital. I don't ever want that to happen again." Many people leap into ac-tion with very little problem. For a lot of folks, though, the pros and cons of changing and not changing are very complicated. If the work you're doing at this stage feels overwhelming, take your time and ask for help, if you can. Talk to other people about their experience with changing any part of their lives. You'll probably feel reassured that you're not the only one having trou-ble. Or talk to a therapist (one who is supportive of the harm reduction ap-proach), someone trained to hold on to and understand all the contradic-tions in a person's mind.

Even though you will move on from this stage, it's what you learn in the contemplation stage that you will come back to, over and over again, when the going gets rough and you need a reminder of why you wanted to change in the first place—or why changing was a crummy idea!

The **preparation** stage is more about *how you want to pace yourself.* There aren't any rules about how long this stage *should* take, just how long you want to spend planning for a change. Many people try a few smaller changes, then wait a while to see how it goes. Others of you will make a decision to try something and do it the next day.

The **action** stage is the shortest of all the stages of change. You decide on a course of action, and you do it! You probably won't be at this stage more than a couple of months, at the most, because you'll either move on or find that your plan of action wasn't quite complete, and you'll end up not following through on it. This is often called a *relapse* and is an indication that you're not quite finished with one of the earlier stages or that your plan wasn't all that it needed to be.

The **maintenance** stage has been called "the grind" for good reason. Most people spend months, if not years, perfecting the skills that are needed to keep the change going. How hard this stage is for you will be determined, in part, by how many stresses and how little support you have in your life. In general, though, if you've had an alcohol or drug problem for many years, it's reasonable to expect to spend many years learning new ways of living.

When you ***terminate*** your problematic relationship with your drugs, it's for the rest of your life. That doesn't mean you don't have a relationship with the drug. Just as you can stop fighting with your girlfriend, or get back together with her years after you broke up, you can continue to live with alcohol, pot, opiates, or cocaine and not use them in the same way you did before.

The bottom line is, change will take as long as it takes. You might get frustrated if you're taking "too long" or if your family thinks that, but nobody can predict how all the factors in your life will conspire to help you or block you. In general, the more help you have, the quicker you will get through contemplation and into action. But all of the evidence shows that most people—even people who are trying to change less serious problems than addiction—circle through the stages at least a few times before they reach their ultimate goal. Harm reduction is about *all* the things you do to reduce the harm that drugs and alcohol are causing in your life. You'll be successful at many steps along the way to your ultimate goal. **Success is defined as "any positive change, any step in the right direction toward health."** If you want to quit drinking, but for the next year you "only" manage to drink half as much as usual, **you've had a success, not a failure.**

If you'd like to identify and track your movement for each drug you use or problem you have through the stages of change on paper, on the next pages are some worksheets to try. Put the name of each substance you use in the top row. Go down the list of stages on the left and decide what stage of change you are at with each drug, then write a few words of explanation in that row.

THE STAGES OF CHANGE WORKSHEETS

Here is an example:

RIGHT NOW	Drug (or other) problem _____	Drug (or other) problem _____	Drug (or other) problem _____	Drug (or other) problem _____
Precontemplation— *who, me?*				
Contemplation— *yes, but*		*Crack—no idea what to do*		
Preparation—*Uh-oh*				
Action—*do it*				*Stop drinking and driving*
Maintenance— *the grind*			*Eating better*	
Relapse—*back to the drawing board*	*Had quit drinking*			
Termination— *I'm over it*				

100

AFTER ONE MONTH	Drug (or other) problem ___	Drug (or other) problem ___	Drug (or other) problem ___	Drug (or other) problem ___
Precontemplation —*who, me?*	*Bad relationship*			
Contemplation— *yes, but*		*Cut down frequency of crack use*		
Preparation— *uh-oh*				
Action—*do it*			*Join Moderation Management for drinking*	
Maintenance— *the grind*			*Eating better*	
Relapse—*back to the drawing board*				
Termination— *I'm over it*				*Drinking and driving*

(cont.)

THE STAGES OF CHANGE WORKSHEETS *(cont.)*

Use this chart to track your own stages and progress for as long as you want, forever even.

RIGHT NOW	Drug (or other) problem _____	Drug (or other) problem _____	Drug (or other) problem _____	Drug (or other) problem _____
Precontemplation—*who, me?*				
Contemplation—*yes, but*				
Preparation—*Uh-oh*				
Action—*do it*				
Maintenance—*the grind*				
Relapse—*back to the drawing board*				
Termination—*I'm over it*				

AFTER ONE DAY	Drug (or other) problem _____	Drug (or other) problem _____	Drug (or other) problem _____	Drug (or other) problem _____
Precontemplation —*who, me?*				
Contemplation— *yes, but*				
Preparation— *uh-oh*				
Action—*do it*				
Maintenance— *the grind*				
Relapse—*back to the drawing board*				
Termination— *I'm over it*				

(cont.)

103

THE STAGES OF CHANGE WORKSHEETS *(cont.)*

AFTER ONE WEEK	Drug (or other) problem _____	Drug (or other) problem _____	Drug (or other) problem _____	Drug (or other) problem _____
Precontemplation —*who, me?*				
Contemplation— *yes, but*				
Preparation— *uh-oh*				
Action—*do it*				
Maintenance— *the grind*				
Relapse—*back to the drawing board*				
Termination— *I'm over it*				

AFTER ONE MONTH	Drug (or other) problem _____	Drug (or other) problem _____	Drug (or other) problem _____	Drug (or other) problem _____
Precontemplation —*who, me?*				
Contemplation— *yes, but*				
Preparation— *uh-oh*				
Action—*do it*				
Maintenance— *the grind*				
Relapse—*back to the drawing board*				
Termination— *I'm over it*				

(cont.)

105

THE STAGES OF CHANGE WORKSHEETS (cont.)

AFTER THREE MONTHS	Drug (or other) problem _____	Drug (or other) problem _____	Drug (or other) problem _____	Drug (or other) problem _____
Precontemplation —*who, me?*				
Contemplation— *yes, but*				
Preparation— *uh-oh*				
Action—*do it*				
Maintenance— *the grind*				
Relapse—*back to the drawing board*				
Termination— *I'm over it*				

106

AFTER SIX MONTHS	Drug (or other) problem ___	Drug (or other) problem ___	Drug (or other) problem ___	Drug (or other) problem ___
Precontemplation —*who, me?*				
Contemplation— *yes, but*				
Preparation— *uh-oh*				
Action—*do it*				
Maintenance— *the grind*				
Relapse—*back to the drawing board*				
Termination— *I'm over it*				

(cont.)

107

THE STAGES OF CHANGE WORKSHEETS (cont.)

AFTER ONE YEAR	Drug (or other) problem ____	Drug (or other) problem ____	Drug (or other) problem ____	Drug (or other) problem ____
Precontemplation —*who, me?*				
Contemplation— *yes, but*				
Preparation— *uh-oh*				
Action—*do it*				
Maintenance— *the grind*				
Relapse—*back to the drawing board*				
Termination— *I'm over it*				

AFTER TWO YEARS	Drug (or other) problem _____	Drug (or other) problem _____	Drug (or other) problem _____	Drug (or other) problem _____
Precontemplation —*who, me?*				
Contemplation— *yes, but*				
Preparation— *uh-oh*				
Action—*do it*				
Maintenance— *the grind*				
Relapse—*back to the drawing board*				
Termination— *I'm over it*				

(cont.)

THE STAGES OF CHANGE WORKSHEETS *(cont.)*

AFTER THREE YEARS	Drug (or other) problem ___	Drug (or other) problem ___	Drug (or other) problem ___	Drug (or other) problem ___
Precontemplation —*who, me?*				
Contemplation— *yes, but*				
Preparation— *uh-oh*				
Action—*do it*				
Maintenance— *the grind*				
Relapse—*back to the drawing board*				
Termination— *I'm over it*				

What to Change?: What Is Necessary, Manageable, and Tolerable

If you don't know what to do, or whether to do anything at all, you're most likely at the contemplation stage. This is the stage that we all spend a lot of time in when faced with pressure to *do* something.

A helpful task at this point is to determine what change, if any, is necessary, what is manageable, and what is tolerable. What is necessary may be what someone else is insisting you do "or else." What is manageable may be something that you can do with relative ease, at least in theory. What is tolerable is what you can stand to do without running off the nearest cliff.

What is necessary, manageable, and tolerable may be in conflict with one another. You may discover that to keep your driver's license, you need to start drinking at 7:00 P.M. (after arriving safely at home) instead of 4:00 P.M. (while finishing your day's work at the office). This may be necessary and even manageable but not tolerable. If it's intolerable, you have to think of another plan. So you consider starting at 4:30 and having only one and a half drinks. At least, you'd probably have an adequately low blood alcohol level while on the road. Or perhaps you could still drink at 4:00 P.M. and not count your drinks but would find it manageable to take public transportation home.

You may find yourself unable to tolerate any changes that have been deemed necessary. If this happens, identify something that *is* tolerable and manageable, even if it's not necessary, and do that. Decide to use blue rolling paper instead of white for your joints. Change the pocket in which you store your cocaine. These changes may seem superfluous, but they are *crucial* to the harm reduction process. Making these small changes sets you on a path toward other changes, more necessary ones. Eventually you'll discover that you're not so rigid and fearful of change. It's like limbering up your muscles. Your change muscle is way out of shape. Loosen it up a little with some inconsequential changes.

What Is Necessary

Necessities are basic to sustaining life. Food, water, shelter, and physical safety comprise the short list. From our observation of babies in some orphanages, we also know more clearly than ever that if we're deprived of love or basic attachment to a nurturing caregiver, we fail to thrive. Do you drink enough water when you use ecstasy? Do you eat—before or after an evening of drinking or at all? Do you have alcohol or GHB blackouts that might leave you vulnerable to assault? Have you emptied your bank account on a cocaine binge and not had enough money to pay the mortgage, rent, or electric bill? Does your nightly glass of wine inflame your hepatic liver? Does anyone ever give you a hug? Even if you have a home, eat regularly, and don't consider your use immediately lethal, it's possible that using substances has some effect on the basic necessities of life. Perhaps it's worth taking a look.

What Is Manageable

It's important to separate what's manageable from what's tolerable. What's manageable is what's doable. Planning to use public transportation as an alternative to driving under the influence when there is no public transportation in your community is not a manageable solution. If you're able to tolerate chain smoking through your urge to snort cocaine but your landlord has a no-smoking policy, chain smoking is not a manageable solution. Discovering what is manageable means educating yourself about your resources and your environment.

What Is Tolerable

Tolerance is the uncut gem of the psyche. It allows you to endure what you don't like. It is also about kindness and understanding. It's the raw material for wisdom and peace. Like change, it's another of those underused muscles. We rely on tolerance, often unconsciously. You probably tolerate things all day long without knowing it. You sit on the train with your pants twisted, too embarrassed to straighten them out, even though they're cutting painfully into your groin. But you sit there anyway, tolerating it. You answer the phone moments before kickoff and tolerate the frustration of being interrupted. You tolerate the burning feeling in your chest when you smoke crack. You tolerate your spouse's anger, or your own despair, about drinking too much. You tolerate plenty. Make no mistake: it is not that you lack tolerance for discomfort or pain; it's that you have not yet learned to apply this tolerance to the pain and discomfort that has become your habit to avoid.

Labor and delivery coaches often tell pregnant women, "You can stand anything for a minute—that's about how long a contraction lasts." Tolerating contractions, like tolerating other physical or emotional pain, is a state in which you're able to feel your discomfort, distaste, disgust, fear, anxiety, outright rebellion, pain, or impatience and just sit there. It doesn't mean *em-*

bracing what disgusts or enrages you. It doesn't mean transforming your distaste into appreciation. It simply means allowing how you feel about something to lurk about, without actually *doing* something to get rid of it.

In practicing harm reduction, your task is to begin to notice what *changes* you can tolerate. Can you live with the churning in your belly when you want to drink at 4:00 in the afternoon but you've promised yourself to wait until 4:30? If you tolerated a delay for one minute yesterday, could you tolerate two minutes today? Tolerating the delay won't stop the churning. It won't make you like the feeling. Tolerance is simply sitting with it. And if you can accept that tolerating discomfort is OK, you might actually find it easier than when you fought against it.

In the words of Mark Twain, "Habit is habit and not to be flung out the window by any man, but coaxed downstairs one step at a time." As you read beyond these pages, feel free to stand on the upstairs landing just as long as you need to, and make sure your footing is secure as you proceed—no matter how slowly that is.

SOURCES AND SUGGESTED READINGS

All about how people make decisions:

> *Decision Making*. Irving Janis and Leon Mann. Free Press. 1977.

On the stages of change:

> *Changing for Good*. James Prochaska, Carlo DiClemente, and John Norcross. Avon Books. 1994.

You can find some helpful worksheets to chart your decisional balance process in:

> *The Addiction Workbook: A Step-by-Step Guide to Quitting Alcohol and Drugs*. Patrick Fanning and John O'Neill. New Harbinger. 1996.
> *Changing for Good*. James Prochaska, Carlo DiClemente, and John Norcross. Avon Books. 1994.
> *Sex, Drugs, Gambling, and Chocolate: A Workbook for Overcoming Addictions*. A. Thomas Horvath. Impact Publishers. 1998.

What happens psychologically when we break promises to ourselves:

> *Relapse Prevention*. G. Alan Marlatt and Judith R. Gordon, Eds. Guilford Press. 1985. (See sections on the "abstinence violation effect.")

6 HOW DO I KNOW EXACTLY WHAT MY PROBLEM IS?

So you've measured your use and decided that it bears more attention. Or you've steered well clear of measuring—goodness knows, you don't want to *count* how many ounces of whiskey were in those drinks, the number of hits you took off the pipe today, or the size of that last shot. But you've considered change, you've played with your decisional balance, you know you're concerned, and you're still reading. What now?

There's another way of measuring. It's more complicated, but it's more real. It takes into account *all* of who you are.

Let's say you use three different drugs: alcohol, pot, and cocaine. You drink socially and on the light side, never more than two drinks a few times a week. You use cocaine occasionally (once a month), and when you do, you party for the whole weekend. Your pot use is more confusing. You smoke just a little every day, and you need it to relax. When you smoke, though, whatever other good ideas you had for the evening—doing your taxes, writing the paper that's due next week, cleaning the garage—vanish. You've been thinking you're addicted. (We hope you're getting used to not labeling yourself as an addict.)

For the moment, you can continue the risk–benefit analysis that is part of your decisional balance. For example, you may think that smoking every night is a problem, but perhaps fulfilling your promises for the evening also would create problems. If you were going to balance your checkbook and your bank account is in ruins, you may have saved yourself some stress and a sleepless night, followed by an unproductive day at work tomorrow. If you were going to have a talk with your husband about the fact that the two of you haven't had sex in a year, you might be grateful to have forgotten that idea in the comforting haze of pot. So might he! If you were going to help your daughter with her math homework, but you failed math as a kid, you just saved her some frustration and yourself some embarrassment. You *should* clean out the garage, but last time you did, you threw your back out. On the one hand, it looks like you aren't taking care of business, but on the other, it looks like smoking is saving you from any number of difficult situations. Avoiding stress and pain is a common and valid reason for a lot of people who use alcohol or other drugs.

In Chapter 3 you were introduced to a few ideas about how drugs can harm you. Chapter 4 gave you the opposing viewpoint: that people use drugs for reasons, and those reasons are often real benefits. Whether a particular drug is a problem or, in fact, a solution to another problem, depends. It depends on virtually all the variables that make you who you are—your gender and age, your body size, ethnicity, culture, physical health, medications, mental health, why you're using, and even where and with whom you use.

It also depends on what the drug is, how it works, how you take it into your body (the "route of administration"), and what else is in it. In the chart here and on the next page, look at how alcohol impacts three different people, depending on their unique situations.

	Person 1	Person 2	Person 3
Drug	Alcohol	Alcohol	Alcohol
Route of administration	Beer—oral administration	Whiskey—oral administration	Wine—oral administration
Gender	Male	Male	Female
Age	21	50	30
Body size	Heavy	Thin	Medium
Race/ethnicity	Black	White	Latina
Culture/ community of origin and affiliation with it	African American from the urban South, close to family and old friends	Irish American from the rural Northeast, alienated from family and their community	Mexican American from rural California
Culture/ community of identity now	Educated, politically active student community	Close to wife. No friends or community	Latin music and dance community in urban California
Physical health	High blood pressure	HIV+, fatigue is primary symptom	Apparently OK
			(cont.)

	Person 1	Person 2	Person 3
Mental health	Anxious and shy	Depressed	Posttraumatic stress and depression (sexual abuse survivor)
Medications	None	Protease inhibitors (for HIV)	Antidepressant
Why it's used	Peer group activity	Relief of boredom, fear of dying	Relaxation in sexual relationships
Where it's used	At bars and parties	At home and at work	In bars and at home
With whom it's used	With friends	Alone	With boyfriends

Harm can come to anyone who uses drugs or alcohol. Let's say you're not addicted to alcohol, but you have diabetes. You drink beer twice a week. Is that safe? Not necessarily—it could be lethal. Let's say you have high blood pressure and you use cocaine just once. Is it safe? Maybe, but stroke is a risk of cocaine *and* high blood pressure. Or you're a student, and you smoke pot once a week or so. Marijuana impairs memory. Is it harmful for a student who is not "addicted" to marijuana to use it? Maybe, maybe not. It probably depends on how much she smokes and when. Look at the results of alcohol use on the three people in the chart above:

Positive impact	Better able to participate in political and social activities.	Able to tolerate long periods at work alone (works as night security guard) and to avoid thoughts and feelings about being HIV+.	Dulls traumatic memories. Able to have sexual relationships.

	Person 1	**Person 2**	**Person 3**
Negative impact	High blood pressure increased—physician's warning that he might need medications. Grades slipping.	Drowsy at work. Got caught drinking at work and was fired. Wife very upset. Impedes absorption of nutrients. Reduced immune function.	Unknown at this point.

To get a clear look how drugs and alcohol operate in *your* life, you must plug in your own individual circumstances. You need to identify all of your unique characteristics to determine how many issues in your life need attention and in what order.

Drug, Set, and Setting

It's always tempting to organize new information in a hierarchy. We like to "get our ducks in a row," see the higher priorities above the lower ones, understand "what came first, the chicken or the egg." But here is the bottom line: your relationship with drugs and alcohol is interactive, not causal or hierarchical. One factor didn't cause your problems. What came first is often incidental. Thinking about what caused what in the first place may be useful and sometimes helps a person figure out where to start, but it is not necessarily the way things are now. Knowing what came first is not essential to working in a harm reduction framework.

Many people who work in substance abuse and 12-Step programs say that people with addictions need things made simple. But simplification leads to black-and-white, all-or-nothing thinking. They usually blame the drugs for all your other problems. But we think people are up to the challenge of complex thinking, at least most of the time. That's why we suggest you allow your drug and alcohol use to be as complicated as it really is, rather than try to oversimplify it.

The danger with simplicity is that the solutions you come up with might leave out important factors, and it is these "wild cards" that cause you to fail in your efforts to change. For example, you might believe that because alcohol is a central nervous system depressant, too much drinking must be the cause of your depression. You would probably think, then, that not drinking would clear up your depression. And, of course, it might. But it might also be true that you began drinking when you were young and unhappy and found that it made you feel better. Over time, drinking too much has caused social problems for you. You tend to get angry when you're drunk, so people have learned to avoid you. Now you're lonely, which makes you feel depressed in a different way.

If you just quit drinking, you may feel better at first just because you've taken away one factor in your depression. People now like being around you, and you feel better, less lonely. You might find over time, however, that you're getting just as depressed without the alcohol. What got left out is the possibility that you suffer from a longer-term depression that needs to be treated by medication or therapy. It's also possible that you left out a different medical explanation. Perhaps, over time, your thyroid stopped working so well, and low thyroid is really the most important factor in your current depression. It's not that any one of these things is *the truth*. It's that if you try to simplify a drug or alcohol problem, you're likely to miss the *interaction and the relative importance* of several different factors. You're then likely to apply the wrong solution or miss one of several solutions.

A model that helps explain how some people get into trouble with drugs and others don't, called "Drug, Set, Setting," is illustrated by the triangular chart to the right. Problems with drugs result from an *interaction* between three things: the *drug* you use, the *set* (this originally referred to your mindset) and the *setting* or environment influencing you. Not only do *problems* with drugs emerge from this interaction, but often the *drug experience itself* is a product of this interaction. Like when your best experience on mushrooms was with your college roommates, and your worst trip ever was with a boyfriend with whom you wanted to break up.

The "Drug, Set, Setting" model was developed in the late 1970s and early 1980s by a psychiatrist, Norman Zinberg. He studied the phenomenon of recreational heroin use to understand why some people did not become "addicted" to this assumed-to-be "addictive" drug. What he found was that recreational heroin users made the same sensible decisions that so-called social drinkers do: there is a time and place for everything, and everything in moderation. Don't use every day (or you will become physically dependent). Use on weekends. Don't use until the kids are in bed. Or get a babysitter and go to someone else's place. Give yourself time to detox before responsibilities loom. He also learned that people's use changes over time, just like our

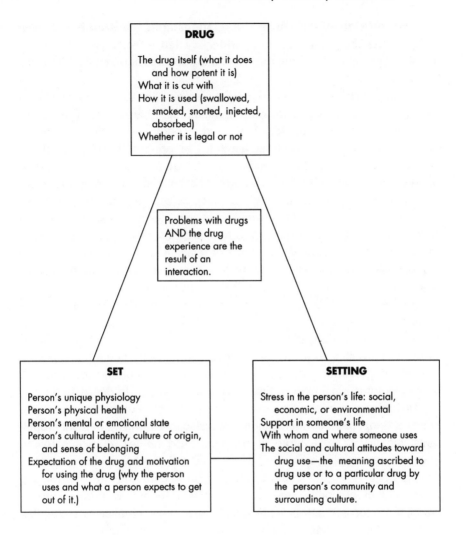

DRUG

The drug itself (what it does
    and how potent it is)
What it is cut with
How it is used (swallowed,
    smoked, snorted, injected,
    absorbed)
Whether it is legal or not

Problems with drugs
AND the drug
experience are the
result of an
interaction.

SET

Person's unique physiology
Person's physical health
Person's mental or emotional state
Person's cultural identity, culture of origin,
    and sense of belonging
Expectation of the drug and motivation
    for using the drug (why the person
    uses and what a person expects to get
    out of it.)

SETTING

Stress in the person's life: social,
    economic, or environmental
Support in someone's life
With whom and where someone uses
The social and cultural attitudes toward
    drug use—the meaning ascribed to
    drug use or to a particular drug by
    the person's community and
    surrounding culture.

eating habits. We eat more from Thanksgiving to Christmas, then watch what we eat for a few months, following that New Year's resolution. Out of studying users' behaviors and decisions, he developed the idea that addiction is not solely dependent on an "addictive" drug. Nor is it entirely dependent on a person's being "diseased." As you can see from the triangular chart, each of the three elements of a relationship with drugs has several subparts, all of which are important.

The DRUG itself influences the relationship. Each drug has its own unique chemistry and produces widely varied effects. (See "What Are These Drugs Anyway?" in the middle of this book for more detailed information.)

A drug's action is the first important element. Sedatives such as benzodiazepines (Valium, Xanax, Ativan, Klonopin, etc,), barbiturates (phenobarbital, Nembutal, Seconal, etc.), GHB, and alcohol; anesthetics such as nitrous oxide and ketamine; and narcotics or opiates (heroin, morphine, codeine, and other synthetic version opiates) are all *central nervous system depressants,** although they all behave differently in your brain and make you high in different ways. They are called *depressants* because they depress, or slow down, brain activity and at high doses can shut down vital functions necessary to sustain life (breathing, heart rate). Generally speaking, the modulated experience is one of relaxation. Withdrawal can cause the opposite—anxiety, jitteriness, restlessness, and sometimes dangerous levels of brain hyperactivity, which is the cause of seizures.

Stimulants such as cocaine, amphetamines (speed), nicotine, and caffeine excite brain and body activity, sometimes to the point of jitteriness, nervousness or anxiety, sweating, or even dramatic effects such as paranoia or stroke. Stimulants provide energy, focus, and a sense of euphoria, power, or well-being. Withdrawal, or the crash, can be uncomfortable to miserable, with symptoms ranging from headache to restlessness to depression.

Hallucinogens, marijuana, dissociative anesthetics (ketamine and PCP), solvents (glue, paint thinner, lighter fluid, gasoline, varnish), aerosol propellants, inhalants (amyl nitrite or poppers, butyl nitrite), deliriants (nightshades, some mushrooms, nutmeg), and alcohol may have relaxing and depressant effects, euphoric and stimulating ones, consciousness-rearranging ones, or all of the above. Some can have uncomfortable withdrawal effects (marijuana, for example), some are dangerous in themselves (solvents), and some lead to dangers like accidents (anesthetics or alcohol).

Finally, some drugs produce physical dependence in *anyone* who uses regularly or heavily, even when used properly for medical reasons. A withdrawal becomes inevitable, and can be either extremely uncomfortable (as in the case of opiates) or dangerous (in the case of depressants like alcohol, barbiturates, and benzodiazepines) and that should be medically managed.

Another important feature of the drug is the **dose** used. Small amounts may create euphoria. Larger amounts may cause "drunkenness" or over-

*Do not confuse this use of the word *depressant* with the depression that refers to mood. People often experience an *elevation* of mood with these drugs because of their relaxing properties. Many also have other unique effects that make them interesting, useful, or desirable.

dose. Whether a drug is in its natural plant form, is the extracted active ingredient of the plant, or is made in a lab (synthetic) affects the dose—extracts or synthesized drugs are much more potent. How a drug is taken—**the route of administration**—affects the experience. How quickly and how dramatically the drug gets to your brain and affects you is different when a drug is smoked, injected (IV), absorbed through mucous membranes, or eaten. (Smoking is the fastest; IV gets the most of the drug to your brain.) The faster the drug comes on, the more compelling it is, which is one reason smoking cocaine has become a larger problem than snorting it ever was. Finally, a drug's **legality** influences our relationship to it. The quality control of illegal drugs is poor to nonexistent, making it hard to monitor dose and impurities. Moreover, one often uses in a hurry to avoid being caught. Rushing your drug use can be dangerous, especially if you're injecting it and don't take the time to test a small amount of your dose for potency.

All of these factors influence the effect of a drug on your body, your mind, your emotions, and your relationships with others. If you're drawn to a particular kind of drug (either depressants, stimulants, or consciousness-distorting or -enhancing drugs), you might get clues about what underlying or coexisting mental, physical, or emotional issues you have. You should also use the chart at the end of Chapter 4 for this—the one that tells you how different classes of drugs affect different feelings, moods, or psychiatric issues.

SET refers to the influence of the characteristics of each individual user on the drug experience.

The set means you, the person using the drug. It originally referred mostly to your mindset at the time of using. We use it more broadly to factor in all of who you are. This includes your unique personality as well as your motivation for using and your hopes for a good effect. Are you a risk taker? Do you love a challenge? This personality trait may make it easier for you to experiment with different drugs than it would be for someone who is a more cautious type. Do you want a new view or understanding of life? A search for meaning and insight may motivate you to try LSD or some other hallucinogen. Are you a rebel? Do you think people in authority are frauds? You might be more willing to use illegal drugs than is the person who has a deeper respect for authority. Is your family life upsetting? Sniffing nitrous oxide will take you away from it all (as will gasoline, and it's relatively cheap*).

---

*We are not recommending gasoline—or any other drug, for that matter. As much as we would like to say "Just Say **NO**" to inhalants such as glue and gasoline, we acknowledge that tens of thousands of children all over the world use them, and just like us adults with our drugs, they use them for reasons.

Your mood, what motivates you to use a drug, and what you expect from it influence the experience you have. People who use marijuana and hallucinogens like LSD probably know this. Your mood and your expectation affect how high you get, whether you get relaxed, silly, talkative, sleepy, or anxious, and whether you have a "good trip" or a "bad trip." This phenomenon has also been studied with alcohol. When given nonalcoholic drinks that they are told contain alcohol, people show many of the same signs of intoxication as people who were actually given alcohol!

Innate characteristics, physical condition, and ongoing mental and emotional issues are important. Are you male or female? (Women have approximately 50 percent less of the enzyme in the stomach that metabolizes alcohol than men do, so women become more intoxicated at a lower dose.) Do you belong to an ethnic group (Asian, primarily) that lacks an enzyme in the liver that metabolizes alcohol? This will cause you to "flush" or get a headache while drinking. Have you used the drug before, and do you have enough of a tolerance to handle the dose you are about to use? Do you have a medical condition that makes certain physical or organ systems more vulnerable (liver disease, high blood pressure, lung disease, diabetes, etc.)? Do you have a mental or emotional condition that makes you more susceptible to the effects of certain drugs? For example, are you normally anxious? Taking cocaine, a stimulant that activates the norepinephrine, the fight–flight neurotransmitter, could make you paranoid. Then again, there are anxious, even psychotic, people who find cocaine paradoxically relaxing. Are you taking medications that might interact with your chosen recreational drugs?

Finally, who you are, your cultural identity, and the extent to which you feel identified and secure as a member of a group are important. Do you feel alienated from your culture of origin, either because you don't like its members or because they've rejected you? Have you taken on another identity about which you feel good? The most common examples are when young people (or adults, for that matter) come out as gay, get involved in an interracial relationship, or develop a radically different political orientation from their family or community of origin. It is then that rejection and alienation can take a serious toll on self-esteem or create feelings of depression or anger.

SETTING—where you use and the larger environmental influences—can be as important as who you are or what you use.
The setting part of the equation refers to the environment in which you drink or use drugs. Who are you usually with and where are you? Alone?

With friends or family? Outside under a freeway overpass or inside a dry apartment with running water? The setting will determine not only what drug you might use but also the effect it will have on you. Shooting heroin in a back alley is not as safe as shooting it at home. Home is usually cleaner, has running water, and, unless you have people there you're trying to hide from, you're not as rushed, so you can be careful to do it right. An important harm reduction fact discovered in recent years is that people overdose more easily on heroin when they use the same drug in an unfamiliar environment. Where and with whom you use psychedelics such as LSD makes a very big difference to whether you have a "good trip" or a "bad trip." Drinking alone is a different experience from drinking with others. It could be anything from more depressing to more relaxing. Most important, if you're using a drug that is prone to lethal overdose or causing accidents—heroin, alcohol, ecstasy, nitrous, ketamine, solvents—using with others around, who have the ability (they aren't too loaded themselves or too afraid to call 911) to take care of you in an emergency, could save your life.

The setting also refers to the stresses as well as the support in your life. Do you have a job and enough money, or are you poor? Do you have family to take care of, or are you responsible only for yourself? What is the quality of your relationships with family members? Are you hiding your drug use from your spouse or kids, parents, or siblings? Are they aware and worried about you? Are they ashamed of you? And what about other relationships—do you have supportive friends or a group with whom you spend time? Do your friends encourage you in healthy or unhealthy choices and behaviors?

The setting refers to the larger context of your life, too—the attitudes and beliefs of your community and the dominant culture around you. Many people define their community primarily by their personal relationships with their families and friends. But *community* can describe everything from your religious affiliation to your local political and social environment. What are some of the unique beliefs, traditions, and activities associated with your culture? Does religion play a big part? How about social activities? Do people in your culture spend most of their time with family, or are friends just as important? Is it expected that you marry and have children to fit in? What if you don't? How do people feel about celebration and fun? Is it part of how life is supposed to be lived, or is hard work more valued? On the one hand, these cultural forces have made you who you are. On the other, you may be alienated from your culture of origin. Perhaps you grew up in a strong Italian Catholic culture but now you're a lesbian, and women in that culture are supposed to get married and have children (with a man). Or perhaps you married young and raised a family, but now you want to travel and not be part of a multigenerational family? The conflicts you feel will certainly affect your tendency to use drugs or alcohol in a way that may be different from those in your family of origin.

Attitudes about alcohol and drugs vary widely in different communities in the United States, so the level of acceptance or stigma also varies a great deal. Do you belong to a group in your society from which you might be hiding your drinking or drug-using habits, or to a group that accepts your habits? Your church might frown on your marijuana use, but your fraternity accepts it. Some attitudes might add stress as you struggle with, or try to enjoy, your use.

How Drug, Set, and Setting Interact

Chapter 4 introduced you to the idea that we all use drugs for reasons. Pulling apart the reasons may be a bit like trying to separate sticky taffy. And, in fact, knowing the reasons may not lead directly to a solution, just more clarity about the problems. We are going to suggest that you assess yourself in the three areas of drug, set, and setting. This will be the place for you to start pulling things apart and identifying *all* the issues that deserve attention. Through this process you will develop a list of the things that concern you most, the things you need most, the things you might think about changing. Some of these things may have nothing to do with your drug and alcohol use; others will.

Let's take Stella for an example, and let's pick the Xanax she's using.

Drug: Xanax is a benzodiazepine, an antianxiety medication. It's legal and must be prescribed by a physician. It helps people calm down when they're upset and helps them not panic. In fact, it's often prescribed for panic attacks. If she's taking it as prescribed by her doctor, it will help in the short run and probably not cause problems. It can be unpleasant, however, when the drug wears off—and it wears off quickly, so you get a sudden drop that can make you feel bad. When taken regularly for long periods of time (months or years), it will almost certainly result in physical dependence and can cause problems for you when you are trying to learn new things. Stella hasn't been taking Xanax for very long or in high doses. She is drinking alcohol, however. Although it takes a lot to overdose on either benzodiazepines or alcohol, you can overdose more "easily"when you combine them. As far as we know, Stella is not using the two at the same time, so she may not be risking that danger right now.

Set: Stella is grieving and depressed and doing the best she can. She mostly wants to avoid falling apart so that she can continue to work. Xanax is a pretty good choice for what she feels like she needs, a quick pick-me-up in the morning to soften those feelings. She's not taking it to get high, to socialize, or to have fun. It's a way to cope, a medicine. Because it calms her and puts aside her grief and her worries, it seems to be a good thing. One problem, though, could be that she really *does* need to think about her husband and grieve the loss of him. If Xanax keeps her from thinking and feeling all the time, then it will probably backfire on her at some point. Avoiding grief usually makes it last longer.

Setting: Stella drinks and uses Xanax by herself. In European American culture, it's normal for people in her situation and her social group to drink. It's also usual for them to take medicine for their "nerves." Stella doesn't feel alienated from her social network, but on the other hand, she's not seeing much of other people right now. She knows she's drinking too much and shouldn't be using pills so often. Her children, her supervisor, and her EAP counselor are all pressuring her. This multisided pressure could ultimately turn out to be helpful support, even lifesaving, if her drinking increases or her judgment slips and she starts driving while intoxicated. The pressure could also backfire if she feels alienated from the only people who know her situation, and starts hiding her use.

Stella is more confused than defensive when her counselor tells her she has a substance abuse problem and has to quit or she'll never deal with her husband's death. From her perspective, alcohol and Xanax are her medicine for grief, and *that's* the problem. From this analysis of drug, set, and setting, she just may be right. What she's going through is normal and natural. Rather than abandoning her to her own sense of how many pills to take, it would be better for somebody to work *with* her during this difficult time, initially demanding nothing of her. We would start by inviting her to talk about Victor and his death. We would evaluate her for a short-term treatment with antidepressant medication. We might switch her to another benzodiazepine that is gentler. We would not insist that she stop drinking. We would educate her about the dangers to avoid, including combining drugs and using in a way that's drawing negative attention at work.

Assess Yourself

The best way to decide if *you* have a problem with drugs, and what exactly that problem is, is to think about all the important parts of your life—your mind and how you think; your emotions and how you feel; your body, physical health, and how well you take care of yourself; how connected you feel to the rest of world; your relationships with parents or children, friends, spouse or lover, brothers and sisters; your sense of belonging in a culture or community; your work; your finances; and, of course, your drugs.

Then think about how your drugs interact with each of the other parts of your life. You don't have to know exactly how they interact. Just focus on how you feel in your body, your mind, your emotions, and your surroundings when you use different drugs in different amounts.

If you answer the questions on the following pages, you'll get a rich picture of your relationship with alcohol and other drugs. Use a journal or the worksheet that follows the questions. Answer the entire set of questions for each drug that you use. Even though some of the answers will be the same (such as your family situation), the information about yourself and the setting will be different with each drug, even if only slightly.

This is a fairly comprehensive set of questions, some of which ask you to concentrate on things about yourself that you don't normally focus on, even the kind and amount of drugs you use. Although it's a useful part of practicing harm reduction, practice harm reduction *while you do it*. Ignore what others say and especially ignore antidrug propaganda. Stop whenever you start to feel bad or overwhelmed. Take breaks even when you don't. Eat plenty of food, drink plenty of water, and get plenty of sleep. Unless you need to make changes in behaviors or lifestyle that are *immediately* life-threatening, rushing this process will not get you faster to your goal.

Alternatively, consider getting help from a harm reduction-friendly therapist, one who will help you neutrally evaluate all the parts of your life without making assumptions about which are the biggest problems or which are the ones you should be taking care of first.

Establishing a Hierarchy of Needs

Instead of worrying about how all of these variables interact with each other (you probably have an intuitive sense of what influences what, and that's good enough), you should just make a list of what issues stood out as you answered these questions. In other words, which things caused you most concern, which got you most excited, which did you feel most attached to, which most alienated from? Which seemed easy to do something about, which made you groan, "I'll never ... "? This becomes your "pay attention" list, the list of things that you want or need to attend to. Ac-

Drug

What drug:

In what form do you use it (*smoke, eat or drink, inject, or absorb by mucous membranes or skin*)?

Where do you get it (*prescription, street, liquor store, known dealer or stranger*)?

Do you know its purity or what it is cut with?

Is it legal or illegal?

How much does it cost?

How often do you use it?

What size dose do you use?

How long do you wait between doses?

How many other drugs do you use at the same time?

Which ones? (*Generally, think about whether you're combining stimulants with stimulants or with depressants.*)

Set (Person—You)

Physical characteristics

Gender*

Body size:

(cont.)

---

*If you're transgendered, you will most likely react to drugs on a physical level in accordance with your birth gender, with the exception of drugs that stimulate estrogen or testosterone if you're taking hormones. In other words, if you were a woman at birth, you are likely to retain the same metabolic relationship with alcohol. Birth gender does not have anything to do with what different drugs evoke emotionally.

Body type:

Race/ethnicity:

Physical health

Known diseases:

Prescribed medications:

Over-the-counter medications (*for example, herbal remedies, cold or flu remedies, diet aids, nutritional or performance supplements*):

Suspected problems—list any pains or other symptoms that make you think you might have a physical problem (*such as shortness of breath, lack of energy, dizziness, etc.*):

Nutrition (how often and what you eat; how much water you drink):

Mental health (*the information in Chapter 4 should help you identify aspects of your mental health, even if you have little knowledge of mental health*)

Known/treated problems:

Treatment/medications:

Known/untreated problems (*maybe you have panic attacks or were given medications for depression in the past, or perhaps you were abused as a child and have trouble sleeping*):

Suspected problems—list any emotions or attitudes that make you think you might have a mental health problem (*for example, do you feel generally, or sometimes, depressed, pessimistic, anxious or frightened, confused or disoriented, overly elated and optimistic, lonely, angry, hostile, suspicious, flat [unemotional], distant from other people, critical?*):

Personality characteristics (*style of doing things, interacting; for example, are you outgoing or shy, do you like to take risks and do exciting things, do you think things over before deciding on a course of action, or do you make up your mind quickly?*):

Specific relationship to this drug

Why you use it:

What specific effect you expect to feel when you use it:

Identity

We have many different ways of describing ourselves and feeling a part of different groups of people. How do you identify yourself in terms of

Race:

Ethnicity:

Gender:

Sexual orientation:

Social/economic class:

Family (*do you currently view yourself as a member of a family? Who are you? Mother, child, aunt, domestic partner, father, significant other, extended family member, etc.? Are you married or with a partner, single, have several relationships, etc.?*):

(cont.)

Sense of self and belonging in the world

Some people might call this area the spiritual sphere. Recognize if you are occupied with any of the following concerns:

How solid and secure do you feel in your existence?

Do you have existential anxieties about why you are here, what you are supposed to do with your life, why your life is so hard, whether you deserve to live or die?

Do you wonder if there is a god and, if so, what he or she intends for you?

Do you have a strong relationship with a religious or spiritual practice? Or do you not concern yourself with any of these questions?

Setting–Environment

The setting of your drug use

Where do you use this drug?

When do you use it (*morning, afternoon, evening, night; before or after major obligations such as work or family responsibilities or operating machinery; before, during, or after stressful or celebratory occasions, etc.)?*

With whom do you use it, or do you use alone?

The stress in your life

Social (*too many people, too few people, the wrong people, family/relationship problems*):

Environmental (*the quality of your housing, your neighborhood, your work-place*):

Occupational (problems on the job, at school, or the lack of work/occupation):

Economic (*too little money, too much money, not enough control over money, too much money spent on drugs*):

The support in your life

It's important to identify the strengths in your environment. Go over the list in the preceding material and focus on how you get support from some of those areas or people and how they might help in your attempts to deal with a substance abuse problem. For example, maybe your family is going through difficult financial problems right now, and that's a source of stress for you. But it could also be that one or more of them would feel glad to help you out emotionally if you asked. In the midst of everyday problems, we often forget that people who care about us usually *want to be helpful.* In addition, consider your community and what sources of support or obstacles it provides.

Community (*this is an extension of your identity in many cases but also includes your town or the particular social, political, or religious groups to which you belong*):

What is the attitude of your community-of-origin to this particular drug?

What is the attitude of your community-of-origin toward your use of this drug?

What is the attitude of your current community toward this drug?

What is the attitude of your current community toward your use of this drug— and do you feel that you have to hide your use?

DRUG/SET/SETTING WORKSHEET

Here's an example:

	Drug	Me	Environment
What's helpful	Wine It's legal.	I'm anxious with people and wine's relaxing. I work so hard, wine's the only thing that helps me unwind.	Lots of chatty people at the bar. I work so hard that I've lost other friends to hang out with and other things to do.
What's harmful	Wine It's kind of expensive if you drink at bars. Fattening.	I have hepatitis C and drinking will make my liver more vulnerable. Headaches the next morning. I've gained weight.	My boyfriend doesn't drink. He hates it that I smell like alcohol and cigarette smoke when I've been at the bar and he won't sleep with me.

DRUG/SET/SETTING WORKSHEET

	Drug	Me	Environment
What's helpful			
What's harmful			

DRUG/SET/SETTING WORKSHEET

	Drug	Me	Environment
What's helpful			
What's harmful			

cording to harm reduction, you can attend to problems in the order in which they concern *you*, not the order in which a counselor or therapist, maybe not even a family member, might be concerned. (You might consider making an exception when someone qualified to do so alerts you to immediately life-threatening danger. Also make sure he or she is not being hysterical about drug use. Ascertain the medical basis of the concern in detail.)

Your list should be ranked according to a hierarchy, with the most pressing problem—the one most important to *you*—coming first, the least important problem coming last. We know we told you that things aren't really hierarchical but rather interactive. That's when it comes to other people telling you there are rules about what came first. That shouldn't stop you from setting your own priorities in a hierarchy of what's most important to *you*. This is *your* **hierarchy of needs**. A hierarchy of needs is simply a list of what you need, which harmful effects are of greatest concern, which problems you need to handle, or which goals you want to accomplish *in order of priority*. If it seems helpful, use the worksheet at the end of this section. Psychologist Abraham Maslow developed a theory about a hierarchy of needs in the 1960s. We humans have needs that differ in their degree of importance. Most fundamental are our basic survival needs for food, water, warmth, and perhaps some love or attachment. Relationship and spiritual needs and work come in along the hierarchy. At the end is our need for what Maslow called "self-actualization," the process of bringing to life our best potentials as human beings. In harm reduction, the idea of a hierarchy of needs is based on the principle that *we can't do everything at once, so we might as well prioritize.*

When we help people establish their hierarchy of needs, we clearly acknowledge that drugs and alcohol aren't their only problem, may well not be the most important problem, or may be the cause of any or all of their other problems. "Take care of the drug problem, and the rest will take care of itself" is not a belief to which we subscribe. Problems can be independent or may well be interactive, but we make no assumptions about the cause-and-effect relationships between drugs and problems until we know the person very well.

Let's go back to Cheryl and Masa. What would they determine as their hierarchy of needs? What would they choose as their most important goals?

Cheryl is not happy and wants to feel better. She is probably considering the following issues: her loneliness and desire for a successful relationship, her history of sexual abuse, her stress before drinking and her moods after drinking, her growing irritability, her tiredness and its effect on her work performance, and the attitude of her friends toward her drinking. Being an organized person, she might look for a structure by which to prioritize her concerns. She starts writing things down:

1. Loneliness
2. Choice of partners and sexual tension
3. Stress after work and my use of alcohol to relieve it
4. Tiredness and irritability
5. Anger toward partners and the connection to my history of abuse
6. Attitude of my friends

At first it seems that Cheryl faces a Catch-22. Stopping one thing (drinking) might exacerbate another (loneliness or sexual tension). At this point Cheryl is confused and not sure what to do.

Masa has been accumulating issues for a few years now. His parents' lack of acceptance of his being gay, his chronic depression, the release he gets from drugs that allows him to dance and have sex, his psychosis, and the fact that he is in school all compete for attention and concern. In his psychology class he is learning that people act in response to their motivations and feelings. He becomes curious about the way he acts when he's on drugs, off drugs, depressed, etc. Masa knows that he is having trouble with many things. If a friend happened to ask him, Masa might prioritize his needs and concerns this way:

1. Avoid depression.
2. Need help to feel uninhibited in groups and in sexual relationships—a reaction to parents' lack of acceptance and isolation as a teenager?
3. Want friends and lovers.
4. Psychosis—is it because of speed, or is it bipolar disorder (manic–depression)?
5. Manage school.

Masa, too, feels like he's in a Catch-22—the only thing that helps him avoid depression and have easy relationships are the very drugs that might cause psychosis. We don't even know what's going on at school.

We hope these examples help you clarify your own hierarchy of needs. We hope you are now comfortable *not* making drugs the first or the only problem, unless that's where they belong. Following is a sample worksheet and a blank one for you to fill in.

HIERARCHY OF NEEDS WORKSHEET

Here's an example:

	Drug	**Masa**	**Environment**
Concerns and needs, in order of priority	*Speed: is it the cause of my psychosis?*	*Depression.* *Inhibited in groups.* *Traumatized by my parents' reaction to my being gay.* *Psychosis—figure out if it's the speed or bipolar disorder.*	*Parents still don't accept me.* *Want friends and lovers.* *Need to manage school.*

	Drug	**Me**	**Environment**
Concerns and needs, in order of priority			

	Drug	**Me**	**Environment**
Concerns and needs, in order of priority			

What Next?

When you take yourself through this process, you will get to know yourself in a more detailed way. Your particular hierarchy of needs might surprise you. You may never have taken a close a look at your whole life. Maybe you didn't look too hard because the only thing you could do about your alcohol or drug use was to feel bad about it. The idea that you can make decisions, plans, and changes based on what *you* want is a whole new idea. Perhaps it never occurred to you before this that you don't have to make any changes at all. It's your life. It's complicated. Or it's a lot of fun and you're not hurting anyone. You need to live with your new awareness and respect the very human tendency to resist change. When you're ready, the next two chapters will give you some guidance about how to change your drug use, whether you want to quit or to use more wisely and safely, and about how to take care of yourself in the meantime.

SOURCES AND SUGGESTED READINGS

About drug, set, setting. This book is out of print, but you might be able to get it at a library:

> *Drug, Set, and Setting: The Basis for Controlled Intoxicant Use.* Norman E. Zinberg. Yale University Press. 1984.

For some good checklists to help you figure out your own set and setting specifics:

> *Sex, Drugs, Gambling, and Chocolate: A Workbook for Overcoming Addictions.* A. Thomas Horvath. Impact Publishers. 1998.

To read the original material on "hierarchy of needs":

> *Toward a Psychology of Being.* Abraham Maslow. VanNostrand. 1962.

To find out more about the impact of expectations on the drinking or drug experience, read

> *Relapse Prevention.* G. Alan Marlatt and Judith R. Gordon, Eds. Guilford Press. 1985. See especially the section on the abstinence violation effect, or the "what the hell" effect (pp. 41–43); and the section on alcohol expectancies—the tendency to experience different effects due to expectation rather than the biological effects of alcohol (pp. 137–150; technical).

WHAT ARE THESE DRUGS, ANYWAY?

General Concepts and Terminology

What Is a Drug?

To quote Andrew Weil, who is much studied and well respected on the subject, a drug is "any substance that in small amounts produces significant changes in the body, mind, or both." A *psychoactive* drug is one that crosses the blood–brain barrier (aspirin, for example, does not) to cause alterations in mood, perception, or brain function. The blood–brain barrier can be crossed only by drugs that are soluble in fat. The range includes prescribed medications, alcohol, stimulants such as cocaine, and common solvents such as gasoline.

What Is the Difference between a Drug and a Food?

Sometimes, very little. We commonly think of tea, coffee, and chocolate as part of our diet, but in fact they contain the world's most-consumed psychoactive substance—caffeine. Sugar is a food, but it is notorious for causing changes in activity level and mood. A recent article in the British journal *Addiction* suggests that our historic use of mind-altering substances may have been, in part, as a source of nutrients—to ward off hunger or fatigue or to replenish neurotransmitters (brain chemicals) in situations where food was scarce or didn't travel or keep well.

Tolerance

Tolerance refers to the process of physiological adaptation, whereby the body and brain attempt to establish homeostasis (balance) in the presence of a new chemical. The body adapts by producing chemical changes and by learning to behave under altered circumstances. Tolerance has developed when consuming the same amount of a drug produces a lessened effect, so that to get the same effect as before, one must consume larger amounts of the drug. Tolerance can develop to some effects and not to others; for example, a person can become tolerant to the sedative, sleep-inducing effects of Valium but not usually to its anxiety-reducing effects.

Cross-tolerance happens when tolerance develops to all drugs in the same class (for example, alcohol and benzodiazepines are in the sedative class; benzodiazepines can be used to help someone go through alcohol detoxification).

Withdrawal

Physical or psychological symptoms appear when the drug is discontinued. Usually these symptoms are opposite of the drug effects. For example, opiates cause constipation, and diarrhea is a symptom of opiate withdrawal. Long-term or heavy use of alcohol and benzodiazepines raises the seizure threshold in the brain by causing neurons to fire more rapidly to maintain balance (homeostasis) in the presence of the depressant effects of the substances; during withdrawal, the risk of seizure is increased during the lapse of time before neurons slow down again.

For more information on the following definitions, check out Chapter 3, where we talk about the continuum of drug use.

Abuse

Abuse refers to the use of a drug for nonmedical purposes that results in health or social problems and/or continued use, despite negative consequences.

Dependence

Dependence is a combination of three factors: continued use, despite negative consequences; psychological compulsion and loss of control; and inability to stop using, despite continued attempts.

Dependence is not the same thing as **physiological dependence**, which is characterized only by tolerance and/or withdrawal and may have nothing to do with suffering harm. For example, if you take pain medicine over a long period of time, you will eventually become physically dependent on it and will have to stop slowly to avoid suffering withdrawal. The same is true of some antidepressant medications, such as Paxil. However, your functioning will remain better than if you didn't take the medicine. So the basic idea is: if a medicine makes you function better, you are not *addicted* to it even if your body becomes physically dependent on it.

Addiction

Most accurately, *addiction* refers to a state of dependence, compulsive use, or chaotic use in which the user's life has become dominated by his or her drug(s) of choice. The term is often used more loosely to refer to any abusive use of a drug, but this is too wide a definition, we believe, and does not speak to the user's relationship with a drug.

How Drugs are Taken

- Oral: By mouth, the slowest way of getting drug effects; the drug has to pass through the digestive system and the liver before going to the brain.
- Smoking: The fastest way of getting drug effects; the drug enters capillaries in the lungs and goes directly to the brain.
- Injection:
    —*Intravenously (IV)*, the second fastest way to get drug effects (one or two minutes)
    —*Subcutaneously (skin-popping)*, an alternative to IV, which is NOT safer or cleaner. In fact, there is a greater risk of infection and abscess this way. However, because it is a slower route to the brain and some of the drug is lost in tissue, there is a lower risk of overdose.
    —*Intramuscularly (IM), the biggest injection risk for disease transmission and infection by introduction of bacteria into the body from needles or the skin, as with subcutaneous* injection.
- Mucous membranes in the nose, mouth, vagina, or rectum: some drugs are applied to the skin and are then absorbed by capillaries close to the surface.

The Action of a Substance in the Brain

Most drugs either stimulate or suppress the activity of neurotransmitters, the brain's chemical information system. Opiates and marijuana, however, act directly on certain neurotransmitter receptor cells. They are so similar to certain natural neurotransmitters that they replace, rather than stimulate, them.

Neurotransmitters Affected by Drugs*

- Dopamine: Responsible for feelings of pleasure and fine motor control; considered to influence the addictive potential of a drug.
- Norepinephrine (noradrenaline): The fight-or-flight chemical that arouses the brain/body when in danger; also facilitates learning and memory processes.
- GABA: The brain's Valium, it depresses or regulates activity in the brain.
- Glutamate: The brain's stimulant, it excites electrical activity.
- Serotonin: Affects mood and aggression (possible that lower levels in abused or neglected children lead to higher levels of aggression and substance abuse); is also related to basic functions such as sex drive, appetite, and sleep.
- Endorphins: The brain's endogenous (naturally occurring) opiates, they sup-

*For more information, see Chapter 4.

press pain and cause euphoria; opiates mimic the action of endorphins and replace them.

- Acetylcholine: The main neurotransmitter in the body, it controls muscle contractions; if blocked, paralysis can occur.

Half-Life

Half-life is the time it takes for half of a substance to be eliminated from the body. In general, the shorter the half-life (short-acting as opposed to long-acting), the greater the addictive potential of the drug. This is partly because the "high" is lost very quickly, which makes both the brain and the psyche a bit "cranky" and leads to cravings for more. Crack cocaine is a good example of this phenomenon; it is very short-acting, leading to a compulsion to use more and more of the drug.

BAC

The acronym *BAC* refers to blood alcohol concentration, measured in grams of alcohol per milliliter of blood: 0.08(%) is the legal limit for driving; 0.50(%) is enough to kill some people.

The Schedule of Drugs

In 1970, Congress enacted the Comprehensive Drug Abuse Prevention and Control Act, which established the Drug Enforcement Agency (DEA). This agency is a branch of the Department of Justice. This legislation, also called the Controlled Substances Act (CSA), requires that all persons who are involved in the manufacture and distribution of medicines/drugs register with the DEA. It also set up five "schedules," or categories, of drugs, supposedly based on a drug's potential for abuse and dependence and whether or not it was deemed to have any medical uses. Since then, every time a new recreational drug hits the streets, it is temporarily legal until the DEA finds out about it. Whether or not there are any studies proving that the drug has medical benefits or if it is addictive, it is usually "scheduled," and always as a Schedule I drug (ecstasy, "designer" hallucinogens, and recently, all analogs of those, even if they haven't been synthesized yet).

- *Schedule I*: High abuse potential, no acceptable medical uses (for example, heroin, LSD, ecstasy, marijuana).
- *Schedule II*: High abuse potential; severe dependence but also accepted medical uses (narcotics, barbiturates, amphetamines).
- *Schedule III*: Less abuse potential and only moderate dependence (primarily nonbarbiturate sedatives and nonamphetamine stimulants, and certain small amounts of narcotics).

- *Schedule IV*: Less abuse potential and limited dependence (antianxiety drugs, nonnarcotic pain relievers, some sedatives).
- *Schedule V*: Limited abuse potential (small amounts of codeine for use in cough syrups and antidiarrhea medicines).

Recreational Drugs, HIV/AIDS, and Medications

The three concerns about the effects of recreational drugs in relation to HIV and treatment are (1) the ability of someone to adhere to treatment regimens while using drugs, (2) the impact of drugs on HIV disease, and (3) the interaction between recreational drugs and HIV medications. One of the main issues is that most drugs and medications are processed by the liver. Some drugs speed up processing, which makes other drugs move through the system faster. Others slow down processing, which makes any other drugs hang around longer. Not a lot is known conclusively because of the lack of controlled studies of illegal drugs, in general. However, to keep up with information and debate, two websites are useful: *www.projectinform.com* and *www.thebody.com*.

Our Position on Drugs and Drug Use

We neither condemn nor condone the use of any particular drug. We simply recognize that people use them and always have, whether we think they should or not. We want people to stay alive, to be as safe as possible, to enjoy their lives, and to have relationships with people who are interested in their well-being. It is with these values in mind that we have taken as much care as possible with the following section.

Accuracy of the Following Information

Many of the sources listed in the reading list give conflicting information. In some cases, research is poor because most of the drugs are illegal. In other cases, the drugs are too new to allow long-term observations of them. We have done our best to select reputable sources, but as in all things, we cannot guarantee either that we have found the best sources or that your individual experience will match what we say here. For many reasons, it is good for each person to do his or her own research. JUST SAY KNOW.

Alcohol

What Drugs

Ethanol is the only form of alcohol that can be consumed safely. Methanol, the product of home distilleries, is dangerous and can cause blindness.

History

Alcohol might be the first intoxicant ever used. Mead (fermented honey) was probably the first alcohol. Evidence of this use of alcohol dates back to 8000 B.C. Evidence of winemaking in Iran dates back to 5400 B.C. Breweries dating from 3700 B.C. have been found in Egypt and Babylonia. Early beer was more similar to a food than a beverage, and it is possible that early agriculture was intended to sustain sources of alcohol as well as other food. Wine as medicine has been recorded since the Sumerians wrote recipes for wine-based medicines in 2200 B.C. The Greek physician Hippocrates recommended wine as a disinfectant, a medicine, and an important part of a healthy diet. The Roman physician Galen treated the wounds of gladiators with wine. And the Jewish Talmud describes wine as "the foremost of all medicines."

The first documented distillation—the conversion of wine into brandy—occurred during the Middle Ages at a medical school in Italy. It was used for medical applications and was believed to cure many diseases. As it was popularized, it was called *aqua vita*, "water of life." In Gaelic, *whiskey* also means "water of life." In the mid-seventeenth century, when gin was distilled, it overtook most of the alcohol consumption in Europe. By 1750, a virtual gin epidemic was creating havoc in London and other European cities. Charles Levinthal explains:

> The epidemic of gin drinking in England during the first half of the eighteenth century illustrates how destructive the introduction of a potent psychoactive drug into a newly urban society already suffering from social dislocation and instability can be. The consequences in many ways mirrored the introduction of crack cocaine into the ghettos of the United States during the 1980's.

Beer was a common drink in colonial America. Indeed, in the Northeast, the tavern was the center of community life. By the early 1800s the average per capita consumption of alcohol was about five drinks a day. Alcohol is the drug that spurred this country's first War on Drugs and inspired the idea of the American disease model of addiction. Two hundred years ago, Benjamin Rush, a physician and signer of the Declaration of Independence, described the dangers of alcohol abuse and declared that alcoholism acted "as if it is a disease. Strong liquor is more destructive than the sword. . . . A nation corrupted by alcohol can never be free." (Note that he did not actually call it a disease.) Rush advocated moderation as the solution to alcohol abuse. As a result of the temperance movement that began in the early 1800s, the average per capita consumption dropped 50 percent, which is still higher than the level of consumption today (less than one drink per day). It was primarily religious and political groups that declared that alcohol led to poverty and civil disobedience. These groups started the Public Hygiene Movement, an effort on the part of middle-class women to reduce the spread of disease from urban ghettos; and the temperance movement (the Women's Christian Temperance Union, the AntiSaloon League, and the National Prohibition Party), which was an effort on the part of the same women to stop public drunkenness. In fact, the Industrial Revolution and the urbanization of American life, along with the westward expansion (primarily of single men), *had* dramatically increased the consumption of alcohol. Coincidentally, there was an increase in the incidence of poverty, disease, and civil unrest. (The union movement is an example of what was deemed civil unrest.) Alcohol was the scapegoat blamed for these social ills. Was alcohol the cause of these social problems, or the perceived relief for the urban poor and single men in a new environment?

The temperance groups succeeded in electing congressmen who ultimately passed the Volstead Act, which, in 1920, became the Eighteenth Amendment that prohibited the manufacture and sale of alcohol in the United States. Increased crime was not the only harm caused by Prohibition. There was an alarming increase in medical problems associated with illegal drinking, especially when methanol was added to "bathtub gin." By 1933 President Roosevelt, supported by people who were appalled at the increase of criminal activity associated with the sale and consumption of alcohol, signed the Twenty-First Amendment, which repealed Prohibition. However, some counties prohibit the sale of alcohol to this day.

A financial advantage of the repeal of Prohibition was the return of taxation on alcohol, which is one of the most heavily taxed consumer products in the United States (42 percent of the price of a bottle of distilled spirits goes to taxes). The presumed effect of taxation is to reduce consumption, the same logic that contributes to the high price of cigarettes today.

Alcohol consumption has declined from the 1970s to the mid-1990s and has remained stable since then at less than one drink per day per capita. Most of the alcohol drunk in the United States is beer, which is responsible for a disproportionate number of problems. In other words, heavy beer drinkers cause and suffer more problems than do heavy wine or distilled spirit drinkers. It is interesting to note that both abstainers and heavy drinkers earn less than moderate drinkers and are less likely to have gone to college. Binge drinking on college campuses has increased dramatically over the past ten years and is now an epidemic with all the associated harmful effects for both the binge drinkers and the nondrinkers who are forced, via proximity, to endure the resulting behavior of their intoxicated peers. For example, 19.5 percent of students in 2001 experienced a sexual assault in which alcohol was involved.

Uses

Recreational (social) use is the primary pattern of alcohol consumption. HOWEVER, alcohol is also used as a sacrament in Christian religions and for medical purposes throughout the world (mixed with other ingredients in liquid forms of medications, etc., and to cleanse wounds when other types of medicines or water are not available).

How It Works

Alcohol normally passes through the digestive tract and is absorbed through the intestines. It then passes through the liver prior to reaching the brain. Food and other mixers dilute the effects and slow absorption. The first drink, however, passes straight from the stomach to the bloodstream without going through the intestine. This means a much more rapid effect for that first drink, especially if you drink on an empty stomach.

In the brain, alcohol releases dopamine in moderate amounts. It increases the supply of GABA (the brain's Valium) and depresses the supply of glutamate (the brain's stimulant). Long-term heavy use causes cell loss in the hippocampus, where new memories are formed, causing problems with short-term memory, abstract thinking, problem solving, attention, and concentration.

Alcohol also crosses the blood–placenta barrier and can put the fetus at risk of birth defects.

Effects

• *Psychological*: Pleasure, euphoria, anxiety reduction, sedation, impaired coordination, impaired concentration and memory, fluctuating moods. Seems to have antidepressant effect in women. Alcohol is renowned for causing disinhibition (loosens you up), which can either make you easier and friendlier or more aggressive, depending on what qualities have been suppressed by shyness or self-control.

• *Physiological*: Slowed heart rate and reflexes, pain relief, possible cardiovascular benefits (in moderate amounts) due to lowering of LDL ("bad") cholesterol. Affects more organ systems than any other drug; stresses the liver, the heart, the stomach and digestive tract, and the pancreas. Can cause blackouts, or loss of memory, while still functioning as "normal." This is due to impairment, while intoxicated, of the part of the brain that records memory.

Dependence, Tolerance, and Withdrawal

Tolerance develops to alcohol's psychoactive effects but very little to its psychomotor or physical effects. In other words, the damage of alcohol is dose-related. If you are a regular drinker, you may have to drink more to *feel* the intoxicating effects, but the more you drink, the more you will suffer both short-term (psychomotor impairment) and long-term (organ damage) risks. This is why you may *think* you are able to drive if you have an increased tolerance to alcohol, but it is your blood alcohol concentration (BAC) that determines your *actual* ability to drive. Long-term, high-dose alcohol use causes physiological dependence. Withdrawal syndrome includes anxiety, depression or irritability, sweating, tremulousness, insomnia, seizure, delirium tremens. Due to removal of the sedating effect of alcohol, blood pressure, pulse, and heart rate rise, which can be dangerous.

Benefits

People have used alcohol for centuries because of its many benefits, physical, psychological, and social. It has often been called a stimulant because it encourages social interaction and creativity. It still is used for "social lubrication" at parties and other social events. It has also been used to calm down anxious or worried states, to soothe teething babies, and to relieve minor pain. Alcohol is used for religious sacraments and other spiritual rituals throughout many different cultures. There is a lot being written about possible benefits to heart health, mostly because of alcohol's ability to lower the levels of "bad" cholesterol. This viewpoint has come under attack as being too "alcohol positive" and encouraging people to drink who otherwise might not. A recently released study, in the *New England Journal of Medicine,* has determined that men who consume alcohol at least three to four days per week have a lowered risk of heart attack. Finally, alcohol is sometimes used to enhance or to smooth out the action of other recreational drugs. Mixing drugs, though often pleasant, can be a serious risk because of drug interactions.

Risks

Long-term use can cause significant nutritional deficiencies, damage to brain and nerve tissues, stomach distress and inflamed pancreas, increased risk of certain types of cancers (especially cancers of the mouth and throat when used with cigarette smoking), and lowered resistance to infection. Some of these effects are of concern to people with HIV and other illnesses. And of course, the most well-known physical effect is on the liver. Many people develop milder forms of liver disease (fatty liver) but may progress to chronic alcoholic hepatitis or the lethal cirrhosis. This is particularly problematic for people who already have hepatitis. Alcohol blackouts can be dangerous because people have interactions with others and make decisions (like about driving or having sex) yet are unaware of what they are doing and have no memory of what they did afterward.

Greatest Dangers

Alcohol can cause death due to respiratory depression, cardiac irregularities, coma, alcohol poisoning, overdose, or choking on vomit. Heavy drinking is more dangerous with marijuana, which inhibits vomiting, thus increasing the likelihood of alcohol poisoning. Withdrawal can be dangerous, with risk of seizure or DTs (delirium tremens), and may need to be managed medically by administering benzodiazepines. Since alcohol slows down reaction time and impairs judgment, driving or operating other machinery when drinking has been the cause of many deaths and injuries. Accidents are the leading risk factor from alcohol. Some people become very aggressive when drinking, and alcohol is a leading contributor to domestic violence.

Other Hazards

- *Cardiovascular disease*: Two or more drinks per day for men increases by 51 percent risk of death by heart attack or cardiovascular disease. In a study in China, one or two drinks per day lowered the death rate by 20 percent; two or more per day increased the death rate by 30 percent. According to Robert Julien, small to moderate amounts of alcohol (up to 2.5 ounces) may reduce the risk of coronary artery disease and ischematic stroke (due to loss of oxygen to certain parts of the brain). Five or more drinks a day may increase risk of stroke.

- *Medical complications*: liver damage or cirrhosis, pancreatitis, brain damage (Korsakoff's or Wernicke's syndromes—permanent or acute cognitive impairment), hypertension, poor nutrition.

- *Fetal alcohol syndrome*: intellectual impairment and physical abnormalities; fetal alcohol effects occur at even moderate (one drink per day) levels.

- *In women*: metabolize less alcohol (25–30 percent) due to lower levels of metabolizing enzyme in the liver. Birth control pills also slow the rate of elimination. Increased risk for breast, liver, and pancreas damage/cancer, and hypertension. Associated with increased risk of domestic violence and sexual assault.

- *Associated (and most common) dangers*: Violence, suicide, auto accidents, burns.

Drug Interactions

In combination with other drugs, the following effects can occur:

- Sedatives—can cause death due to increased sedation.
- Anxiolytics—extreme drowsiness.
- Antibiotics—nausea, headaches, vomiting, seizures; most dangerous: Furoxone, Grisactin, Flagyl, Atabrine.
- Anticoagulants—decrease blood clotting.
- Antidepressants—Increase sedative effects of tricyclics. No evidence of problems with SSRIs.
- Antipsychotics—increase sedating effects.
- Antihistamines—increase sedating effects.
- Antidiabetic meds—acute drinking prolongs the medication effects. Chronic drinking decreases medication availability. Also nausea and headache.
- Antiseizure medications—acute drinking increases dilantin levels. Chronic drinking lowers dilantin levels.
- Narcotic pain meds—increase sedation.

- Nonnarcotic pain meds—increase stomach irritation and bleeding.
- Acetaminophen taxes the liver and should not be used by heavy drinkers.

Harm Reduction

The key principle is "Less is More" (that's the same principle with a lot of drugs). You'll get more enjoyment and suffer fewer harms if you moderate your drinking. This means, first and foremost, not bingeing. When you drink a lot of alcohol at once, even if only once a week, it can cause more problems than regular moderate drinking. Even with moderate drinking, though, it's good to eat enough and take vitamins! But, if you do want to party with alcohol, there are some things you can do to stay safer. Drink lots of water and eat food before and while you're drinking. Limit your use of other drugs at the same time, especially sedatives or opiates, to reduce the risk of oversedation and overdose. Drink beer rather than hard liquor. Count your drinks and pace yourself. Before drinking, make arrangements for transportation home. If a friend has had way too much to drink, don't just let him "sleep it off." He may just sleep himself to death, either by alcohol poisoning or choking on vomit. Stay with your friends until they sober up or at least until they throw up. When in doubt, call 911. We know this can be scary, since the police might show up too, but it is your friend's life. . . . *Times to avoid drinking or at least getting drunk*: when you're in a bad mood; if you have hepatitis or otherwise compromised liver; on a date or at a party where you might end up in a sexually vulnerable situation; when driving; before having sex; when taking other sedating drugs or any other drugs, if you can help it.

The other greatest danger, besides overdose and accidents, is severe withdrawal. If you've been drinking heavily for months or years, or for some people even weeks, you might suffer from tremors, seizures, or delirium tremens. Withdrawal can be dangerous or fatal. If you're more than a little tremulous (shaky), get medical help to withdraw safely. A physician can prescribe benzodiazepines such as Valium or Librium for a few days, although some would prefer that you go to a residential detox center for this treatment so you can be observed medically. If you don't have access to medications or a detox center and you become too tremulous or have a seizure history, a little alcohol will stop the withdrawal process. In fact, you can detox yourself by drinking ever-decreasing amounts of alcohol. Heavy drinkers might find this discipline challenging, but a little less alcohol is better than dangerous withdrawal, at least in the short term, until you can get medical help.

Sedatives/Hypnotics and Anxiolytics

What Drugs

- Chloral hydrate
- Barbiturates (Nembutal, Seconal, Amytal, etc.)

- Meprobamate (Miltown)
- Methaqualone (Quaalude)
- Benzodiazepines:
  —Chlordiazepoxide (Librium)
  —Diazepam (Valium)
  —Flunitrazepam (Rohypnol, or roofies)
  —Others: Ativan, Dalmane, Halcion, Klonopin, Paxipam, Restoril, Serax, Tran-
  xene, Versed, Xanax.
- GHB: Gamma-hydroxybutyrate (Liquid X, Easy Lay, Grievous Bodily Harm)
  and GBL (Gamma-butyrolactone), which converts to GHB when ingested.

General Information

The term *sedative/hypnotic* refers to the combined sedating and sleep-inducing effects of these drugs (*hypnosis* comes from the name of the Greek god of sleep). *Anxiolytic* refers to the antianxiety effects of these drugs, the reason many were developed.

History and Uses

Chloral hydrate was the first of these drugs, developed in the mid-1800s for use in treating insomnia. A few drops in whiskey is a Mickey Finn. Unfortunately, effective as it was, it irritated the stomach. *Barbiturates*, developed in 1903, were so effective for sedation, anesthesia, and seizures (they depress electrical activity in the brain), and were so easy to modify to create different effects, that 2,500 types were synthesized. All barbiturates depress vital functions, especially respiration, so overdosing is easy, and they became the most common method of suicide in the United States. *Meprobamate* (Miltown) was developed in the 1950s in an attempt to create the ideal sleeping pill. It became the first drug marketed as an antianxiety medication, but in fact it mostly produced relaxation and sedation. (It is no longer sold in the United States due to its side-effects and the availability of more effective and less harmful alternatives.) *Methaqualone* was developed in the 1970s as an alternative but became a recreational drug of abuse (Quaaludes) because of an unfounded reputation as an aphrodisiac. When reports of overdoses started appearing, it was made a Schedule I drug in 1984 and is no longer manufactured in the United States. Barbiturates became recognized as dangerous for general use, and *benzodiazepines,* first developed in 1957, became a safer substitute. They too cause sedation but without the effects on vital functions such as breathing and heart rate, making them the safest of the anxiolytic medications.

Originally produced as an anesthetic, *GHB* was imported from Europe. It has also been used for bodybuilding because it stimulates a growth hormone, but was banned from over-the-counter sales because of increasing use as a party drug. GHB is a naturally occurring substance that is similar to GABA. It is used in clubs and raves as a party drug and is sometimes associated with date rape, because it creates sedation and amnesia for the experience. *Rohypnol (roofies)* is most often associated with date rape, and it also creates amnesia for whatever is experienced while intoxicated.

How They Work

Barbiturates, one of the original classes of sedatives, are central nervous system depressants. They act on the reticular activating system, which induces sleep, slows respiration as well as heart rate, and lowers blood pressure. They also increase the activity of GABA, which slows down brain activity. These drugs can be fatal if taken in too large a dose or mixed with other depressants such as alcohol. Different barbiturates have different major effects—sleep, anesthesia, or antiseizure. Because they also have a significant effect on liver enzymes, barbiturates can cause serious interactions with other drugs and medications as well as produce a quickly increasing tolerance.

Anxiolytics, the more commonly used antianxiety drugs nowadays, increase the function of GABA, which reduces the excitability of brain activity. A major group of anxiolytics belong to the *benzodiazepine* classification. Because they work on GABA only indirectly, they cause sedation and relaxation without inhibiting respiration or significantly slowing down the heartbeat. Different brands of benzodiazepines have different half-lives (length of action), so some are more useful for sleep (Klonopin, for example), whereas others are useful for panic attacks or short-lived anxiety-producing situations such as flying (Xanax, for example, although Xanax has a very unpleasant withdrawal effect). Still others are so sedating as well as short-acting (Versed) that they are used only during surgery.

Effects

These drugs create sedative, sleep, anxiety reduction, anesthetic, and antiseizure (by reducing electrical activity in the brain) effects. Relaxation, some mild euphoria, lightheadedness, vertigo, drowsiness, slurred speech, and muscle incoordination are common experiences. Some people have what is called a "paradoxical reaction" and become agitated instead of calmed (especially the elderly). The effects of GHB are unpredictable dose by dose.

Dependence, Tolerance, and Withdrawal

Tolerance and physical dependence develop rapidly with barbiturates and can lead to potentially dangerous withdrawal symptoms, including seizures. Psychological dependence to these drugs can develop as well, especially because a person usually becomes tolerant to the sedation and needs to take increasing doses to get that effect. Benzodiazepines tend to produce significant tolerance and dependence only with high-dose, long-term use. Once dependence develops, however, a withdrawal syndrome similar to that with barbiturates can occur. These drugs should be discontinued under medical supervision to prevent serious withdrawal symptoms, which can lead to death. GHB has euphoric effects, so it may release dopamine. Not much is known about dependence on GHB, though it certainly can cause a psychological dependence.

Benefits

Medical uses such as sedation, detoxification from alcohol, and relief from anxiety are one type of benefit. For recreational use, these drugs create a feeling of being at ease and often facilitate social interaction. They are also used in combination with stimulants to decrease some of the negative effects stimulants produce, such as muscle tension. Benzodiazepines are more easily available today than are barbiturates.

Risks

Barbiturates interfere with cognitive functions such as judgment, impulse control, and new learning. They also greatly affect muscle control and coordination, leading to accidents and injury. It is very easy to become dependent on these drugs. Benzodiazepines cause these types of problems less often, but dosage is the key: "Less is more." In general, except for the short-acting benzodiazepines (which are used for medical sedation or as a sleeping aid), these drugs are relatively safe in small doses for recreation. Tolerance and dependence can occur, but only with regular use at higher-than-usual doses. Alcohol mixed with any of these drugs dramatically increases the risk of serious problems.

Greatest Dangers

Barbiturates and GHB can cause fatal overdoses, preceded by drowsiness, nausea, headache, loss of reflexes, loss of consciousness, and suppression of breathing. They are especially dangerous when mixed with alcohol or other sedative drugs. Eighty percent of GHB deaths have involved alcohol. Benzodiazepines do not, by themselves, result in fatal overdoses; the deaths that have been studied were related to use in combination with other drugs. Long-term use of benzodiazepines can inhibit new learning and short-term memory and may also cause amnesia (especially roofies).

Drug Interactions

- Mixing sedatives with other central nervous system depressants (alcohol, opiates, ketamine, and other sedatives) increases risk of overdose.
- Protease inhibitors (antiretroviral medications for HIV such as ritonavir) may

increase the effects of GHB. Take a small dose and wait thirty to sixty minutes to see what happens before taking more.

Harm Reduction

Again, the motto is "Less is More." It is really tempting to overuse these drugs, especially benzodiazepines, because they make you feel good and rarely have unpleasant side effects. Doing them only occasionally is the best way to enjoy them and avoid problems. One teaspoon is usually a standard dose of GHB. Start with that and wait for thirty to sixty minutes before taking more. Remember, the dose lasts for up to four hours. Mixing these various drugs, because they belong to the same class, is not a good idea, for all of the above reasons. If you do take these drugs to counteract stimulants that you are using, be aware that you will not be able to feel the full effect of the cocaine or speed so easily, and you might be tempted to use more than your body can handle. It's best to wait until the end of your speed run or cocaine use to take these drugs. That way, you're not adding a drug that will confuse the picture. As with alcohol, don't drive when using any of these drugs, unless you're using regular, appropriate amounts prescribed for anxiety or for a seizure disorder.

Opiates and Opioids

What Drugs

- *Opium* is the basic opiate substance, derived from the sticky resin in the seedpod of the opium poppy.
- *Laudanum* is opium mixed with alcohol.
- *Morphine* (MS Contin and Roxanol) and *codeine* are opium's active ingredients.
- *Hydromorphone* (Dilaudid), *oxycodone* (Percodan), *hydrocodone* (Vicodin), are chemically modified substances from morphine or codeine.
- *Heroin* is a chemical modification of morphine to speed absorption in the brain.
- *Meperidine* (Demerol), *methadone, fentanyl,* and *propoxyphene* (Darvon) are synthetic opiates.
- *Oxycodone hydrochloride controlled release* (Oxycontin) is a time-release chemical modification of codeine.

Efficacy

How effective these drugs are, in order of strength:

- Morphine, Dilaudid, Demerol, Fentanyl, Heroin
- Vicodin, Percodan
- Codeine, Darvon

History

Earliest references to opium come from Babylonia/Assyria 4,000 years ago. Morpheus, the Greek god of dreams, is often depicted with poppies in his hands. Pipes for smoking opium date between 100 and 30 B.C. in Asia, Egypt, and Europe. Opium was imported to China by Arab traders between A.D. 600 and 900. England imported opium from India to China as a major source of trade in exchange for the many Chinese products England wanted. China's concerns about opium dependence led to the Opium Wars in the early nineteenth century, when China banned the import of this drug. Opium use in Europe has been popular since the Middle Ages. Paracelsus developed laudanum (a tincture of alcohol and opium) in the early sixteenth century, and it was the most common painkiller used in Europe through the late nineteenth century.

Opium has been used throughout the history of the United States as a major ingredient of many tonics and medicines, including "Mrs. Winslow's Soothing Syrup," a teething formula for babies, and paregoric, also used for teething babies and for diarrhea. Morphine was isolated from opium around 1805 and used in hospital settings once the hypodermic syringe was invented in 1853. Chinese immigrants introduced the smoking of opium to the United States, where it became popular and then became the first banned drug in this country in 1906. Opiates have been controlled substances since 1914. Today, only heroin is a Schedule I drug (unavailable for any medical use)—even though it was developed and marketed as a medicine by the Bayer company in 1898, two years before they marketed aspirin. The latest opiate drug scare has been the increased use of Oxycontin, sometimes referred to as the "poor man's heroin." Oxycontin is a long-acting, time-release form of codeine that is excellent for chronic pain. However, some people are crushing the pill and shooting the powder, thus canceling out the time-release function and leading to potential overdose.

Uses

Opiates are unparalleled in their medical applications for analgesia (decreased pain sensation), cough suppressant, antidiarrhea, and sedation.

How They Work

Opiates are easily absorbed by many routes:

1. Orally—slowest; has to go through intestine to blood to liver, where some is metabolized and discarded.
2. Intravenously (IV—very rapid and also cost-effective since the whole dose is absorbed).
3. Smoking—fastest, but some goes up in smoke.

4. Snorting—only heroin can be ingested in this form.
5. Subcutaneous injection—skin-popping; perceived as easier and safer than IV, although this is not true.

How fast these drugs get to the brain depends on the particular drug and the route of administration. Fentanyl is fastest, then heroin. The user generally doesn't experience a rush if taken orally. Most effects after the rush last four to six hours, except methadone (twelve to twenty-four hours) and fentanyl (one hour).

In the brain, opiates initially release dopamine, especially if injected, then bind to endorphin and enkephalin receptor sites. Endorphins regulate mood, digestion, body temperature, breathing, and create calm when the organism is under stress. Enkephalins communicate messages in parts of the brain that process pain sensation and regulate breathing, and in parts where the reward system (dopamine) operates. The main opiate receptor ("mu") provides analgesia, euphoria, and respiratory depression.

Effects

In addition to the preceding medical uses, opiates cause sedation, euphoria, decreased sex drive, respiratory depression, and pinpoint pupils.

Dependence, Tolerance, and Withdrawal

Tolerance develops to the euphoric, analgesic, and respiratory effects, which means higher doses can be tolerated the longer one uses. However, tolerance does not affect the symptoms of constipation or pinpoint pupils. Tolerance is partly setting-dependent, meaning that one's tolerance can be different (higher or lower) depending on where and with whom one is using. This variability is possibly due to the body's response of "readying" itself to counter the effects of drug, a process that is initiated by the cues in one's familiar using environment. It is possible that people who use opiates for intense or chronic pain, not for recreation, do not develop tolerance to the analgesic effects as quickly as those who use recreationally. Cross-tolerance develops with all opiate drugs.

Physiological dependence due to tolerance causes a withdrawal syndrome of flu-like symptoms: cramps, chills, sweating, nausea, increased pain sensation, insomnia, increased heart rate, restlessness, diarrhea, and dysphoria (depression). The worst effects occur from twenty-four to seventy-two hours after last use and can last up to a week.

Opiates have moderate addiction potential, *but* most people who are opiate-dependent are not addicted (that is, most opiates are used by people for medical reasons, and they don't develop the behavioral signs of addiction).

Benefits

There are as many ways to use opiates as there are opiates! Even with all of this variety, though, people who use opiates usually report very similar feelings. Opiates make you feel warm and safe, give you a pleasant floating sensation, and reduce worries. If you're depressed, they make you feel better, and if you're uptight, they make you looser. To get other, more intense effects, people use different doses by different routes of administration. In lower doses opiates can enhance the experience of being with friends or make you forget your loneliness. Higher doses might separate you from the world and from your feelings, putting you into a more dream-like state. Shooting opiates results in a "rush" of euphoria from dopamine, and many people use this method just because of that rush. If you are using occasionally, these effects are more deliberate and controlled by you. Once a person starts using regularly, though, the timing and amount that he or she uses is often controlled by increasing tolerance and dependence rather than a conscious effort to create an experience. "Less is More."

Risks

These drugs can induce nausea and vomiting. If you are already high, vomiting could put you in danger of choking. Tolerance can develop rapidly and take you by surprise. You could end up using a lot, spending a lot of time and money buying the stuff, and having less fun.

Greatest Dangers

OVERDOSE: *opiates in combination with other drugs that depress respiration, such as alcohol, benzodiazepines, GHB, or barbiturates, can be deadly.* Overdose is due primarily to respiratory depression. Sedation leads to coma. Warning signs are (1) respiration lower than 12 breaths per minute, (2) unconsciousness or extreme drowsiness, and (3) unresponsiveness to pain. Overdoses can happen to naïve users who take a dose larger than their tolerance can handle; to regular users in unfamiliar surroundings; or to former users who have detoxed, then return to using their usual dose. Of course, unless you know your dealer very well, you may be buying drugs of unknown strength (heroin is often stronger today than in the past, and East Coast heroin is generally a lot stronger than what's available on the West Coast).

Regular opiate use shuts down production of our own endogenous opiates, so for several weeks or months after stopping, people are more sensitive to pain and depressed. Research suggests that the longer one uses opiates, the less likely these internal opiates will regenerate, but this long-term effect remains unclear. Another possible explanation for dependence on opiates is that many people who become dependent on opiates do so because they never had good enough endorphin systems—perhaps due to early-life trauma—and therefore opiate drugs become a very effective way of self-medicating.

There are no other major detrimental effects due directly to the drugs; opiates are generally benign substances and cause little or no direct damage to the body. Most of the dangers—HIV, hepatitis, tuberculosis, abscesses, vein damage due to injecting particles or large/damaged needles, severe bacterial infections, poor nutrition, legal problems—are associated with contaminants, lifestyle, and unsafe use practices. Many of these consequence are deadly.

One of the least understood dangers for opiate users is getting inadequate pain treatment when they need it. Because of increased tolerance, people who use opiates regularly will require larger doses of medicine for postsurgery or for injuries, etc. However. these people often try to hide their opiate use from their doctors (realistically, for fear of being treated badly or refused pain medication) and thus end up suffering when they need increased dosing.

Drug Interactions

• Mixing opiates and opioid drugs with other central nervous system depressants (alcohol, benzodiazepines, barbiturates, GHB, and ketamine) increases the risk of overdose.

• Mixing with stimulants masks the effects of opiates, so you might take more than you intend of either.

• Protease inhibitors (for HIV) may decrease the effects of heroin. Before you take more than your usual dose of heroin, check out how you feel.

Treatment

• Overdose—*naloxone* (Narcan) blocks opiate receptors and reverses drug effects. It acts quickly because it is administered by injection.

• Deterrence—*naltrexone* (ReVia) also blocks opiate receptors so you can't get high, but it is taken orally, so it acts more slowly and is not useful for emergency use to interrupt overdose.

• Withdrawal—*clonidine* (Catapress) lowers heart rate and eases restlessness.

• Detoxification or maintenance—opiates other than *methadone* are not generally used in outpatient settings for detox. Using methadone for detox or maintenance unfortunately puts the person into a "system" of care in federally controlled clinics rather than under the care of a private physician who can make decisions based on less restrictive federal guidelines. Office-based methadone treatment is under consideration in some areas of this country, and buprenorphine has just been approved by the FDA for treatment of opiate dependence.

Harm Reduction

Much of the harm caused by opiate use could be prevented by public health interventions: (1) making clean syringes available (so people wouldn't have to share their "works," thus spreading HIV, etc.), (2) teaching people safer injection techniques (including how to test their dose for potency), (3) teaching people how to perform rescue breathing, (4) making Narcan available more readily, and, of course, (5) offering a wider range of treatment options for those who want to quit or cut back. All of these services are available, but the federal government and most states do not sanction them, so they operate underground or are at constant risk of being shut down.

In the absence of these needed services, you'll have to do what you can. Is there a syringe exchange in your area? Use it not only for needles but for educating yourself about other safety measures. If you can't figure out any way to get clean syringes, follow the bleach guidelines that people have been using (clean syringe and *all* works, with bleach, then water, three times, then a final rinse with water). It is not wise to crush up pills and shoot them—yeah, we know, sometimes that's all that's available—but pills contain a lot of fillers that are OK passing through your stomach acid but can cause damage to veins and serious damage to the smaller blood vessels in your lungs. Even the best "cottons" might not filter out all the gunk. Specific information on all of these safer-use techniques can be found at the Harm Reduction Coalition website and by pamphlets that are available (see these references in our Sources and Suggested Readings section).

You also might want to consider not shooting your drugs. Snorting may not get you off as quickly and you may waste a little of the drug, but it might work better for you in terms of your overall health. Smoking is a very rapid way to use many opiates and carries little of the risks of shooting. Some opiates can be eaten or taken in pill form. You generally don't feel a rush this way, but, again, it's safer.

Another way to increase both your pleasure and your safety is to use less frequently. It takes only a few days of not using to decrease your tolerance and to prevent physical dependence. That way you can still get high, not use as much drug (or money), and not get hooked. Start by not using on a day when it will be easy. If you are dependent, though, quitting all at once for a few days will put you into withdrawal, so you need to assess where you are first.

Finally, although opiates don't usually cause serious medical problems by themselves, many of the pill forms also have acetaminophen (Tylenol) in them. This drug is hard on your liver, so taking large quantities can be dangerous, especially if you have hepatitis C. Switch to a pill that doesn't contain acetaminophen (look at the drug books in our Resources section or call a pharmacy).

Major Stimulants

What Drugs

- Cocaine—*powder*: cocaine hydrochloride, a crystalline distillate of coca leaves, snorted or dissolved for injection; *crack*: cocaine boiled with bicarbonate of soda to precipitate cocaine base.

- Ephedrine—active ingredient of the Chinese herb ma huang.
- Amphetamine—a family of ephedrine-based stimulants; brand name Benzedrine.
- Methamphetamine—a chemical derivative of amphetamine (speed, ice, or crystal); brand names Desoxyn, Methedrine.
- Methylphenidate (Ritalin), dextroamphetamine (Dexedrine), and Adderall (Cylert)—prescribed for attention deficit disorder.
- Khat—mild stimulant from leafy plant in East Africa and southern Saudi Arabia; used for centuries; cathinone is the active ingredient; methcathinone is synthetic and more potent than khat.

Other Stimulants

There are many other plants and seeds that have stimulant properties and are widely used in local areas around the world. Betel seeds (India) can be chewed, and yohimbine, from the bark of an African tree, has been used as an intoxicant, an aphrodisiac, and a medicine.

General Information

Cocaine is both a central nervous system stimulant and an anesthetic. It is the active ingredient derived from the coca leaf found in the rainforests and fields of the upper slopes of the Andes. The coca leaf contains no more than 2 percent cocaine, whereas refined cocaine is almost 100 percent pure and crack cocaine, when not purposely cut, is about 75 percent pure cocaine. It takes about 250 pounds of coca leaves to produce 1 pound of cocaine.

Amphetamines and their derivatives are synthetic forms of ephedrine, the active ingredient of ma huang. Ephedrine does not have the psychoactive properties of amphetamines. Methamphetamine, the most popular form for recreational use, is a chemical derivative that allows quicker passage across the blood–brain barrier.

Methcathinone is the synthetic form of khat, which has been chewed in Yemen and other Middle Eastern countries for centuries. Heavily used in the former Soviet Union in the seventies and eighties, methcathinone once represented 20 percent of all illicit drug use in that country. In the United States, labs were set up in Michigan starting in 1989, and its use has spread into the upper Midwest. Its effects last up to six days.

Ephedras are plants that grow mostly in desert areas. Ma huang is such a plant in China. In the United States, the Mormons, who are not allowed to use caffeine or take other intoxicating drugs, discovered a bush containing ephedra and learned to make a stimulant tea from its leaves, commonly referred to as "Mormon tea."

History

History of Cocaine. Cocaine has been used for at least 5,000 years in South America. Coca leaves were chewed for alertness and endurance at high altitudes in the Andes. The Incas, who operated coca plantations, believed coca to be a gift from the gods. A journey in the Andes was measured in the number of mouthfuls of coca chewed along the way. Spanish conquerors tried to ban the use of coca, until they realized that silver miners could work harder when chewing coca leaves—then they kept their forced laborers well supplied. Addiction to coca leaf chewing is generally unknown in South American cultures, yet about 90 percent of Peruvians who live in the mountains chew coca, thus demonstrating that "addiction" is, at least in part, a function of refining the drugs. For example, street kids in the urban areas of Colombia, Peru, and Brazil inhaled ether fumes to get high, until ether was outlawed in cooperation with the American Drug Enforcement Agency in the early 1970s. Since then, *basuko* (crack cocaine) has been used. Since coca was readily available, it was transformed into crack. Addiction to crack is now rampant in these urban areas, whereas coca leaves are still chewed without problem in rural areas.

Coca was exported to Europe and purified in the 1850s by a German chemist. A wine made with cocaine extract from the coca leaves, Vin Mariani, was created in Italy and became the first recreational use of cocaine. It was loved for its invigorating properties. The French sculptor of the Statue of Liberty said, "If I had been drinking Vin Mariani while designing it, it would have been three times taller." The U.S. pharmaceutical industry took notice, and Parke-Davis produced a cocaine-containing tonic. Then an Atlanta pharmacist developed a syrup made from an extract of coca leaves, added caffeine, and Coca-Cola—also touted for its ability to energize—was born. This is likely why soda fountains became a fixture in drugstores. (One Coca-Cola imitator called his soda Dope Cola.) The active cocaine was taken out of Coca-Cola in 1901, but the formula still contains decocainized products of the coca leaf.

In Europe, synthetic powder cocaine was given to the German Army and found to increase the endurance and mood of troops. Freud, at the time practicing as a neurologist in Vienna, heard about this use and its use in plant form in the Andes. He obtained cocaine from the Merck drug company, took it himself, and gave it to others. He praised its many virtues, including its use as a cure for depression and for morphine addiction. His description from his paper "On Coca," sounds very familiar today:

> Cocaine brings about an exhilaration and lasting euphoria which in no way differs from the normal euphoria of the healthy person. . . . You perceive an increase of self-control and possess more vitality and capacity for work. . . . In other words you are simply normal, and it is soon hard to believe that you are under the influence of any drug. . . . The result is enjoyed without any of the unpleasant after effects that follow exhilaration brought about by alcohol.

A friend, at his suggestion, used cocaine for his morphine addiction, ended up a very heavy user, and became psychotic, becoming the first recorded case of cocaine psychosis. Freud was eventually criticized for his publication of the value of cocaine, thereby contributing to its popularity as a prescription medication. In the meantime, he had also noticed its anesthetic properties, and his publication of that use of cocaine contributed to its eventual use as local anesthetic.

Finally, until recently, the Brompton Cocktail, named after the hospital in London that developed it, was administered to terminally ill patients in England as a soothing and reviving mix of cocaine, morphine, and alcohol.

The presence of large amounts of cocaine in therapeutic tonics led to toxic effects in many people, which in turn led to the Pure Food and Drug Act of 1906, which required labeling of all medical substances, and the Harrison Narcotic Act of 1914, which limited the use of both opiates and cocaine and restricted any prescription to "addicts." Cocaine now has very limited medical uses. Synthetic alternatives that are cheaper to produce and lack the psychoactive properties of cocaine (procaine and its derivatives) have been developed. Cocaine fell into disuse until the 1970s, when there was a resurgence in its use, followed by the development of freebase, which was the first smokeable form of cocaine, and then crack in the eighties. In 1999, 11 million people in the United States admitted to using cocaine, and 25 percent of those had used crack cocaine. In the month prior to that household survey on drug abuse, 700,000 had used cocaine, 200,000 of them crack. Currently, young people are using crack cocaine much less than in the 1980s and less than older people. Indeed, it has fallen into disrepute among young people. Despite a drop in cocaine use in the 1990s, however, medical emergencies were on the rise, presumably due to the chronic nature of the remaining cocaine use and the associated problems that develop over long-term use.

History of Amphetamines. Ephedrine, the active ingredient of ma huang, has been used for 5,000 years to treat asthma, because it stimulates the nerves that dilate bronchioles. It works like epinephrine (adrenaline), the body's own stimulant, but epinephrine cannot be formulated to be taken orally. Epinephrine is administered by injection, which meant that a person having an asthmatic attack had to be rushed to the hospital to be treated. Now people with asthma can carry it and the injection equipment with them. Ephedrine was isolated in 1887 by a German chemist. It was in short supply, however, so amphetamine was developed by a U.S. chemist as a synthetic alternative. It was available in inhalers (Benzedrine) and became popular due to its stimulant and euphoric effects. It was not long before people discovered that they could remove the drug from the inhaler and take it orally.

Amphetamine was also noted for its appetite-suppressant qualities. It was given to soldiers for alertness and energy during World War II by the German, Japanese, and British armies. (At that point, it had not been determined in the United States whether the drug was dangerous, so U.S. troops often got their amphetamines from the British Army.) At the end of the war, the largest amphetamine epidemic in history was under way in Japan, where 5 percent of the population was dependent on the drug (its use had been encouraged for productivity of the workforce at home). Since the Korean War, and especially since the first Gulf War and the recent invasion of Afghanistan and Iraq, amphetamines, or "go pills," have been given to U.S. pilots and other combat service personnel to help them adjust to long hours and nighttime duties.

A study of the effects of amphetamine on students at the University of Minnesota popularized its use among students and then among long-distance truckers. Its euphoric effect on mood, much like cocaine's, popularized its recreational use. Like cocaine, it was advertised and recommended for treatment of depression, but the rebound depression that occurred after usage was discontinued rendered it ineffective in that application.

In the 1960s, the medical supply of amphetamine tightened, so illegal labs were created. But its popularity waned as interest in cocaine picked up again. Not until the 1990s did amphetamine, or methamphetamine (which is both easier to make and more effective in its psychoactive properties), come into more common usage, not only in urban areas, especially in the West, but in rural areas where "meth" labs can be easily operated undetected. Pharmacies have had to limit sales of Sudafed and other remedies containing ephedrine or pseudoephedrine, which are used to synthesize methamphetamine.

Uses

- *Cocaine*: Local anesthetic, especially in eye surgeries.
- *Amphetamine or amphetamine-like drugs*:
  —Attention-deficit/hyperactivity disorder (ADHD), in both children and adults: Ritalin, Dexedrine, Adderall, Cylert, and occasionally Methedrine
  —Obesity: Bontril, Prelu-2, Adipex-P, Fastin, Ionamin, Meridia (Acutrim and Dexetrim have been withdrawn, because they contain actual amphetamines, which physicians are concerned about prescribing).
  —Narcolepsy: modaninil (Provigil)
  —Nasal congestion: ephedrine (Primatine); pseudoephedrine (Sudafed, Comtrex, others); Afrin, Dristan, Privine, 4-Way Fast-Acting Nasal Spray, Neo-Synephrine, Vicks Sinex

How They Work

Both cocaine and amphetamine (more commonly, methamphetamine) increase the amount of norepinephrine in the brain. Norepinephrine is the neurotransmitter that controls the fight-or-flight response and is a part of the emergency response system. As such, it controls the sympathetic nervous system, increasing heart rate and respiration and constricting blood vessels and increasing blood pressure—all necessary to mount an emergency response, but very stressful to the system if activated on a regular basis. Cocaine and amphetamine also dramatically increase levels of dopamine, more than any other recreational drug, making them the most "rewarding" of all drugs. They work in slightly different ways; amphetamine more closely resembles the norepinephrine and dopamine molecules, making it better understood. Cocaine's mode of action is less well understood. But they are similar enough to be discussed together. The most dramatic difference is the duration of effect: cocaine's effects last from a few minutes to an hour, while amphetamine's effects can be felt up to 12 hours.

Effects

- Euphoria and increased energy, attention, concentration, alertness, motor activity, sense of well-being, sexual desire, and sociability; injected or smoked produces most intense feelings of euphoria.
- Increased heart rate, blood pressure, body temperature, respiration.
- Increased blood flow, leading to prolonged erection and delayed ejaculation.
- Dilated bronchioles, which allows for more oxygen to the lungs.
- Suppressed appetite, which allows for dietary decreases.
- With long-term heavy use, motor activity can become repetitive, and stimulant psychosis can emerge.
- *Ephedrine* has weak psychoactive properties (doesn't enter brain well) but amphetamine-like effects on the body (heart rate, blood pressure, etc), making it potentially dangerous for people taking it to get high. *Ritalin* has opposite effects (primarily stimulates norepinephrine, which increases attention).

Dependence, Tolerance, and Withdrawal

Cocaine and methamphetamine are compelling due to a euphoric "rush" from the release of dopamine. This effect makes them intensely pleasurable and reinforces their continued use—rats will die trying to get more (unlike their less compulsive response to alcohol, nicotine, or heroin). There has always been debate about whether or not stimulants cause physiological dependence. Suffice it to say that they create enough changes in the functioning of the norepinephrine and dopamine systems that they produce powerful cravings and other reactions that make up what is basically a tolerance and withdrawal syndrome.

Tolerance develops to stimulant effects, making it more difficult to get high, but reverses with a few days of abstinence. Repetitive motor activity and paranoia get more exaggerated with long-term use.

Withdrawal or crashing creates symptoms of depression and anhedonia (inability to feel pleasure), probably due to a deficiency of dopamine, which leads to craving, irritability, and possibly aggressiveness for up to several months. Exhaustion is also experienced, probably due to a depletion of norepinephrine and lack of sleep during a long cocaine or speed run.

Benefits

The euphoric and energizing effects are the most attractive features of stimulants for recreational use, and the medical benefits can be lifesaving for some people. Relief from narcolepsy (uncontrolled falling asleep) and attention-deficit disorder enhance a person's quality of life as well as his or her basic functioning. For people with depression or schizophrenia (whose depression-like negative symptoms of anhedonia and social isolation are quite intolerable), stimulants provide relief and a sense of being able to participate in the world. Stimulants counteract the flattening effects of some antipsychotic medications (the older types) for schizophrenia and mood-stabilizing medications for bipolar disorder (manic–depression).

Risks

- Headaches, nausea, vomiting, chest pains, dizziness.
- Erectile dysfunction and delayed ejaculation (constricts blood vessels in penis).
- With heavy, prolonged use, repetitive movements that can be bizarre or self-destructive, such as skin picking.
- Because they release dopamine, stimulants also can cause psychotic symptoms in people who use a lot, or in vulnerable people (those with schizophrenia, in particular). Paranoia, hallucinations, and delusions may sometimes lead to violence as the person tries to protect him- or herself from "attacks by enemies." These symptoms usually resolve with discontinued use.
- Mood swings from euphoric to depressed.
- Snorting can damage the interior of the nose, causing lesions.
- Regular use restricts blood flow to the capillaries, causing gum deterioration, in particular.
- Regular use often leads to poor nutrition (stimulants interrupt digestion as well as interfere with appetite).
- Lack of moisture in the mouth results in dental cavities.
- Chronic activation of the "fight–flight" response can impair immune function due to repeated release of stress hormones (cortisol, etc.).
- Poor nutrition and fatigue from speed use can further compromise a weakened immune system for people with HIV.

Greatest Dangers

- *Overdose*: increased heart rate can cause irregular heart rhythm and extremely elevated blood pressure, leading to stroke or heart attack.
- Stimulants that are used at *closely spaced intervals*: the effects on the brain diminish long before the body eliminates the drugs, so with frequent dosing the body can accumulate toxic levels. It is possible to overdose with a single dose. Speedballs

(a combination of speed or cocaine and heroin) reduces sensation of both the opiates and the stimulant, thus increasing the chance of overdose.

- Long-term use can lead to *atherosclerosis* (fatty buildup in blood vessels) or damage to the heart due to lack of oxygen.
- *Body temperature* rises, sometimes to dangerous levels (this is rare; also, section on ecstasy).
- *Seizures* can occur when blood levels of stimulant are high: all emergency room admissions for seizures are checked for cocaine when the patient has no seizure history.
- *Ephedrine* can be toxic to the cardiovascular system at two to three times the recommended dose (which is often recommended for recreational drug effect).
- *Methamphetamine* causes actual damage to dopamine and norepinephrine neurons: nerve endings are cut back, causing deficits in amount of these neurotransmitters available; longer-term consequences on movement and mood disorders are unknown at this point.

Drug Interactions

The protease inhibitor ritonavir may slow the clearing of speed from your system, causing a buildup that could lead to overdose if you keep using.

Harm Reduction

- Don't dose on the high—there is still stimulant left in your body. If you have to take more the same day, dose on the half-life (the time it takes for half the drug to leave your body): two to four hours for cocaine, eight to twelve hours for speed.
- Dilute when possible: if you snort, snort with water—it's easier on the nose.
- Maintain regular sleep and eating habits.
- Don't combine, either with other stimulants, which potentiate the effects, or with depressants, which mask what's happening to your body and mind.
- Don't use to get through your usual activities of the day.
- In other words, use purposefully—know why you use and use for only that purpose.
- Antipsychotic medications can be used to treat stimulant psychosis; these should be withdrawn after symptoms disappear.

Nicotine

Nicotine belongs to drug class, although it has many stimulant properties.

General Information

Nicotine is a toxic substance (that is, a poison) found in tobacco. Sixty milligrams of nicotine would be enough to kill an adult. Cigarettes contain from half to two milligrams, however, and only 20 percent of that amount is ingested while smoking. A little more is ingested by chewing or snuff.

History

Tobacco has been used in religious and magic rituals by native North and South Americans for thousands of years. The belief is that the smoke carries prayers to the gods. When not smoked regularly, it causes a significant high. Introduced to Europe by the Spanish invaders of the "New World" in the 1500s, it was too harsh to be smoked regularly, as it is today. So it was also used there intermittently to alter consciousness. Tobacco became associated with witchcraft and with excessive Westernization (in countries such as Russia and Japan) and was considered an evil new drug. It was banned in many European countries in the early 1600s, especially vigorously in Russia, where the most severe penalty for smoking was death. When it became clear that tobacco use continued nevertheless, and tobacco could be a source of tax revenue, it was legalized by the end of the 1600s.

Tobacco was chewed or snuffed until the mid-1800s, when cigars were developed, then cigarettes. The practice of spitting chewed tobacco became a major source of the spread of tuberculosis. (It was also a most unpleasant practice in the public rooms of taverns, etc.) Cigarettes were brought from Turkey by the British. Cigars were developed in the United States, where North Carolina became the dominant tobacco-growing region. Cigarettes, more delicate than cigars, made smoking more attractive to women.

In the first half of the twentieth century, tobacco use was encouraged in the United States as an aid to concentration and relaxation—both of which it does very well, in fact. It was advertised for its weight-control benefits—also not an inaccurate claim. Although women did smoke, it was some time before it was acceptable for them to smoke in public. By the1960s, 40 percent of Americans smoked. Now, about 28 percent do. In the 1990s there was an increase of young people smoking, from 28 percent of twelfth graders in 1991 to 34 percent in 1995.

Uses

Nicotine currently has no use beyond recreational.

How It Works

When smoked, nicotine goes immediately from the lungs to blood to brain, where it stimulates acetylcholine neurotransmitters, otherwise known as *nicotinic re-*

ceptors, in the brain. These release dopamine and increase activity in regions associated with memory and physical movement. The release of dopamine and the speed of action in the brain make nicotine extremely reinforcing. The effect peaks in ten minutes or less, and nicotine has a half-life of twenty minutes.

Effects

- Subjective reports of the calming, antianxiety effects of tobacco are probably due to the fact that nicotine reduces muscle tone, thus relaxing muscle tension.
- Most people do not enjoy their first cigarettes; they must learn to accommodate to the toxic effects while paying close attention to the positives. Peer pressure is important in this process.
- Elevates heart rate and blood pressure.
- Suppresses appetite, for unclear reasons (also happens in animal studies).
- Found to increase learning, memory, attention, and concentration.
- Associated with depression in young people. Unclear if this is caused by nicotine or due to a preexisting depression, which a person may be attempting to medicate.

Dependence, Tolerance, and Withdrawal

Tolerance develops to both the physical and mental effects of nicotine. The first cigarette after a period of abstinence is the most potent and can cause dizziness, nausea, and sometimes vomiting. Since nicotine stimulates dopamine, it is reinforcing and therefore has great addictive potential. Withdrawal consists of extreme cravings and irritability for at least two to three weeks. Some people report nausea and vomiting in withdrawal. Many people who have successfully quit other addictive drugs report that they have the hardest time giving up cigarettes. Others seem to just walk away from them once they decide to quit.

Benefits

Nicotine has shown potential greater than amphetamines to enhance memory, concentration, and focus. It is being researched for use with ADHD and Alzheimer's disease. The current delivery systems (cigarettes and cigars, as well as chewable), however, are so toxic that the associated dangers outweigh the benefits. In some peer cultures, smoking is encouraged, and participating allows you to be accepted. People feel like they have a place where they belong. In addition, once you can overcome the nausea or throat irritation, smoking does offer a feeling of well-being and relaxation, while not dulling the senses.

Risks

- Ingestion of carbon monoxide and tar, which deprive the body of oxygen and stick to the fibers in the lungs, respectively. The combination of carbon monoxide and oxygen deprivation may counteract the potential good effects on attention and memory.

- Secondhand smoke, also called passive smoke, is thought to be responsible for about 40,000 deaths per year.
- Because nicotine is easily available, many people try it, and many quickly become dependent on it. Greater reported difficulty stopping this drug than any other.

Greatest Dangers

Tobacco is the psychoactive drug responsible for more deaths in the United States than all other drugs, including alcohol: 450,000 per year versus 125,000 caused by alcohol versus 10,000 caused by all other drugs combined.

- Lung diseases (chronic obstructive pulmonary disease, chronic bronchitis, emphysema) and cancer to the lungs, mouth, throat.
- Cardiovascular damage: increased heart rate leads to need for increased oxygen supply, which is depleted and replaced with carbon monoxide. This depletion causes stress and damage to the heart. Furthermore, arteriosclerosis, hardening of the arteries, and artherosclerosis, the buildup of fatty deposits in the arteries, are associated with smoking. Up to 30 percent of cardiovascular deaths are due to smoking.
- Thinning of the skin, possibly due to oxygen deprivation.
- Nicotine passes through the blood–placenta barrier, causing lower birthweight in babies and possible learning deficits.
- Men who smoke have increased risk of children who will get cancer, possibly due to damaged sperm and altered DNA.

Harm Reduction

Although few tobacco users limit their smoking to occasional use, this would be the better way of reducing harm. Quitting, however, seems to be the best way of reducing harm, since the drug is so reinforcing that controlling use is very difficult and stressful. Smoking cessation programs can be helpful and they are often free at local public health centers or at the Lung Association. Your doctor can prescribe Zyban, which has been shown to assist a person by reducing cravings. (This drug is the same as the generic drug buproprion, which would be a lot cheaper). You can also get a prescription for nicotine patches, which administer nicotine through your skin and help reduce your reliance on cigarettes.

If you don't quit:

- Don't smoke where you can affect others.
- Avoid using at times when you don't really need or want a cigarette (don't use automatically).

- Try to decide on a certain number of cigarettes a day (such as 5 or 8), and smoke only that much.
- Don't smoke at all one or more days a week.
- Switch to a lower tar and nicotine brand.
- Use a nicotine patch or gum in place of some of your cigarettes (be careful, though; too much can make you sick).
- Manipulate your environment: spend more time in places where you can't smoke.
- Don't smoke while pregnant.
- Don't smoke while trying to become pregnant (women *and* men).

Caffeine

What Drugs

Found in coffee, tea, soft drinks, chocolate, kola nuts from Africa, over-the-counter pain relievers, stimulants and performance drugs, and some prescription medications.

General Information

Caffeine belongs to a class of stimulant drugs called *xanthines*, a family that includes caffeine, theophylline, which is found in tea, and theobromine, found in chocolate. Theobromine is only one-tenth as potent as the other two. For unknown reasons, the effects of coffee and pure caffeine differ—coffee seems to be more potent than pure caffeine or other caffeine-containing plants. *Note*: There are two species of coffee in the world: arabica and robusta. Arabica is the original coffee and is grown all over the world. Cheaper robusta coffee is grown primarily on the island of Java and in Africa and is used as a filler in commercial blends. Robusta has more caffeine than the more high-quality arabica.

History

- *Tea* can be traced back to 2700 B.C. in China. It is the world's oldest caffeine-containing beverage. It was thought to have medicinal properties. It was introduced to Europe by the Dutch in the early 1600s, but it was the British and Russians who adopted it as a national drink.
- *Coffee*, called "the wine of Islam," originated in Ethiopia, and cultivation spread to Yemen and Arabia between the eleventh and fifteenth centuries. Religious leaders opposed it—they believed that it encouraged treachery and was as much an intoxicant as alcohol. Coffee won, however, and has been the regional drink for centuries. When it spread to Europe in the 1600s, coffeehouses became popular places

for intellectual conversation. Coffeehouses were banned in England, as the discussions held there were associated with sedition and political unrest. Furthermore, the beverage was believed to be a strong intoxicant and was attacked by the temperance movement. The ban was brief, and coffee grew in popularity. Coffeehouses served the same function in the United States—as the locale wherein the leaders of the American War of Independence planned their rebellion. By 1830, coffee had replace alcohol as the national drink of America, and by 1860, Americans consumed about three-quarters of the world's coffee.

- *Chocolate*: Cacao is native to Central America and Mexico and was used in religious ritual by the Aztecs. Legend has it that it was a gift to humans from god to give us a taste of paradise. In the early 1500s Cortez took cacao back to Spain, where the royal family added sugar to it. It became a secret recipe until it was unveiled to the public at the wedding of a princess a hundred years later. The Dutch developed a method to refine it by removing fat. The fat was made into chocolate bars. Today the average annual per capita consumption of chocolate in the United States is twelve pounds, whereas in Switzerland it is twenty-two pounds.

- *Colas* are made from the African cola nut, which is very bitter and is chewed for its stimulating effect. Little cola is left in sodas, but it is one of the original ingredients, along with extract of cocaine, of the original Coca-Cola.

- *Guaran'a*: The national drink of Brazil, made from the seeds of a bush, contains more caffeine than coffee and is made into sodas.

- *Mate*: The national drink of Argentina, sometimes sold as a herbal tea in the United States, it *does* contain caffeine.

How It Works

Caffeine's main action is to block adenosine, which sedates brain activity. Two cups of coffee stimulate brain activity.

Effects

- Increases alertness and euphoria.
- Increases heart rate and blood pressure.
- Increases adrenaline.
- Causes nervousness and tremulousness at high doses.
- Has diuretic effect (causes the kidneys to release urine—can result in dehydration from fluid loss).
- Increases urinary excretion of calcium and slows absorption of calcium.
- Stimulates breathing (tea, especially, has been used to treat asthma).
- Relaxes the smooth muscles in the bronchioles.
- Enhances physical performance and endurance.
- Restricts blood vessels, which is useful for treating headaches.
- Releases fat into blood.

Amount of caffeine in different substances (in milligrams):

- Coffee   65 (instant), 150 (drip robusta) per cup
- Tea   20–100, depending on brand; 70, iced
- Chocolate   20 per one ounce of dark chocolate
- Sodas   38 (Pepsi), 116 (Red Bull) per can
- Pain relievers (per pill the recommended dose is usually two)
  —Anacin   32
  —Excedrin   65
  —Goody's   33
  —Midol   32
  —Vanquish   33
- Over-the-counter stimulants (per pill)
  —Caffedrine   200
  —No-Doz   100 (two is the recommended dose)
  —Vivarin   200
- Diuretics
  —Aqua-Ban   100 (two is recommended dose)
- Cold remedies (per pill)
  —Coryban-D   30
  —Dristan   16
  —Triaminicin   30

Benefits

Many of the above effects are considered benefits by at least some, which is why caffeine is an ingredient in some medications. Flavonoids, compounds that act as antioxidants in the blood and prevent the development of arteriosclerosis and atherosclerosis, are found in cocoa. Three tablespoons of cocoa powder, or a 1.5-ounce piece of chocolate contains approximately the same amount of flavonoids as a 5-ounce glass of red wine. *Warning: milk chocolate contains milkfat and other saturated fats that can negate this good effect.*

Dependence, Tolerance, and Withdrawal

People become dependent on coffee quickly. Tolerance to and dependence on coffee are common in Western societies. Withdrawal symptoms begin about twenty-four hours after the last dose and include a vascular headache that can be severe, irritability, nausea, and lethargy. Withdrawal tends to last up to three days.

Risks

Note to parents of young children: The effects of caffeine listed above reflect adults doses. These effects will be compounded in children.

- Osteoporosis risk increased at levels of three cups of coffee or five cups of tea (due to caffeine's effect on calcium elimination and absorption).
- Irritates the stomach lining, causing indigestion (in the United States, there are as many brands of antacid as there are coffee).
- Irritates women's bladders.
- Common cause of headaches, heart palpitations, and problems with sleep.
- Increases high blood pressure and the body's stress response and is sometimes associated with anxiety and panic attacks (consumption of four to five cups of coffee a day can precipitate a panic attack in those with a history of anxiety or panic).
- Increases LDLs (the bad cholesterol) except when filtered through a paper cone.
- Contributes to dehydration if used for, or with, exercise.
- Some studies report low birthweight of babies of coffee drinkers. At the end of pregnancy or while taking oral contraceptives, caffeine is eliminated more slowly, and a buildup can occur that causes symptoms of caffeine intoxication.
- Restricts blood flow in eyes, decreasing nutrients and clearing of waste.
- Smokers eliminate coffee twice as fast as nonsmokers, thus increasing the risk of drinking more caffeine beverage to prolong the caffeine effect.

Greatest Dangers

Caffeine is generally not dangerous; however, eight hundred milligrams of caffeine could be toxic in a small child (about eight cups of coffee or two pounds of chocolate). Toxic symptoms are upset stomach, vomiting, extreme nervousness, and nervous system stimulation, which could lead to seizures.

Harm Reduction

Since caffeine products are legal and pleasing to many, a general harm reduction advisory should suffice. As is always the case when thinking about risk from a harm reduction perspective, the poison is in the dose, and the risks depend on the person and the situation. Don't be fooled by decaf—it contains small amounts of caffeine and all of the other irritants to the gastrointestinal, cardiovascular, and urinary systems. If you suffer from anxiety, nervousness, trouble sleeping, heart palpitations, or upset stomach, try cutting back or eliminating caffeine as a first experiment. You'll be surprised by how much it helps.

Marijuana (Cannabinoids)

AUTHORS' NOTE: *An equal number of people pointed out the benefits of marijuana use as pointed out the potential harmful effects. The only consistent statement is that marijuana does not seem to cause serious psychiatric or medical* *problems in the vast majority of people who use it (forget* Reefer Madness*!) and is definitely not associated with violent behavior. In addition, pot use is so widespread in the United States that many people actually tend to forget that it's illegal! Typical statements are "It's not like I'm smoking crack" and "It's a lot better for you than alcohol" (which happens to be true). What we have learned from our clients and colleagues seems to relate to short-term versus long-term effects and to the idiosyncratic nature of an individual's response to this drug. This makes general statements and harm reduction techniques difficult to formulate. For example, in the short run a person might get positive or negative effects. People with underlying psychotic disorders may subjectively feel better, even if their symptoms increase over time. Other people might feel anxious or nauseated when they use, even though that is not a typical response. The good news is that if people experience negative effects when they first start using, they almost always stop using.*

The tricky part really comes when trying to evaluate the benefits versus harms over a longer period of time. Many people are now using pot as a drug substitution medicine. They claim that it keeps them from going back to heroin or alcohol. Other people seem to manage anxiety and muscle tension by smoking pot and are extremely productive in their work and stable in their personal lives. Since the only licensed drugs effective for this type of anxiety are the benzodiazepines, which can have long-term negative effects, who's to say that they haven't chosen wisely? Those who are using "medical marijuana" for pain control, to increase appetite in chemotherapy or HIV disease, for glaucoma, etc., are especially strong believers in its safety and efficacy. The medical benefits do not seem to decrease over time, nor does the person's functioning tend to suffer. We do see many people, however, who come to us after having been regular pot smokers for twenty to thirty years, telling us that it is a problem for them. They think their pot smoking has impaired their intimate relationships and contributed to disorganization, low self-esteem, and a lack of motivation. They feel these problems "snuck up" on them over time.

What follows in this section is as much information as seems accurate and consistent with general scientific research, clinical observation, and many conversations with people who use marijuana.

What Drugs

- Marijuana
- Hashish

General Information

Cannabis is the general botanical name of the plant that produces marijuana and hashish. All parts of the plant are usable. Most commonly, the stems are used for hemp fiber, the resin-covered leaves and flowers of the unfertilized female plant are dried and cured for marijuana, and the resin itself becomes hashish when scraped from the leaves and dried.

Marijuana falls into no drug category; it is considered to have hallucinogenic qualities but is not a hallucinogen. There are four hundred active ingredients in the cannabis plant, THC (tetrahydrocannabinol) being the most potent. THC was first isolated in 1964. Typically these days, marijuana has a THC concentration of 4 percent, compared to the 1–2 percent concentration in the marijuana generally imported from Mexico in the sixties and seventies. The concentration of THC in hashish is 8–14 percent. THC in hashish oil can range from 20 to 70 percent. The receptors in the brain that respond to marijuana were only discovered in 1990. The natural analog to THC (the neurotransmitter) is called anandamide.

History

In the East, the first recorded reference to marijuana occurred around 300 B.C. in China, in which an emperor from almost 3000 B.C. was reputed to have praised it as medicine for rheumatism, gout, malaria, and (ironically) absent-mindedness. It was also grown for its durable fiber, and hemp pots have been found in China dating to the Stone Age. It was used for paper there beginning in 100 B.C., but was primarily used as a food grain. Its intoxicating properties were noted but not discussed in those early days.

In India, marijuana, referred to as *bhang*, *ganja*, or *charas*, depending on which part of the plant is used, was and is used ritually and recreationally for its intoxicating properties. By A.D. 1000, Egyptians were using marijuana recreationally.

In the Muslim world, marijuana was cultivated as an alternative to alcohol, which was discouraged by the prophet Mohammed and banned in the Koran. Marijuana was also used in paper production from 1150.

Hashish was developed in North Africa: the hot climate causes the production of large amounts of resin, which protects the leaves from excessive heat.

In the West, the first mention made of hemp used for psychoactive purposes was by Herodotus in 450 B.C. Moving swiftly forward in time, crusaders brought back word of hashish in the thirteenth century, as did Marco Polo. Despite the fact that the pope condemned it along with witchcraft in 1484 (merely eight years before the Spanish Inquisition and the expulsion of the Jews from Spain and the funding of Columbus's voyage to the "New World"), marijuana remained a staple of apothecaries, herbalists, and priests throughout the Renaissance. Presumably, then, it was known for its intoxicating properties. As in the Middle East, it was used in paper production. Early nineteenth-century Europeans popularized the use of hashish brought from Egypt by Napoleon's troops. In the 1840s a group of intellectuals formed the Club of Hashish-eaters, where they gathered and talked and ate hashish (mixed with butter, sugar, and flavorings). In the second half of the nineteenth century many papers were published in Europe on the medical uses of cannabis. It is also listed in the U.S. pharmacopoeia as a medicine for various ailments.

Hemp was imported to the New World in the 1500s and 1600s by the Spanish and English. Like tobacco, it was a major cash crop and used for fiber. George Washington grew hemp to avoid relying on British supplies, and, in fact, farmers were required to produce a certain amount of hemp, which was used for barter throughout the colonies and for production of sailcloth, military cordage, and uniforms. Only in the twentieth century, however, did recreational use in the United States become noticeable. The Spanish word *marijuana* was introduced when it was brought into this country primarily by Mexican migrant workers in the Southwest. During Prohibition in the 1920s, when alcohol was outlawed, marijuana use became more widespread. Jazz musicians went to marijuana clubs, called *tea pads*. There were more tea pads than speakeasies in Harlem. The drug was tolerated because it was not illegal, and there was no disturbances of the peace by marijuana users.

Marijuana was demonized in the 1930s by the first chief of the newly created Federal Bureau of Narcotics (FBN), Henry J. Anslinger. Having been introduced by, and associated with, Mexican immigrants, it became a convenient target of hysteria, fed by the economic stress of the Depression and hostility toward immigrant labor. Inaccurate information about its effects was circulated, much of it by the FBN, and much of it focused on the Mexican population (primarily fabricated episodes of violence and insanity, to tarnish the idea that it had legitimate medical uses). Although several states had already banned marijuana, in 1937 marijuana was effectively driven underground by the Marijuana Tax Act.

Since then there has been much debate about the benefits versus the risks of marijuana, with the most hysterical fears of violence being retracted. Generally, by those not directly involved in carrying out the War on Drugs, marijuana is considered one of the most benign of the recreational drugs, and its medical uses far outweigh its problems as an intoxicant. Possession of small amounts for personal consumption has been decriminalized and/or its medical use has been legalized in several states. But the battle continues.

Uses

- Nonmedical: Hemp for fiber, seeds for oil and animal feed, and food; hemp is an extraordinarily durable fiber used for ropes and other products such as ship sails and shoes.
- Medical: Appetite stimulant, reduces nausea, reduces pressure in eyes caused by glaucoma, relaxes muscles; useful for multiple sclerosis and other disorders that cause muscle spasticity, seizures, migraines, chronic pain, and asthma (when taken orally).

How It Works

Marijuana is generally smoked or eaten. If smoked, it goes from lungs to heart to brain in a few seconds, peaks in ten to twenty minutes, and lasts up to a couple of hours. When eaten, it goes through the liver first. Its effects may not be felt for an hour, but the high lasts longer because of the slower route, and eating it is more likely to induce a hallucinatory experience than smoking.

There are receptors in the brain for cannabinoids. It is unclear what their purpose is, but there are two compounds discovered so far that bind to cannabis receptors–anandamide (*ananda* means "bliss" in Sanskrit) and 2-AG. THC receptors are found mostly in the hippocampus, which controls new memory formation (learning); in the cerebellum and basal ganglia, which coordinate fine motor movements; and in the nucleus acumbens, which contains dopamine. There are few cannabis receptors in the brainstem, which controls vital functions, so there is no risk of overdose or death.

THC's psychoactive effects last only a few hours; however, it can be detected in the blood after 20 hours, and it accumulates in the tissues of the liver, kidneys, spleen, and testes. It is also stored in fatty tissue and released slowly. Thus a large dose or regular use can be detected for three to four weeks, particularly in a person with a lot of body fat. THC crosses the blood–placenta barrier, but the evidence of any impact on the infant (lower birthweight among mothers who used) is confounded by the often corresponding use of alcohol and tobacco.

Benefits

Marijuana effects are very sensitive to set and setting, more so than most drugs. Some people experience relaxation and sedation, others stimulation, still others agitation and anxiety. In general, marijuana is used to intensify sensory experiences. It creates the sensation of greater creativity, greater connection between mind and body, and/or lightness and hilarity with other people. It fosters an open, relaxed state, reduces stress, alters time perception, and lowers aggression. It relaxes muscles and relieves pain from headaches and cramps. It reduces nausea and increases appetite, both useful for treatment of AIDS and chemotherapy patients.

Risks

Marijuana impairs attention, concentration, and ability for linear thought (although, to some extent, these can be relearned while under the influence). Difficulty with short-term memory, but no evidence of long-term cognitive damage, has been reported. It may cause drowsiness, dry mouth, increased heart rate (no evidence of adverse effects on the primarily young people studied), anxiety, dizziness, confusion, paranoia, and panic. It blocks airflow in heavy smokers, contains some of the same carcinogens as tobacco, and can cause coughing and upper respiratory problems. There have been no credible, replicated studies that support the idea that marijuana lowers testosterone levels and sperm count, nor that it suppresses the hormone necessary for the implanting of fertilized eggs. If this were true, we certainly would have noticed it by now. In fact, many excellent studies conducted since 1839 (W. B. O'Shaughnessy) indicate the medical benefits of marijuana.

Addiction, Tolerance, and Withdrawal

Tolerance does develop (and some control can be gained over effects on coordination and concentration). Marijuana is thought to have low addiction potential, due to its relatively mild activation of dopamine. Many people struggle to control or stop their marijuana use, however. Psychological dependence can develop in regular users. Withdrawal is nothing like an opiate-type syndrome, however. It is generally mild, with irritability, restlessness, insomnia, bad dreams, sweating, headaches, and mild nausea possible for a day or so.

Greatest Dangers

New memory formation (learning) is impaired. This effect may last for two days after using. Mental flexibility and problem-solving ability may be impaired in heavy users. There is an increased risk of accidents while driving, and psychomotor retardation can last for at least twenty-four hours after using. "Amotivational syndrome," referring to the loss of motivation to set goals or accomplish tasks, has been pretty well disproven. Lack of motivation may be observed more in people who are still users. There is no danger of overdose.

Hallucinogens

What Drugs

Serotonin-related (chemically similar to serotonin):

- LSD (lysergic acid diethylamide), synthetically derived from ergot, a fungus in moldy rye
- Ololiuqui (morning glory seeds)
- Psilocybin (mushrooms)
- Dimethyltryptamine (DMT), found in the bark of some trees and nuts in Central and South America
- Harmine, found in the bark of a South American vine
- 5-MeO-DMT and bufotenine, found in the venom of certain toads

Norepinephrine-related (similar to norepinephrine):

- Mescaline, found in the peyote cactus in Mexico and U.S. Southwest
- Dimethoxy-4-methylamphetamine (DOM or STP), a synthetic mescaline-like compound, not much used because it is very potent, dosages are not well-controlled, and toxic reactions are common.
- 2C-B (4-bromo-2,5-dimethoxyphenethylamine), synthesized by Alexander Shulgin and considered an *entactogen* ("touching within") like ecstasy more than a hallucinogen
- MDMA (ecstasy) and MDA, also synthetic compounds and also considered entactogens, not strictly hallucinogenic (discussed in the next section)

Acetylcholine-related (similar to acetylcholine):

- Atropine and scopolamine, found in bella donna or deadly nightshade, mandrake, henbane, and datura plants (including jimsonweed)
- Hyoscyamine, found in mandrake, henbane, and datura plants
- Ibotenic acid, found in *Amanita mascaria* mushrooms and the iboga plant

History

Some of these compounds are the products of plants found in different parts of the world and have been in cultural or religious use for hundreds or thousands of years. The synthetic compounds were all developed in the twentieth century for a variety of reasons, usually unrelated to their current recreational use. See each individual drug for a brief history.

How They Work

In general, these drugs either stimulate or suppress the activity of the neurotransmitter most similar to them. The serotonin-related drugs and the norepinephrine-related drugs tend to *stimulate* one of the serotonin receptors that causes hallucinations when it is not stimulated in balance with the others. The acetylcholine-related drugs *block* acetylcholine, which slows the heart and helps to form memories. For more information on each drug, the website The Vaults of Erowid (*www.erowid.org*) is a good place to go, as is the book *Buzzed*.

Effects

The term *hallucinogenic* refers to the ability of a drug or substance to produce hallucinations, which are perceptions of visions, sounds, or smells that are not real. Hallucinogenic drugs more often intensify or alter perceptions rather than creating ones that are not there. However, the power is in the dose. At very high doses, these drugs can actually produce true hallucinations. The most popularized term for this tupe of experience is *psychedelic,* referring to the drugs' positive abilities to create "mind-expanding" experiences.

Serotonin-Related Hallucinogens. Effects vary depending on which drug is used, the person's expectations, and the setting. Hallucinogens are among the most set- and setting-dependent of drugs. Mild effects include detachment and an altered sense of space and time. Higher doses cause visual disturbances and hallucinations, depersonalization, intense feelings of insight, a sense of being very focused, and "synesthesia" (confusion of senses—"hearing sights" or "seeing sounds"). They do not cause a real psychotic experience, but they can trigger psychosis in a vulnerable person.

- LSD was developed in the 1940s by Albert Hoffman, a chemist in Switzerland. He was interested in the ability of the ergot acid to reduce blood flow and increase smooth muscle contractions, especially in the uterus, with the goal of finding a non-toxic chemical that would help in childbirth. He accidentally swallowed some LSD that was on his fingertips and proceeded to have a "trip," about which he wrote extensively. LSD is the most potent of the psychedelics, and a trip lasts for many hours, up to 12 for some people.
- Ololiuqui, or morning glory seeds, have been used for centuries by Central and South American native peoples for spiritual communication. The active ingredient is similar to LSD. The side effects of nausea, vomiting, headache, increased blood pressure, dilated pupils, and drowsiness are fairly prominent, so it is not popular as a recreational drug.
- Psilocybin mushrooms grow in Mexico and Central America. They were praised by the Aztecs and used for healing physical and spiritual ailments. Two to four mushrooms is an average dose. Effects are similar to LSD. These mushrooms seem to produce visions of shapes and colors similar to those of Aztec designs, suggesting that the designs might have been prompted by the use of mushrooms. At high doses, they can cause anxiety, numbness, sweating, and nausea.
- DMT, from Central and South America, is a short-acting hallucinogen, causing a trip of just an hour–the "businessman's lunch." It is so quick, it is more likely to cause anxiety. DMT is metabolized by monoamine oxidase (MAO). (If you are taking an MAO inhibitor antidepressant medication, DMT metabolism will be slowed.)
- Harmine is a compound found in the seeds of a vine native to the Middle East but also found in South America. It creates a dream or trance-like state during which a person sees visions. When mixed with DMT into a brew called ayahuasca, it produces more potent visions. Because harmine is an MAO inhibitor, it slows the metabolism of DMT. Ayahuasca is made in the Brazilian and Peruvian Amazon basin and is considered a very sacred brew. It is a legal religious sacrament, used in controlled rituals, much like peyote. There are religious groups now in North America who use ayahuasca.
- Bufotenine and 5-MeO-DMT: Bufotenine is found in the venom of a toad and in

trees in Haiti and South and Central America. Bufotenine, as well as DMT, is used in snuffs in South America. It has been identified in various powders used in voodoo rituals. It produces a brief high and some unpleasant side effects: increased blood pressure, blurred vision, cramps, and temporary paralysis. It is also metabolized by MAO. A trip lasts for about two hours.

Norepinephrine-Related Hallucinogens

• Peyote has been used for at least 3,000 years in Mexico. It was used by the Mescalero Apaches in the nineteenth century, thus the name of the active ingredient *mescaline*. Peyote was officially incorporated into the Native American Church of North America in the early twentieth century and is used as a sacrament. The cactus buttons are sliced, dried, and then eaten. Otherwise, a tea is made from them. The sacrament lasts two days, Saturday and Sunday. Although peyote, or mescaline, is listed as a Schedule I drug (meaning there is no acceptable use), federal law has made an exception for use in the Native American church. Physical effects are similar to those produced by amphetamine. Psychological effects are similar to those experienced on LSD, and a trip lasts almost as long. Nausea is a common effect.

• 2C-B has the effect at lower doses of making people feel "in touch" with themselves. At higher doses, it produces vivid hallucinations but with more mental clarity than other hallucinogens. It is usually taken orally in tablets or gel caps. It is very dose sensitive, and it is difficult to know the dose in a tablet, so be careful. There have been some reports of nausea, chills, and trembling. How it actually works is unknown.

Acetylcholine-Related Hallucinogens

• Belladonna or deadly nightshade: Historically, this substance has been used as a poison, as a medicine to treat asthma, as a beauty aid (it dilates the pupils, considered appealing in women), and ritually for thousands of years. Recreational use is recent. It was used in female deity worship in pre-Christian Europe. Women using it were called witches by Christians. Some historical accounts say that it was used in satanic rituals. Atropine and scopolamine are the active ingredients. Atropine can give the feeling of flying, possibly contributing to the idea that witches can fly. It causes a bizarre dream-like state and increased heart rate and temperature. It is a bronchodilator and causes amnesia.

• Datura or jimsonweed: Causes a hypnotic, hallucinogenic experience, as well as disorientation, confusion, and amnesia. It is toxic at high doses.

• Mandrake: Historically, mandrake was considered an aphrodisiac. At low doses it is a depressant and has been used for anxiety and sleep. At higher doses it causes bizarre hallucinations and muscle paralysis.

• Henbane: Means "harmful to hens" and is also a poison (Hamlet's father was murdered with it). Lower doses have anesthetic and painkilling properties.

- Amanita Muscaria (mushroom):, from the northern hemisphere, is at least a 3,000-year-old intoxicant that causes muscle spasms, dizziness, hallucinations, and increased aggression. It was believed used by Vikings before they set off for battle, causing their reputation for savagery. It may also be the divine substance referred to in an ancient Hindu text and the "nectar of the gods" of Greek mythology. The mushroom looks like the dancing mushrooms in Disney's *Fantasia.*
- Ibogaine, related to ibotenic acid, from the iboga root in Africa, has been used in tribal ceremonies in Gabon and the Congo as an aid in seeking advice from ancestors. The root is chewed, and intoxication can last for thirty hours. Ibogaine is now being researched as a therapeutic drug to help reduce cocaine, alcohol, nicotine, and opiate dependence.

Dependence, Tolerance, and Withdrawal

Tolerance to the effects of some of these drugs develops, but since there is little to no stimulation of dopamine, there is low dependence/addiction potential.

Benefits

The benefits have been detailed above. When used respectfully and in the right circumstances, these drugs give a sense of expansiveness and connectedness as well as visions or insights that would otherwise be unattainable.

Risks

- Accidents and physical injury during bad trips or due to disorientation from some drugs have been reported.
- Anxiety and nausea due to high doses are not uncommon (sometimes nausea is a normal part of the experience).
- Flashbacks may be related to memory changes. There is some evidence that the brain responds to stimuli and recalls stored memories. Up to 60 percent of heavy users experience flashbacks; they are not usually dangerous.
- Underlying psychosis can be triggered by use of hallucinogens.

Greatest Dangers

Beware of all of the acetylcholine-related drugs. *All can be lethal at doses that are not much higher than the recreational dose. All are toxic at any dose.*

Harm Reduction

- Know your dose.
- Plan your trip—it's most enjoyable then—and allow plenty of time. You'll also be tired the next day.
- Use one drug at a time.

- Don't pick mushrooms unless you are experienced.
- A full stomach will increase the likelihood of getting nauseous, so eat just a little, if at all.
- Anxiety can be treated with reassurance or benzodiazepines.
- Drugs exist that can stop a trip by blocking serotonin receptors.
- Do not drive or try to operate other machinery.
- Use with people you know and with whom you feel safe. Keep an eye on each other. Some people tend to wander off while under the influence and can get lost either in an urban setting or when using out in the countryside.

Ecstasy

What Drugs

- MDMA (3,4=methylene-dioxy-methamphetamine)
- MDA (hallucinogen)
- MDEA (variation on MDMA, but lacks empathic quality—is not manufactured, so is not really "out there")

History

Developed in the 1930s as an experimental amphetamine to be used as a compound in other drugs, MDMA was never used, nor was it studied. It was revived in the 1980s for use as an empathy enhancer in couples therapy. According to the federal government, it was toxic and had no proven medical effect, so it was placed on the Schedule I list. Its most popular use now is in dance clubs. It is taken in pill form—fifty to two hundred milligrams—and is sometimes cut with caffeine, ephedrine, or dextromethorphan.

Uses

It is used in therapy to enhance communication, particularly between partners/spouses, and recreationally, as a mood-enhancing drug, to foster openness and communication and as a dance and party drug.

How It Works

Ecstasy increases levels of serotonin, which creates feelings of well-being. As an "excitatory" neurotransmitter, it causes the release of dopamine and norepinephrine. Ecstasy floods the synapses with serotonin, which explains its dramatic effect on mood.

Effects

Ecstasy peaks in one hour and can last three to six hours. It is considered to have the stimulant effects of amphetamines and the hallucinogenic qualities of mescaline.

It creates a sense of empathy and openness, lowers fear and defensiveness, and decreases one's sense of separateness, aggression, and obsessiveness. It can stimulate sexual interest as an offshoot of the sense of openness, although serotonin itself can actually decrease sexual drive. Ecstasy has amphetamine-like effects, with increased heart rate, blood pressure, temperature, bronchodilation, dilated pupils, increased blood flow to muscles, and lowered appetite. It does not cause real hallucinations, but time perception is distorted.

Dependence, Tolerance, and Withdrawal

Ecstasy is generally used in specific circumstances and not in a typically addictive pattern of compulsive use. In fact, overuse is difficult, since it depletes the brain's store of serotonin molecules and "down-regulates" the serotonin receptors, thus making it impossible to get "high" after a few doses. Withdrawal involves the experience of depression, since serotonin neurotransmitters are exhausted. It takes ten to fourteen days to regenerate one's supply of serotonin.

Benefits

The experience of warmth, empathy, and closeness with others are viewed as the benefits of using ecstasy.

Risks

• Ecstasy pills can be cut with other substances, such as caffeine and dextromethorphan, both of which can increase the stimulant effect and body temperature.

• In withdrawal, there is a dramatic undersupply of serotonin, so depression is common.

• Overuse can lead to chronic undersupply of serotonin, and thus depression.

• Postecstasy panic attacks, which may be due to a preexisting anxiety disorder, have been reported.

Greatest Dangers

• *Hyperthermia*: Ecstasy raises body temperature at high doses (only two to three times a single dose), which causes dehydration, muscle breakdown, and kidney failure. Some people have died as a result. Increasing doses produce symptoms of jitteriness, teeth clenching, cramping, nausea, paranoia, dizziness, crankiness, weakness, and lack of coordination.

• *Neurotoxicity*: A "serotonin syndrome" occurs when there is an oversupply of serotonin and is characterized by hyperthermia, muscle rigidity, tremulousness, nausea, and confusion; it can ultimately lead to loss of consciousness and death.

According to animal studies, ecstasy destroys serotonin nerve cell terminals, the ends that release the serotonin. Once serotonin is depleted, the reuptake transporters start taking dopamine into the serotonin cells. Dopamine is converted into hydrogen peroxide by MAO, which metabolizes serotonin, dopamine, and norepinephrine. The hydrogen peroxide then burns the serotonin nerve endings. This process has not been studied adequately in humans, but we may see longer-term mood problems in people who use ecstasy frequently. It does seem that the nerve endings grow back, but they grow back thicker—whether this is good or bad thing is unknown.

Drug Interactions

- MAO inhibitors (MAOIs, one type of antidepressant medication) increase the supply of serotonin and, in conjunction with ecstasy, increase the likelihood of serotonin syndrome.
- Any drugs that increase heart rate, blood pressure, temperature, or dehydration—for example, stimulants, alcohol, dextromethorphan.
- Ritonavir, a protease inhibitor or antiretroviral medication used in the treatment of HIV, raises levels of ecstasy and can contribute to overdose.
- Alcohol increases the dehydrating effects of ecstasy.

Harm Reduction

- If you can, check your pills for purity. DanceSafe, a harm reduction organization, can be found at some clubs, where workers offer pill-testing kits.
- Drink *water*, not alcohol, when using ecstasy.
- Stay cool—wear cool clothes and avoid headgear; dab the back of your neck and your wrists with cool water.
- SSRIs, most notably Prozac because it has a long half-life, can stop dopamine from being taken up into the serotonin nerve cells by plugging the reuptake transporters. This works up to six hours after the last ecstasy use.
- Tryptophan, found in milk and turkey, can help regenerate serotonin within twenty-four to forty-eight hours.
- Take vitamin C and antioxidants, as they may avert some of the damage of hydrogen peroxide. (This is a theory and, as with most illegal drugs, little has been studied.)
- CALL 911 IF YOU SEE ANYONE SHOWING SIGNS OF HYPERTHERMIA, CONFUSION, NAUSEA, OR UNCONSCIOUSNESS.

Dissociative Anesthetics

What Drugs

- Phencyclidine (PCP)
- Ketamine

- Dextromethorphan (DXM)
- Nitrous oxide (laughing gas)

These drugs are also classified as hallucinogens or psychedelics, but their physical effects are so different from those of the other hallucinogens, and there are such specific risk factors associated with their use, that we have separated them here.

- *PCP (angel dust)* was developed in 1963 as a surgical anesthetic that had the advantage of not depressing respiration or blood pressure or causing heart irregularities. By 1965, however, almost half of all patients administered PCP had experienced delirium, disorientation, hallucinations, anxiety, and agitation. PCP can be smoked, taken orally, or injected intravenously. It creates a sense of disconnection by blocking glutamate receptors. It also releases dopamine, with the pleasure and excitement that go along with it, and acts on the sigma opioid receptors, which block pain as well as cause hallucinations. This combination of actions causes PCP to have more unpredictable effects than any hallucinogen. PCP's effects look like a combination of those of alcohol, amphetamines, and hallucinogens. Signs of PCP intoxication include slurred speech; impaired coordination; increased heart rate, blood pressure, and temperature; a dissociative state; and lowered sensitivity to pain and increased belligerence.

- *Ketamine* ("Special K," "Vitamin K") is a PCP-like substance used in anesthesia. It was used for emergency surgeries in Vietnam and in situations where gas anesthetic could not be used, such as short surgical procedures around the head and neck and in the case of facial burns. However, there was a problem with patients jerking and having bad dreams during surgeries. In fact ketamine does not cause unconsciousness, so it is not really an anesthetic (it is currently used primarily as a veterinary tranquilizer). Rather, it causes a dream-like state and an inability to move or feel pain, so it is more often used on patients who cannot report discomfort (such as infants) or who cannot tolerate the cardiovascular effects of other anaesthetics. It also causes hallucinations, disorientation, delayed nightmares, dizziness, confusion, slurred speech, and amnesia. Since the 1980s it has been used as a club drug in both the gay and straight party scenes. Ketamine can be taken orally, snorted, or injected intravenously or intramuscularly. Like PCP, it causes a sense of disconnection by blocking certain glutamate receptors. The "K-hole," the ultimate ketamine experience, is a dreamlike state, hallucinations, and an inability to move or feel pain.

- *Nitrous oxide* was developed in 1798 by a British chemist who noticed a very pleasant effect of lightness and giddiness. By the early 1800s, it had been nicknamed "laughing gas" and was used recreationally at parties as a nonalcoholic intoxicant in Britain and the United States. In the 1840s, a dentist using it recreationally noticed that people felt no pain while high. He started using it in his dental practice. When used recreationally, it is dispensed from tanks diverted from medical usage and then used to fill balloons to breathe from, or in the form of "whippets," the gas delivery system in cans of whipped cream. A mild anesthetic, the action of nitrous oxide, like the other gas anesthetics, is not clear. It may dissolve membranes between nerves in the brain. Nitrous creates feelings of euphoria, behavioral disinhibition, and pain reduction for a few minutes, as well as a feeling of well-being for several hours. Occasional loss of consciousness is followed by sensory distortion and nausea. It deprives the brain and body of oxygen in proportion to how much is breathed.

- *Dextromethorphan (DXM)* is a nonnarcotic cough suppressant in several over-the-counter cough syrups. It prevents the reuptake of dopamine. It stimulates heart rate, blood pressure, and sweating. The "third plateau" is the high that people usually seek. It takes at least four ounces to get high, and the high can last ten hours.

Dependence, Tolerance, and Withdrawal

Tolerance develops to some of these drug effects. PCP is the only one of these drugs that causes laboratory animals to compulsively take more and more of it.

Benefits

These drugs dissolve self-consciousness, create a sense of detachment, of increase tolerance of physical pain, and decrease fear and anxiety.

Risks

- *PCP* can cause psychosis, accidents, and fights; it is an unpredictable drug that may be added to other drugs, so be careful.
- People on *ketamine* can fall if they try to move around; they may also experience nausea and vomiting, breathing problems, racing heart, and confusion. Ketamine can cause psychosis in vulnerable people.
- *Nitrous* is very cold and can damage the lungs, cause accidents when movement is attempted, and deplete the body of vitamin B_{12}, which can cause neuropathy (damage to the peripheral nerves) over time; damage also can be caused by expanding gas—overinflating lungs or trachea or mouth if not well regulated.
- The cough syrups containing *DXM* can cause nausea.

Greatest Dangers

All dissociative anesthetics can cause *Olney's lesions*, holes in the brain in the areas responsible for socialization, memory, evaluating one's own behavior, learning in new situations, visual perception, understanding metaphors, and pairing emotions to experience. It is possible that the longer you use, the greater the risk. There is some evidence that the use of benzodiazepines can prevent these lesions, but that is only laboratory evidence, not tests done on real people.

- *PCP* can cause general anesthesia at two to five times the recreational dose, very high temperature, increased blood pressure (which can cause stroke), seizure, coma, decreased respiration, a psychotic state, extreme agitation, belligerence, and traumatic injury.
- *Nitrous* can cause suffocation due to carbon dioxide buildup, especially when the nitrous in a balloon is recycled.
- *DXM* can cause nausea and an extremely elevated temperature.

Drug Interactions

- Yohimbine, antipsychotic medications, and antihistamines can increase the risk of Olney's lesions.
- Any drugs that lower the seizure threshold (for example, the antidepressant Wellbutrin, GHB, stimulants) increase the risk of seizure because the brain is already stimulated.
- Any drugs that decrease respiration increase the risk of overdose, with coma being the most dangerous point.
- Antidepressant medications (MAOIs and SSRIs) and ecstasy increase levels of serotonin and increase the risk of serotonin syndrome (the brain and muscles overheating).
- Protease inhibitors (antiretroviral medications for HIV such as ritonavir) may increase ketamine levels, thus increasing heart rate, blood pressure, and difficulty breathing.
- Ritalin and ketamine may create a condition called *chemical hepatitis* (see *www.thebody.com*)
- Stimulants further increase blood pressure and heart rate and cause risk of stroke.
- Marijuana at high doses may increase the dissociative experience.
- Other hallucinogens may tend to make the drug experience too intense.

Harm Reduction

- Valium or other benzodiazepines can alleviate the effects of PCP overdose and may protect the brain against Olney's lesions. However, benzodiazepines also block the interesting experience of ketamine and cause respiratory depression.
- We need a mix of at least 21 percent oxygen in the air we breathe. It is important to breathe in between doses of nitrous. It is also best not to breathe directly from a tank. Do not recirculate nitrous in the balloon; doing so causes a buildup of carbon dioxide.
- Take extra vitamin B_{12} if you use nitrous.
- Use as little as possible of these drugs. Try to limit your use to no more than two times a week and space the use so that you have a couple of days in between.

- Do not drive or operate other machinery. Watch out for your friends and yourself. Use somewhere that is safe and comfortable.

- If you are responsible for someone's care (child, elder, or person with serious illness), avoid using these drugs at that time. It's just too hard to pull it together when on these drugs.

Inhalants

What Drugs

- *Nitrites*: butyl or amyl nitrite (poppers)
- *Anesthetics*: nitrous oxide, ether, halothane—nitrous oxide, the main recreational drug in this category, is discussed in the preceding section.
- *Solvents*:
  —*Glues* contain acetates, acetone, benzene, hexane, methyl chloride, toluene, and trichloroethylene.
  —*Paints, spray paints, paint thinners, and removers* contain acetone, butylacetate methanol, and toluene.
  —*Sprays*, such as hair spray, deodorants, and air fresheners, contain butane and propane.
  —*Nail polish remover* contains acetone.
  —*Lighter fluids* contain butane and isopropane.
  —*Fuels* such as gasoline contain petroleum products.
  —*Cleaning solutions* contain carbon tetrachloride, petroleum products, and trichloroethylene.

Most of the preceding compounds in the various household and industrial products are made from petroleum, as is ether.

- *Nitrites* have been used for medical purposes since the mid-nineteenth-century. They have the same effects as nitroglycerin (1846), an explosive also used to dilate blood vessels in heart patients when the heart spasms. Amyl nitrite (1857), very short-acting, is used only when rapid absorption is needed for cardiac procedures. It turned out to be too short-acting for heart pain caused by blocked blood vessels, so nitroglycerin remains the medication of choice. Although nitroglycerin is taken orally (dissolved under the tongue), amyl and butyl nitrite should be inhaled. Nitrites relax smooth muscle tissue, which regulates size of blood vessels, the bladder, and the anus (thereby facilitating anal sex). They both lower blood pressure, increase heart rate, and create a sense of warmth, lowered inhibition, euphoria, exhilaration, and acceleration before orgasm.

- *Solvents* are not intended for human consumption. They are volatile compounds developed for household and industrial use as cleaners and solvents. Because they are cheap or free and easily available, they are used by the youngest of drug users, particularly in Latin America. Of all psychoactive substances, they are the most destructive. They have effects similar to those of alcohol and anesthetics: euphoria and initial stimulation, followed by central nervous system depression. In addition, solvents cause incoordination, hallucinations, delusions, flushing, double vision, suppression of vital functions like respiration and heart function, and impaired judgment.

Dependence, Tolerance, and Withdrawal

Tolerance develops to *nitrites*, and cardiac problems can occur in withdrawal as the blood vessels contract in the absence of the drug. The same symptoms appear as when one started using—headaches, dizziness, and weakness.

Benefits

As with all psychoactive substances, the ability of inhalants to alter experience and get one "out of it" is attractive and often fun. In the case of *solvents*, this is all that can be said of their benefits. *Nitrites* are more specific in their recreational effects, particularly with regard to enhancing sexual pleasure and creating feelings of well-being and stimulation.

Risks

Nitrites can cause headaches and risk dizziness and loss of consciousness if one tries to move rapidly. All of the risks of *solvents* really fall into the category of dangers, but it is worth noting that accidents are common due to loss of muscle control. Accidents can be avoided by practicing harm reduction. Poppers also may suppress the immune system for several days after use, a serious consideration for people with HIV. They are not recommended for people with low or high blood pressure.

Greatest Dangers

• *Nitrates*: If swallowed, they prevent blood from transporting oxygen, which can lead to death. Nitrites have been suspected of suppressing the immune system and increasing the chances of opportunistic infections in those who are HIV positive, but as is the case for many illegal substances, very little solid research has been done.

• *Solvents*: Cause nothing but damage, especially to the cerebellum, which controls fine motor skills. Anecdotal evidence indicates that memory, attention, and concentration are affected and that 55–65 percent of patients admitted to emergency rooms suffer neurological damage. The long-term effects are unclear. Twenty-six percent of deaths by inhalants are from accidents and 28 percent by suicide. Twenty percent of these deaths are in first-time users.

"Sudden sniffing death" occurs when sniffing gaseous substances such as freon, butane, or propane. These probably interrupt the heart rhythm and increase its sensitivity to adrenaline.

Drug Interactions

When using these inhalants, the most important drugs to avoid using simultaneously are central nervous system depressants such as alcohol, sedatives, or opiates.

DO NOT MIX POPPERS WITH VIAGRA—THE INTERACTION MAY LEAD TO DANGEROUSLY LOW BLOOD PRESSURE.

Harm Reduction

Use nitrites as seldom as possible. Plan your use, enjoy it while it lasts, but put your heart through these changes as little as possible. CALL 911 IF YOU SWALLOW POPPERS.

It is tempting to say JUST SAY NO to solvents. — Since, as harm reductionists, we can't just tell you what to do and expect that you'll do it—and given that at least 15 percent of U.S. high school kids have tried them, and millions of children in Latin America use them—at least try to minimize some of the risk:

- Use as little as possible.
- Remember that other drugs can get you high and do far less damage than these.
- Move around as little as possible to avoid accidents.
- If you feel suicidal, get your friend(s) to help you find someone you can trust to talk to.
- Don't drive or operate other machinery.
- As with any drug that causes disorientation, if you are a parent or a caretaker, plan your use for times that you don't have to take care of anyone.

SOURCES AND SUGGESTED READINGS

All of the books in the Alcohol, Drugs, and Pharmacology section of the Sources and Suggested Readings in Harm Reduction in the appendix, and all of the informational websites and harm reduction organizations in the Resources section in the appendix contain the above information and much more. For a very readable book about drugs, you might try Buzzed. *For a more dense and excellent guide to drugs, read Robert Julien's* A Primer of Drug Action.

You might also be interested in reading Mike Gray's Drug Crazy *and David Musto's* The American Disease *about the history of drug-related attitudes and legislation.*

For the article on the latest study of the effects of drinking on heart health:

"Roles of Drinking Pattern and Type of Alcohol Consumed in Coronary Heart Disease in Men." Kenneth J. Mukamal, et. al. *The New England Journal of Medicine, 348*(2), 109–118, 2003.

7 PRACTICING
HARM REDUCTION
Substance Use Management

If you have not yet decided to be abstinent, or have decided to quit but you're just not ready, if you've decided to keep using but want to manage your alcohol and other drug use better, the resources available to you are pretty slim. That's the point of this chapter (actually, that's the point of this whole book!). This active involvement with managing your alcohol or drug use is called, not surprisingly, *Substance Use Management.* You can use it, according to the information in this chapter, by yourself or with the help of friends, a family member, or a therapist. This information may help you manage your drug use. It may also save your life. But it is not a guarantee.

Remember, harm is relative. As the Renaissance physician Paracelsus pointed out, "The poison is in the dose." This is just as true for botulin (now used to reduce facial wrinkles) as it is for nicotine, alcohol, or ketamine. The history of drug use dates back to the earliest civilizations, when few were concerned that people should avoid psychoactive substances. Using drugs was a normal part of many cultures. When physicians, philosophers, and the general public did express concern, however, it had to do with the amount of alcohol or drugs a person used, the "dose." Eventually, how much a person used *over time* became just as important as how much he or she consumed at any *one* time. This is the attitude of those who use Substance Use Management. It's not *what* you use necessarily, but how, when, where, and how much you use that contributes to either harm or safety.

Substance Use Management (SUM) is a term widely used in the harm reduction movement to describe any steps taken to control your use of, and the harms associated with, alcohol or other drugs. SUM relies on your ability and willingness to *observe* yourself. It also assumes that you, and only you, are responsible for what you put into your body. The suggestions offered here are derived from books about drugs, websites, public health pamphlets, harm reduction videos, professional books and lectures, our clients, and our experience as therapists. It is general information that is publicly available. It is unlikely to cover all that might be involved in your particular drug use patterns. That would take half a library, but we'll give you several other resources to check out.

This chapter is meant to give you a structure to guide you through your own decision-making process and to offer a few specific ideas for how to use more wisely and more safely. The information on each class of drugs in the center of the book is more detailed and can be used in conjunction with the methods described here. If you've decided to quit but want to take it slow, you can use the suggestions in this chapter as steps toward abstinence.

We are not medical doctors and therefore are not qualified to give medical advice or prescriptions. It's a good idea to talk with a medical professional about your drug or alcohol use. Read Chapter 9 for some suggestions on how to talk to your doctor. If you don't feel comfortable talking to him or her, we understand. It's hard to find a doctor who can talk with you about drinking and drug use without immediately telling you that you should quit. If you don't have access to professional advice, you'll have to put together a plan for yourself. Look for other drug users to talk to, but *only those you think do a good job of taking care of themselves and who seem to be educated about the drugs they use*. There are many people in the harm reduction movement you can talk to—just call the Harm Reduction Coalition office in New York or Oakland. A needle exchange program is a good place to go, too, even if you aren't an injection drug user. People there know a lot about most drugs.

SUM is based on three principles: (1) being **honest** with yourself about your drug use and the impact of drugs in your life; (2) being **willing** to make some changes; and (3) learning the **skills** to help you make concrete, beneficial changes in your alcohol or other drug use.*

Hopefully you have already used this book to help you face your drug use honestly. At this point you've probably decided that *something* has got to change. There are many options to consider. Specific SUM techniques include:

---

*Special thanks for the information in this section goes to Edith Springer, to the Harm Reduction Coalition, and to Dan Bigg of the Chicago Recovery Alliance, for extensive details and perspective. Thanks also to the many syringe exchange workers and clients who keep perfecting these suggestions. You can order pamphlets from the Harm Reduction Coalition in New York and a video on safer injection techniques from the Chicago Recovery Alliance.

- Changing the amount of alcohol or drug used.
- Changing the numbers/types of drugs used together.
- Changing the frequency with which you drink or use.
- Changing the route of administration (how you put the drug into your body).
- Changing the situation (using alone versus with others, etc.).
- Planning your use.
- Making drug substitutions.
- Taking overdose prevention measures.
- Quitting altogether.

Most people find it difficult to believe that these are viable options for them. So much is said about a person with alcohol or drug problems being "out of control" and "powerless" that the idea of exerting control over any part of the experience seems ludicrous. But we know many people who can and do control their use. We don't even know you, and we're pretty sure you do, too. Otherwise you wouldn't be reading this book right now.

Many factors determine how easy or hard it will be to make changes, to control your use. Some of these are psychological, some social. Some are actually created by the physical effects of a specific drug. SUM pays particular attention to these physical barriers to change. We'll use the structure of drug, set, and setting to help you go about changing. It's important to think of each drug separately, as you did when you answered the questions in Chapter 6. It is then important to think about the combinations that you use. Using the drug, set, setting model, we'll explain how each area of change works. You will notice that we might not talk about your particular drug in one or more sections. That's because some drugs lend themselves to certain kinds of changes better than others. For example, it's easier to change the amount of heroin than crack cocaine, which people tend to use compulsively. But it's easier to change the frequency of crack cocaine than heroin, which requires regular planned dosing.

Changing the Amount

Drug

Less is more. You are more likely to actually *enjoy* your drug experience if you don't do it all the time or in large quantities. This is because of tolerance. If you've been drinking or using for a while, chances are you're using a lot more now than when you started. Your body has gotten used to some of the effects and made changes to keep the drug from having too dramatic an effect on you. So you continue to need more to get high, as your body tries to balance out your use. This is tolerance.

If recreation is your goal, and you're drinking or using heavily, it makes sense to reduce the overall amount you use. If you can reduce the amount, you'll become more sensitive to a smaller dose. To decrease the amount, you'll have to deal with the fact of tolerance. Your goal is to decrease your tolerance so that you can actually control your use without suffering. If you're not totally physically dependent, the best and easiest way to decrease tolerance is to quit using for a while. Even a few days can make a difference, but a few weeks is a better length of time. This time off will give you a chance to decide how much you will use once you start again. If you've been using for a long time, you might have trouble maintaining your new dose level. Don't be discouraged. You may have to quit and restart many times to get used to a lower level of use (for example, regular or even occasional instead of heavy).

If you *are* physically dependent (you get sick or shaky when you try to quit), lowering your tolerance will be harder and may actually be dangerous. The point is to lower the amount enough to make a difference without causing you too much discomfort. If you try to "tough it out," your chances of succeeding go down, and your risk of medical problems goes up. If you're dependent on alcohol, benzodiazepines (such as Valium, Xanax, Ativan, Klonopin), or barbiturates, you run the risk of serious medical problems—convulsions or death—if you quit abruptly or drastically cut down. Going "cold turkey" or "kicking" is a very stressful thing to do. It creates a biological crisis, never mind a psychological one. There is some evidence that this stress can actually impair your immune system. You might be better off going the traditional medical detoxification route until your tolerance is safely lowered, especially if you have HIV, diabetes, a heart condition, or other problems that are made worse by stress. If you have a physician or nurse you could talk to about this (professionally or even a friend), it would be a good idea. Of course, finding a doctor who will help you with this approach might be tough. At the very least, talk to a friend who has some experience with the drugs with which you're dealing. Call poison control or a local drug hot line for information. Talk to someone at a needle exchange program. Go to different websites for tips.

A lot has been written lately about the use of acupuncture for both detoxification and managing cravings. Dr. Michael Smith of the Lincoln Hospital Acupuncture Program in the Bronx was one of the people to develop "AcuDetox," an acupuncture method that consists of placing five needles in points in your ear. This method has been shown to be useful for most people. You might also try massage, yoga, and other types of nurturing activities to help manage your withdrawal.

Whether you've decided to lower your tolerance on your own or with a friend, you first have to know exactly how much you are using! This is easy for alcohol and pills. For heroin, cocaine, marijuana, and party drugs, it's harder to know how much is in each dose you take. You know how many hits you're taking, or how large a hit, but not the potency until you see how high you get.

For alcohol, the general rule is that each official "drink" contains either 1.5 ounces (a shot glass) of distilled spirits, 5 ounces of wine, 8 ounces of malt liquor or wine cooler, or 12 ounces of beer (a regular can or bottle). When you start drinking, have a pen and paper handy, use your Palm Pilot or other PDA, or write on your arm. Put a penny on the bar for each drink. Count the number of "drinks" in each of the drinks you consume (if you put two shots of vodka in orange juice, that counts as two drinks).

For pills that are legal pharmaceuticals, the dose is standard (five or ten milligrams of Valium, half or one milligram of Klonopin, etc.). All of the drugs in one class are equal, meaning that the doses sound different but are actually equivalent in potency. Count either the number of pills you are using daily or the total dosage.

Once you know how much you're drinking or using, you can begin a reduction plan. You might want to start by writing the details of your current use in a journal or notebook—how much, how often, etc. Keep track for a week or two. That way you will know how much you typically use and then can really keep track of your progress. The general rule of thumb is *"Start low and slow until you know."* This means cutting down a little at a time so as to reduce the stress on your body. Stay at each new level until it feels comfortable or normal to you. You might notice that as you cut down more and more, you won't be able to do it as quickly as you could at the beginning. It's like dieting—it's easier to lose the first ten pounds than the last five. You'll know if your efforts are working not only by how you feel, but by checking back with your journal to see the difference in your use over time.

A slow reduction process looks like a staircase that you're walking down. Start by cutting down by one to three doses. For example, if you typically have eight beers when you go out, try having only seven (or five). If you drink Manhattans, try what a friend in New York calls a "reverse Manhattan" (reverse the measures of the whiskey and the vermouth). Start with a large glass of water or juice before your first drink. Have some food. Then drink a glass of water after each alcoholic beverage. Drink slowly. You probably like to drink that first drink fast, though, because it hits you harder. If you really enjoy feeling the first drink, go ahead and gulp it. You can do your controlling later, but it'll be harder. If you feel really shaky the next day (when you're detoxing from the night before), you're reducing the amount too fast. Go back up for a day or so.

If pills are your thing, count the number you take at any one time and reduce it by one or two pills. Pay attention to how you feel. If you're physically dependent, you won't get as high and you may feel a little shaky and anxious. A little shaky is probably not dangerous, but if you start to sweat or feel nauseated and you're shaking quite a bit, or if you feel confused or panicky, you need medical assistance. In fact, if you feel confused or are nauseated, you should go to an emergency room. Then you'll have to rethink your decision to try this on your own.

If heroin is your drug, a slow reduction might mean starting off at your usual eight-bag day, then using only seven and a half bags tomorrow. See how you feel. If you're not too uncomfortable, try doing only seven the next day. As with any drug, stay at the new level until it feels almost normal to you. That's how you'll know that you can reduce some more. This may take a while. As you reduce your dose, your body has to get used to the change. The more you reduce, the longer it might take for the adjustment. You may find that for the first few weeks you can reduce a little each day, but then you find that you have to wait three days or a week at a new, lower dose before you start feeling normal again. *Low and slow until you know.*

One tip from pharmacology: It's hard to reduce the amount of a drug that has a rapid onset (hits you fast) and is short-acting (doesn't last long). Your body hates it when things change fast, and it reacts by making you feel lousy when the drug wears off (crashing) and by creating cravings so you'll use more to make it feel better again. So, once you start a run of cocaine (or cigarettes, for that matter), it's hard to stop until you run out. It's easier to control a slower-acting drug such as alcohol or heroin. So if you are a binge user and can't get control of the amount you use, and if it's a short-acting drug, you might want to look at the section on changing the frequency of your use. In the meantime, be extra good to yourself in between binges. Do things that make you happy or more relaxed. Go to a movie. Eat chocolate. Whatever. Beating up on yourself when you're not even using just doesn't make sense!

Set

The *set* is you—your personality, emotional strengths or problems, as well as your motivation and expectations. Maybe you've smoked marijuana for the past ten years. You might realize, after reading this book, that you increased your smoking only after your sister was killed in a car accident or after you had an abortion. Chances are that your increase in pot use was your attempt to medicate feelings of anger, loss, or helplessness. To change the amount of pot you smoke, you're probably going to have to deal directly with those painful events and feelings. Read a book about grief. Go to a support group. Get into therapy. Write in a journal. Talk to a friend about it—all of it. A lot of different kinds of therapy are out there now, ones that don't require that you spend a million years talking about your childhood. These include cognitive–behavioral, solution-focused, and narrative styles of therapy. All of these can be useful. Look at Chapter 9 to learn more about finding the help that is right for you.

The best way to reduce your consumption is to know what you want out of the experience. What is your motivation and what are your goals? Do you want to have fun, bury feelings of loss, get completely out of it? Or maybe you really do want to do damage to yourself. Many people use alcohol and other drugs just to get high, for the pleasure of it. Is that truly how and why you started using and why you use now? If so, you're very motivated by pleasure. Then pay attention to how you feel. Paying attention to your experience while using—the music, the sounds, your peace of mind, etc.—will help focus you on controlling the amount. Are you using more than you need to achieve the experience you were looking for? Are you getting as much out of your drug as you did when you first started using, or has it just become a routine? If you were happy with your drug experience, you wouldn't be reading this. So, what do you need to do to make your use pleasurable again? If you want to get pleasantly high, less is more! Of course, if your goal is to get wrecked, you really *don't* want to reduce the amount. Try a different SUM technique.

Go through the same exploration with other motivations and personal characteristics. How big are you, what gender are you, and how much drug can you tolerate? Are you using for a particular medical or psychiatric effect—pain, anxiety, depression, or grief management? You'll have a hard time changing the amount you use until you take care of those issues in some other way—by talking, taking the right medication, practicing meditation, receiving acupuncture treatments, giving yourself hot baths, going for satisfying walks, or in some way attending to your suffering.

Setting

Setting includes all sorts of things in your environment—the people, the places, and the situations in which you use. If you want to reduce the amount you're using, see how difficult this might be to manage in your particular environment. Do you go for happy hour after work? Or, if you use on the streets, does everyone drink out of the same bottle or smoke the same rock, so it's hard to know how much you've had? When you go to a club, are you sharing a bottle of GHB or a bag of heroin? A lot of drug and alcohol use is social. If your friends are big consumers, it could be anything from awkward to virtually impossible to control how much you use. Try avoiding these situations until you've reduced your use. That way, you will have some success under your belt, and you can transfer your learning to your old situation. Beware, however, if you are a heroin user. More overdoses occur when regular users use in unfamiliar environments. If you switch settings, use a smaller dose at first.

On the other hand, if you're a loner when you drink, smoke, or shoot too much, and you're more moderate in public, consider restricting yourself to social situations to reduce the amount you use. Or if you use more heavily in situations that make you feel bad—Sunday dinners with your quarreling family, for example—avoid them for a while, if you can.

In general, look around at your surroundings and see how they might contribute to your drug experience. If you use equipment, do you have a place to clean it and keep it sterile? If you use outside, are you safe from the police so you don't have to rush your hit? Is your home depressing, making you want to get higher?

Changing the Number/Types of Drugs You Mix Together

Drug

Many of the *short-term* harmful effects of alcohol or drugs are related to interactions when you take more than one drug at a time. Some drugs cancel out the action of another. Other drugs may actually slow down the metabolism of another drug, which means more of the drug hangs around in your system, putting you in more danger of overdose, even if you haven't taken much. Still other drugs speed up the metabolism and get rid of the drug effect much faster. For example, regular use of barbiturates causes certain liver enzymes to increase. It's these chemicals that break down (metabolize) the drugs you take. If the enzymes are forced to increase, that means your liver is breaking down things more quickly. For barbiturates, that means that you'll develop tolerance and have to use more to get the same effect. But if you're using other drugs as well, something like antibiotics, which are broken down by the same enzymes, then you're probably not getting enough of the medicine. The biology can get really complicated. The *Physicians' Desk Reference (PDR)* has a companion volume for nonmedical folks that describes all of the possible drug interactions of prescribed medications and usually of alcohol as well. It's not a particularly good reference, though, for illegal-drug interactions. Check out the Resources section in the appendix for some good informational websites.

If you use cocaine for recreation, for example, and then add alcohol on top of it to take the edge off or to help you sleep, you're more likely to run into problems. The combination of cocaine and alcohol creates a substance called *cocaethylene,* which is much harder for the liver to metabolize than either alcohol or cocaine alone. Some drugs that are relatively safe even in large quantities—say, a benzodiazepine such as Valium—can turn deadly when mixed with another drug, such as alcohol. Alcohol overcomes the natural limitations of the action of the Valium (or any benzodiazepine) in your brain, making it easier to get too much sedation. Some HIV antiviral medications and protease inhibitors (Norvir is one example) are notorious for not mixing well with street drugs, alcohol, and some other legal drugs. Medications that help control blood pressure can be made less effective with excessive use of stimulants (coffee, too, not just things like speed) or too effective with some of the sedatives, so you experience a dangerous lowering of blood pressure.

Why do you mix different drugs together? It's important to know. If you mix just because all the stuff is there in one place, you might want to be a little pickier. Exactly what *is* this pill? Ask someone. If nobody can tell you any more than "upper" or "downer," then you have to decide: either you'll be a human guinea pig and figure it'll turn out all right, or you don't care if it's safe or not. But maybe you are conscious about the drugs you mix. You shoot heroin for the warm rush of pleasure and deep relaxation and smoke just a little crack to add a spark. Or you snort speed, and a few drinks take the speedy edge off so you can enjoy the speed more.

You can reduce the harm of mixing drugs if you do *one at a time*. Snort some speed (a little less than your usual dose) and wait for the dose to settle to see if you really need to take the edge off. If you pay attention to your first drug and control it, you might not feel the need to counteract one with another. Shoot heroin and wait a while. You may not need to add a stimulant, but if you do want to, you'll know how much if you wait for the full effect of the heroin to hit. If you really like your combo, and you're not getting into trouble with what you combine in a planned way, then try to eliminate *other* drugs. Don't take other things someone might hand you. Tell them you'll try it later, once you've enjoyed this experience. Don't smoke pot with your usual combination (some people don't think pot counts as a drug, but it does!). Or don't drink coffee if you're going to do speed that day.

In general, stimulants and depressants counteract each other and can cause you to use more than you should of either or both. There are certainly idiosyncratic combinations that are dangerous (some antibiotics and alcohol, for example). But the most dangerous drug combinations to beware of involve drugs that are *similar*. Central nervous system depressants do roughly the same thing—the biggest danger is respiratory failure and possible death. Stimulants overexcite the brain and body—stroke and heart attack are the biggest risks. Antidepressant medications are not recommended in combination with stimulants. Some over-the-counter cold remedies are also stimulants. See "What Are These Drugs, Anyway?" in the middle of this book: just say "know."

Set

It's all about you. What are you trying to achieve with your mixture of drugs? Sometimes chaotic mixing of drugs is a way of expressing hopelessness. Some users of a large variety of drugs and drug combinations call themselves "garbage can users." This is a telling phrase. If you don't really care and are just looking to get as high as you can, it might be interesting for you to know why you want that experience. Do you feel as if you are a part of this world, or that you don't really belong anywhere? Do you feel like you don't really deserve to have good things in life? Do you not care if you live or die? Do you think no one else would care either? Or do you feel invulnerable and just assume you'll be okay, no matter what you do? For different people, the reasons are different. If you had a rough childhood, full of fighting or sexual abuse and fear, mixing drugs might be a way of blocking out all of the different kinds of feelings bouncing around inside of you. Recent studies have found that up to 85 percent of women who abuse drugs have a history of childhood abuse and victimization. For these women the world is not a safe place, and they expect to be hurt. Taking drugs is often a way of coping with this pain and fear, even though it may cause harm, including abuse from current drug-using partners.

Some drugs make some feelings worse, while others do a pretty good job of calming you down. Alcohol can numb many feelings; some people have a great time when they're drunk, while others become sad and tearful. Ketamine or PCP, which give a feeling of floating or dreaminess, might really freak you out if you have memories of abuse that come streaming by when you're high. Check out "What Are These Drugs, Anyway?" in the middle of the book to help figure this out. If these are any of the reasons that propel your mixing of drugs, you'll probably need help—some form of therapy, however brief—to deal with underlying issues. Your drug use is protecting you at the same time that it might be harming you. Taking care of yourself might start with just paying attention to yourself.

Setting

A lot of times you might mix drugs because you're in a social scene where people are sharing their drugs with each other. It's a bonding experience, a way of being a good friend. You might be able to talk to your friends about limiting the mix *together* and actually deciding, as a group, which drugs each of you will do when. Have a "designated driver" even if you're not using a car, someone who can watch out for all of you this time. If, however, it's not really a friendship thing, then you might try coming late to the party—after people have done most of their drugs. Or you might use before you go so you're already high and aren't looking for any more drugs. You could also practice refusal skills. That is, practice your lines for saying no. "I've had plenty, thanks," or just "I'm good" often works. Chances are that people won't pressure you to do more drugs; they're just being friendly. Even though your friends might not be pressuring you, just being with them might trigger you to use more. If that's the case, you might have to see them less or add some new friends to the mix.

Changing the Frequency

Drug

If you've tried to cut down on the amount you use and haven't had consistently good results, changing how *often* you use might be more satisfying. The fact is, the less often you use, the less chance you will have to experience harm over the long run. Daily use causes a number of problems, but perhaps the most insidious is that you get used to the *behavior* of using, so that it becomes an automatic habit and you stop paying attention to whether it's doing what you want (bringing pleasure, numbing pain, etc.). Think about drinking coffee in the morning. If you do it every day, you probably could prepare it in your sleep, right? **Paying attention is the fundamental rule of harm reduction. If your drug use is automatic (a habit), you're not thinking.**

Another problem with daily use is that you often develop tolerance and physical dependence, so that going without becomes difficult or impossible. To change the frequency, *just start changing something*. If alcohol is your drug of choice and you usually start with a couple of drinks at lunch, then end up drinking most of the rest of the day and evening, try delaying that first drink for an hour. Or stop drinking at lunch for a week or two. Now you're drinking only at night. The next step is to pick a day that would be the easiest for you not to drink at all.

If you use speed every day, going without is not going to feel good. You'll feel run down, hungry, and depressed. Pick a day when you don't have to do anything, don't use, and just let yourself complain and be miserable. *You don't have to be brave about this*. Or try the opposite. Pick a day that'll keep you busy and sufficiently distracted. Being home alone with nothing to do can make it harder to stick with your plan. If you use multiple drugs, cut out the one that will be the easiest to do without for a day. Once you get used to going for a day without alcohol or drugs, you can add another day until you reach your goal.

Some drugs lend themselves better to changing frequency than others. If you are a maintenance heroin or other opiate user, this is a ridiculous suggestion. You can't change your frequency—you dose whenever the last dose is running out. You should go back to reducing the amount gradually. If you're a daily heavy drinker, depending on the level of your physical dependence, it may be impossible to stop for a day. You, too, might have to reduce the amount or be medically detoxed. On the other hand, if you are a binge drinker—every weekend all weekend or every two and a half weeks—you could try spacing out your binges. If you're a regular cigarette smoker, you also aren't going to quit for a day, although it's a good idea. But you could cut down from twenty to seventeen cigarettes a day. Crack cocaine and speed, on the other hand, are particularly difficult to control amount-wise. Once you start, they create a compulsion to keep on going till you run out of money or collapse. Reducing frequency is usually the best way to get some control. Whatever your pattern is, find something to interrupt it.

Some drugs (well, all drugs) are probably best used in moderation. But some cause brain changes that lead us to be concerned not just about the amount but also about frequency of use (since dose is often controlled by the user of some of these drugs). Ecstasy's effect on serotonin nerve cells is becoming a concern. Ketamine and other dissociatives (dextromethorphan—the stuff in cough syrups—nitrous, and PCP) have been discovered to cause brain lesions (holes, like Swiss cheese, in the brain) called Olney's lesions. The less you do these drugs, the better. However, they provide many users with wonderful experiences, either of closeness to others, hallucinatory visions, lessening of self-consciousness, or insights into self or the world. If you don't want to give up those experiences, try treasuring them more and pursuing them less.

Inhalants such as glue and gasoline cause brain damage, too. And not just sometimes. We'd like to tell you not to use them at all, but they might be your only way to get out of your head. So use as little as possible, since no one knows of any really safe way to use these drugs.

Set

If you're drinking or using daily, it probably means that there are a lot of other things that you're *not* doing—things that you actually *want* to do! What might some of these things be? Do you like watching old films on TV but find that, by the time they come on at 8:00 P.M., you're too loaded to pay attention? Do you like to walk around and window-shop or people-watch? If you find that you just can't get yourself to do anything or even make a list, you might actually be depressed. A symptom of depression is not being able to enjoy anything. If this is the case, start by getting treatment for your depression. If adequately treated, you might find it easier to do other things to change the frequency of your drug use. Try making a date with someone who depends on you, which might increase your motivation to stick to that other activity. Promise to stop by after work and help someone fix her car. Ask a friend to go grocery shopping with you. Establishing a list of pleasures, projects, or experiences gives you substitutes for using. Make a schedule of activities to keep you distracted. Maybe you have a big project due at work and could stay there with coworkers to finish. Volunteer to do some work for a group that meets in the evening.

One of the major obstacles that you'll run into is called *impulse control.* When you decide not to use for a day, then get tempted by the smell of weed and find your plan dissolving, it's difficult to control the urge to use. Some people experience drug cravings, and others just feel out of sorts, lost, or anxious, not knowing what to do with themselves. Often people feel horribly deprived when they try to cut back or not use. That's why we keep saying to take it easy, go slow. Although distractions might work, it does finally come down to controlling your impulse to use. Pure and simple. Impulse control, if not readily available to you, requires skills and practice. It does *not* come naturally. It is easier for some people than others, for sure, and people with drug problems often have a harder time controlling impulses. But practicing will get you over the hump.

There are many great techniques for impulse control. Most involve either distraction or location change. One that we like is timing the impulse. When you first feel the wish to use, check the time and write it down, if you can. Then just stand still. Don't do anything. Or if it's easier, move around, adjust the window shades, get a drink of water. Distract yourself for a while. *The impulse will go away.* As soon as you notice that you temporarily forgot about using, check the time. Was it one minute or ten? This is your time frame for controlling yourself. You can say to yourself, "If I can wait ten minutes, this urge to use will go away." Now, of course, the urge will come back, maybe right away, maybe not for another hour. Check the time again and do it over. The point that you're trying to teach yourself is that *"This urge will go away whether or not I use!"*

Setting

It's harder at first to change yourself, so try to change your environment. Sometimes you just have to get away from the source of your drugs or alcohol to be successful at using less frequently. Happy hours and TGIF parties are notorious for encouraging heavy drinking. Try going out to eat one day a week instead. Or, if you're a solitary drinker, go out to a movie with friends. If you end up doing coke every time you go to a club, rent videos instead for a night. Reducing the cues for use is important in controlling cravings and urges. One of the best ways to cut out a day is to do it with a friend, whether or not the friend is a drug user. The support really helps.

Changing the Route of Administration (How You Take the Drug)

Drug

There are as many ways to get a drug into your body as there are creative people to think about it! Some are considerably riskier than others. You can swallow a drug, smoke it, snort it, put it in other mucous membranes, inhale the fumes, rub it on your skin, or use a needle to put it in a vein, a muscle, or under your skin. Some drugs are "naturally" taken only in certain forms. Alcohol is swallowed. Nitrous oxide is a gas, so it is inhaled. Other drugs cannot be taken in oral form because stomach acids eat them up. Suppositories are inserted only into the anus. Most drugs, however, can be prepared in several different ways and used by various routes of administration. *In general*, eating a drug is the safest route, and shooting up into a vein is the most dangerous. Smoking isn't very good either, since hot smoke irritates the lung, and some drugs are mixed with tobacco first, so you get all the health risks of cigarettes as well. Any way you use can be made more or less safe.

If you use needles, what do you like about this route? Do you like the rush that comes with it, the second most rapid way of getting a drug to your brain and the best way to get *all* of it there, or do you also get off on the needle itself? This might make it hard for you to decide to smoke your dope. Smoking is not a very efficient use of your drug, since, well, a lot of it goes up in smoke. Thank goodness for that, since a cigar contains enough nicotine to kill you, but most of it ends up as a greenhouse gas. But it *is* the fastest. You might try snorting it, but some drugs don't cut up very well into a fine powder (heroin), and some burn more than others (speed). Some ways of shooting are always dangerous. For example, does your drug of choice come in a pill form? Opiates often do. Eat pills if you can, but don't crush pills to inject—the particles are often too big and cause abscesses in your veins or in the smaller vessels in your lungs. Oxycontin, an oral opiate, is time released when it's in pill form. Crushing and shooting that one will give you a *much* stronger dose than swallowing it and can easily cause you to overdose. Cocaine can only be injected into a vein—you can't "skin pop" it or put it into a muscle without risking a toxic skin infection. Can you do your drug by some other route and save the IV for special occasions? If so, your body will like it. Doing this will slightly lower your tolerance, and you'll get more out of the shot.

If it comes down to your liking to shoot because it gets you off better, then safe injection is the harm reduction practice for you. There are numerous pamphlets and a good video that teaches how to make your injections safer (for example, *Getting Off Right,* put out by the Harm Reduction Coalition in New York). The first thing to put into practice is using a clean needle for each shot. Not only the needle, but the cooker and cotton and tie must be absolutely clean to prevent the spread of diseases such as HIV and hepatitis, and also to prevent nasty skin and heart infections. It's always risky to share any of your equipment with others. If you don't have a choice, remember that sharing needles requires careful hygiene with bleach and water to prevent problems. Rotate injection sites to let puncture wounds heal. A *new* needle for each shot is ideal but often impossible to manage. Each use of the needle makes it duller and causes more damage to your veins. A rule of thumb: **if it hurts, pull out the needle**. An IV injection should not cause pain (the needle itself shouldn't hurt, but the particular drug might burn). If it does, you've missed the vein and may be in a nerve, an artery, or just sensitive tissue. If you're using an unknown potency of drug, test a little of it before you give yourself the whole shot. It'll act like an early warning signal if it's too strong or mixed with junk. The bottom line: Shoot safe.

If you smoke, be aware that for short-acting drugs like cocaine (and, of course, nicotine), smoking is the fastest way for it to get to your brain, but the drug doesn't last long. That will make you want to do more and more, faster and faster. This is where overdose becomes a problem. Try slowing down your use. Set a schedule. Distract yourself. The point is to stay high, not to have muscle spasms and heart attacks. You'll have more fun and stay safer if you limit your smoking to no more than once an hour. Also, it's best if you don't mix your dope with tobacco—why have *that* in your system if you're not a regular cigarette smoker?

If you snort, take care of your poor nose. Heroin is not abrasive, but cocaine and speed are. Mix the powder with a little water and spray it in. Or rub the inside of your nose with vitamin E oil before using. Crushed pills won't pass into the blood vessels in your nose very well, so you might as well just swallow them or mix them in water and drink.

If you drink or eat, what you have in your stomach can make a lot of difference. If you drink alcohol on a full stomach, it will take longer to be absorbed. This is a good thing, because your judgment isn't as impaired by getting high fast, so you can make better decisions about the next drink. But sometimes you just really want a quick buzz, and you end up drinking more than you intended. Try having the first drink on an empty stomach so it hits you faster. Enjoy the buzz. But have food on hand and start eating after you begin to feel the effects, to slow down the process for the next drinks. Don't worry. It's not true that food makes you less high. It just slows it down.

If you're eating marijuana, figuring out how much is enough will take a bit of experimenting. Ask your dealer about the potency. Share recipes with your friends. When in doubt, eat just a little (a quarter of a brownie, for example) and wait an hour to see how you feel. Then do a little more. If you want a smooth high to last all evening, this is a great way to do it. If, however, you don't have much time, or you want to get a blast, smoking is the best way. Eating it just takes too long to absorb and feel the effects.

If you're taking pills, the important thing is to know whether they are standard legal drugs or have been manufactured in a home lab. You can look up standard drugs in textbooks and online to see what you've got and how strong they are. You can also research how a particular drug interacts with others. For homemade pills, such as ecstasy or LSD, you'll have to ask around. Does anyone know what it is and how strong it is? Has anyone taken this particular pill before? Take only one if you're not sure. You can always do more later.

If you feel weird or sick after taking something, don't go off by yourself. Find someone fast. Sometimes just talking to someone will calm you down and help you assess whether you're really in danger. Don't worry about your pride or the cops or anyone's opinion. Take care of yourself. If you don't want anyone to know, call 911. Call poison control. And next time, try to use unknown drugs only when you're with people who can take care of each other if things go bad. Never leave a person who is clearly overly intoxicated or sick. He might not sleep it off. He might just die.

Set

Some people have trouble changing the route of administration for personal or emotional reasons. You might not be very assertive, so you have trouble saying no to a particular activity. You might not have enough information about how else to take drugs. A lot of young women do not know how to shoot their own drugs and are dependent on someone else to do it for them. This is potentially very unsafe—you can't control anything if you're not in charge. Learn how to shoot up yourself.

When you develop a relationship with a drug, you usually also get attached to all the rituals involved in using it. So even if you're still using the same drug, just in a different way, it may not feel as pleasurable at first. You might miss the *way* you used. This reaction often goes away over time, but in the short run you'll have to be gentle with yourself. You've just lost a part of your experience, and it'll take some getting used to. Go ahead and grieve for your loss. It's real. It may help to remind you, each time you use, that you're doing it this way so that you *can* continue to enjoy the drug.

Setting

You may not have much of a choice about the route if only one option is available where you live or with whom you do drugs. If you don't have a stable place to live, the process of preparing a drug to smoke instead of shoot might be more difficult. On the other hand, if you're shooting up on the streets or in a bathroom at a club, you often don't have the time, the light, or the space to do it cleanly or safely. Changing where you use may make a huge difference to your safety. Maybe you'll decide to shoot only at your own place and snort or smoke when you're out. Be aware, if you are shooting heroin, that your tolerance may not be as high if you use in a new situation.

Test your shot to avoid overdose! Know your dealer. Try to use the same one every time. He or she probably doesn't want to cause you harm, and you can probably trust what he or she says about the potency of the cut.

Changing the Situation

Drug

If you're in a bar, the drug that's available is alcohol! If you are at a certain street corner, whatever the person is selling is what you can have. Sometimes changing the situation will automatically change the drug you use. Decide what you want, and don't want, to use. Decide what effect you want to have. Make sure you have what you want and so are less tempted by whatever else is offered. Most people have a drug of choice. Don't settle for second choice!

Set

This is about you, again. It's amazing how your beliefs and wishes can affect the basic pharmacology of the drug and your response to it. As mentioned earlier, experiments have been done that show that if people want to get high on alcohol but are given a fake beverage unknowingly, they'll get high anyway, even though there's no alcohol in the drink! They were in a drinking *situation,* and they *wanted and expected* to get high, and so they did.

Another factor to consider is how well you stand up for yourself. Being assertive about what you do and don't want to do can be extremely difficult for some people. Chances are, if you have trouble setting limits or saying what you want in relation to your drug use, you probably have the same problem in other areas of your life. The good news is that there are a lot of resources out there to help people increase their assertiveness and self-confidence. Books, therapy, classes at the local college—all can make a difference. You don't have to tell anyone that you're really interested in managing your drug use, just that you want to be more in charge of your life or more assertive. You can avoid the stigma—one of the hugest harms of being a drug user—by just not talking about it in some situations. No one has to know your business.

Setting

This is all about the environmental factors surrounding your drug use. Where you use and with whom can either increase or decrease the riskiness of using the very same drug. As we mentioned before, shooting drugs under the freeway or in a bathroom makes it harder to take your time and use good hygiene. Try to arrange places and times when you can have some privacy, light, access to water, etc. Make sure you can *see* what you're taking. Swallowing a bunch of pills that you can't even see and drinking out of a bottle that you haven't been in control of are sure ways to let the setting control you rather than the other way around.

Setting is just as important with alcohol as it is with drugs. You might drink at home and be fine, but if you drink when you're out, you have a tendency to get into fights. Or you find that if you drink with friends, it's a pleasant experience and you don't drink as much. When you're home alone, you tend to get weepy and drink too much. Get to know yourself in different situations. You'll find it easier to manage your drug or alcohol use if you're in charge of *where* you use.

Planning Your Use

You can make some simple rules for yourself that will certainly reduce harm and might even save your life. Planning when and where and with whom to use is actually something you can learn to do pretty easily. Most people think people who use alcohol and drugs, especially people who have problems or abuse these substances, can't possibly think rationally or control themselves in any way. You might even believe this about yourself. But we have learned that people can and do plan how to use to maximize the benefits and minimize the harms. Some simple guidelines that you might make for yourself include:

- **Designate a driver:** either literally have someone to drive you and others who are using or have someone to guide the experience and make sure no one gets hurt (and to call 911 if someone does).
- **Clean your equipment:** pack up your stuff ahead of time if you're going out, or get extra syringes at the exchange when you go. Make sure you have enough cotton, cookers, pipes, etc., before people come over so no one has to share.
- **Choose who you're with and where (especially for psychedelic use):** being with friends or being alone in a place that feels good to you can make an enormous difference and save you from a traumatic trip.
- **Have enough water and food:** start out with some food and water and keep more handy. But if you're using psychedelics, don't eat so much that it makes you vomit—it's pretty uncomfortable.

You can probably come up with a lot more ideas that are particular to you and your situation. Be creative about your health and your fun!

Drug Substitution

Methadone, a synthetic opiate that lasts for twenty-four hours per dose, is the most successful drug treatment in the United States. It has resulted in dramatic improvement in the quality of life, health (HIV prevention is a major success of methadone treatment), and productivity for heroin-dependent people. Unfortunately, there are not nearly enough methadone treatment programs to help all the heroin-addicted folks out there, and the stigma of methadone and the inconvenience factor (methadone is dispensed only on a daily basis by federally controlled clinics) put off many people. Nevertheless, it's remarkably helpful and has saved many lives.

Buprenorphine is another medication treatment for opiate-dependent people that has just been approved by the FDA. It is similar to methadone in that it prevents craving and withdrawal, but it does not create any euphoria. It is best for people who are not dependent on high doses of opiates, as it only partly replaces the effect of opiates. A big advantage is that it can be prescribed in a doctor's office, so you don't have to go to a methadone clinic.

Naltrexone has been used for a long time to treat opiate addicts. It blocks the effects of opiates so you can't get high. You have to want to not get high to use this drug! Naltrexone has also been found effective in reducing the craving for alcohol in alcohol-dependent people.

Marijuana, because it is less harmful than many drugs, might be a consideration for people who are getting into trouble with other drugs but can't face life without something to alter their consciousness. We realize this kind of drug substitution is highly controversial because of the legal status of marijuana, but if you're going to use something, you could do worse than using pot. There are many medical marijuana organizations around the country that you can contact for specifics.

Other medications for conditions that you are trying to medicate are worth considering. Most of the people we work with have problems with anxiety, depression, or posttraumatic stress disorder. Antidepressant medications and a few antianxiety medications are increasingly helpful and targeted to specific symptoms. Do check out this possibility and then see how you feel about your other drugs.

Overdose Prevention

We hope we've addressed overdose liberally throughout this chapter. But no one can give you absolute assurance about safety. Even if you follow guidelines from this book, from a doctor, from professional books and websites, every high might be different, for all the reasons (drug, set, and setting) we've talked about. If you choose to use alcohol, tobacco, or other drugs, you are choosing a certain amount of risk.

Here we offer a few overdose prevention points. You are at greatest risk of overdose if you:

- Mix drugs.
- Don't pay attention to the drugs you're using.
- Shoot drugs but don't do your own shot or test your shot.
- Forget that alcohol can kill you and just try to sleep it off.
- Let people give you drugs that you don't know about.

One other medication to mention is **naloxone** (brand name Narcan), another opiate receptor blocker that is injected and is therefore fast-acting. It actually interrupts a high (so you'll be in withdrawal when you come to), but it's better than dying. Beware that naloxone can wear off before your opiate dose, so make sure you remain under observation and that another naloxone dose is administered if you start to become unconscious again. Narcan is now being distributed by some county public health departments to users, so that friends can take care of friends. Some emergency medical technicians also carry it, as do hospital emergency rooms.

Don't be afraid to call 911 or take your friends to a hospital! Getting in trouble is better than dying. But if you're going to get the law involved, dump your illegal drugs and minimize the harm.

Finally, If You Want to Quit

We won't repeat the advice of the many sources of information about quitting. What we do want to share with you are three ideas by William Miller, a psychologist in New Mexico, who has come up with great innovations to help people who abuse drugs and alcohol. We have mentioned them already in this chapter, but not by name. Miller suggests, in an article about alcohol called "Warm Turkey: Alternative Routes to Abstinence," that you try any one or all of the three strategies. *Tapering* is what we were talking about in changing the amount or frequency. In this case you do it until you aren't drinking anymore. *Sobriety sampling* is a technique where you try abstinence for a while—first to see how attached you are to your drugs by how hard it is to do without, and then to see what you need to do to stay sober. *Trial moderation* is what it sounds like, and the rationale is the same as for sobriety sampling, except that you are not testing your relationship with alcohol by quitting but by seeing if you can drink moderately. If you can't, he says, you should probably quit. We will list a few other books at the end of this chapter that will help you if you want to quit.

Putting It All Together: Practice Makes Perfect

We hope the information in this chapter has been helpful and not too overwhelming. It's a lot to think about because it is a lot to ask of yourself to make significant changes in your alcohol or other drug use. But you've determined that you really are in the preparation or action stage of change, so now's the time. One trick to help you out now is to plan some specific changes and then recheck your willingness to do the things on your list. You may be in a different stage of change with each idea on your list. It might look something like this:

Change the amount of pot that you smoke

1. Don't smoke alone (setting).
2. Don't keep pot in the house (setting).
3. Buy stronger pot (drug).
4. Only smoke when you really need to (set).

Now take a look at your list and see how you feel about it. So *maybe* you could easily not smoke alone, but if it's there in your apartment, it's harder to resist. But if you *don't* keep pot in the house, you may not be able to find it when you need it, and that makes you feel anxious. So #1 isn't possible without #2, and #2 doesn't look like such a good idea to you right now. You are really in either the precontemplation (you can't even think about it) or the contemplation (it's a good idea if you could tolerate it, but you can't right now) stage of change regarding keeping yourself away from your pot. With pot, amount is hard to quantify because there is the volume of marijuana itself as well as the amount of the active ingredient, THC. You might be able to reduce the amount of marijuana that you smoke simply by buying stronger pot. That way, you'll get high without using a lot and burning up your lungs. (On the other hand, if you smoke a lot partly because the activity is soothing, buying stronger pot will not reduce the amount! In that case, buy weaker stuff. You can smoke frequently but still be reducing the amount of active drug you're taking in.) Perhaps buying stronger pot (#3) isn't financially practical or available where you live. That goes off the list for now as well because it's not manageable. You figure that you can tell when you really want to smoke alone—usually it's when you've had a stressful day at work or an argument with your girlfriend or your boyfriend—as opposed to when you just do it out of habit, so #4 seems like a good place to start making a change. Now you need to make a plan for how to do that. Congratulations! You've arrived at the preparation stage.

Cut down on the frequency of your ecstasy use

1. Go to fewer parties (setting).
2. Go to "sober" dances (setting).
3. Switch to alcohol (drug).
4. Try antidepressant medication (set).

It's a great idea to go to fewer or to "sober" dance parties. It would sure stop you from using E. But it's your world, the dance scene. Not only do all your friends meet there, but you love to dance. It's your favorite way to move your body, especially since you aren't into any sports. You're not going to contemplate those ideas—talk about depression! That *would* be depressing, and you HATE it when your mother tells you she wants you to see a doctor because she thinks you're depressed. You consider alcohol. You definitely want a buzz when you're dancing, and a few beers would do it and be refreshing at the same time. On the other hand, you've heard that alcohol is more dangerous in the long run than E, so you're not sure it's a good switch. Still, you're contemplating it as a good possibility. Well, you do know that you get pretty moody, although you wouldn't admit it to anyone else. So you're reluctantly contemplating trying medication, too.

Change the route of administration

1. Snort instead of shooting heroin (drug).
2. Talk to other users at a needle exchange about your love of needles (set).
3. Stay away from people who shoot (setting).

"No way," you say, "am I going to give up shooting." You know you're careless and share works. You know you have friends who have HIV and hepatitis C. But *nothing* beats the feeling of shooting dope. So forget that one. Nor are you going to leave your community and look for other people. Guess that means you are in the precontemplation stage for both of those ideas. Yet you think you *should* stop shooting. It would also help you taper off your dependence on the intense rush you get. All that's left is for you to just talk to people. Talk to people who have tried switching from needles to snorting and see how disappointing it was. Talk to people about needles. Really get into what you love about them. Talk until you can't talk anymore. Then see how you feel. Talking is a way of contemplating, too.

Working on these changes with someone else—whether or not he or she has a problem—is often very helpful. Be careful, though, not to make promises to other people. You are making promises only to yourself and only about *trying* to change. The other person is a witness, a coach, a support— not a nag or a judge. He or she is *not supposed to hold you to your promises!*

Every time you come up with what seems to be a good idea about how to make healthier choices or changes in your drug use, do the same thing. Test out your idea according to how you feel about it, which will tell you the stage of change you are in. Trial and error will tell you best what works for you. You're the expert.

None of us likes to hear that practice makes perfect, but it actually does make a difference. You're trying to change important behaviors. Ways of being and relating to alcohol, drugs, people, and places get ingrained over time. Remember, change is slow. Start with the idea that seems the easiest to accomplish. Success increases our sense of being powerful and makes other changes a bit easier. Or, you might want to start with a change that will make a *huge* impact right away—like never driving if you're using or always cleaning your works. That way you're more likely to stay alive, healthy, and out of jail as you prepare to make other changes.

SOURCES AND SUGGESTED READINGS

There are a number of good resources to help you with practicing harm reduction and substance use management:

The Straight Dope Education Series. Harm Reduction Coalition. 2001.
Getting off Right: A Safety Manual for Injection Drug Users. Rod Sorge and Sara Kershnar. Harm Reduction Coalition. 1998.
Responsible Drinking: A Moderation Management Approach for Problem

Drinkers. Frederick Rotgers, Mark Kern, and Rudy Hoeltzel. New Harbinger. 2002.

Buzzed: The Straight Facts about the Most Used and Abused Drugs from Alcohol to Ecstasy. Cynthia Kuhn, Scott Swartzwelder, & Wilkie Wilson. Norton. 1998.

From Chocolate to Morphine. Andrew Weil and Winifred Rosen. Houghton Mifflin. 1993. (Has excellent suggestions about harm reduction at the end of each chapter).

Uppers, Downers, All Arounders (4th ed.). Darryl Inaba, William Cohen, and Michael Holstein. CNS Publications. 2000.

The Users Voice. The John Mordaunt Trust, c/o Drugscope, 32–36 Loman Street, London, SE1 OEE. Or e-mail them at *usersvoice.jmt@drugscope.org* (This is a newsletter that gives specific information on drug use, policy, and drug safety. See the March–April 2002 issue for marijuana tips.)

Naltrexone and Alcoholism Treatment. SAMHSA Center for Substance Abuse Treatment. Treatment Improvement Protocol #28. 2002.

Take Control Now! A Do It Yourself Blueprint for Positive Lifestyle Success. Marc Kern. Life Management Skills Publishing. 1994.

Look in the Resources at the end of this book for other websites that will give you information about drugs and safer use.

For help with quitting:

Sober for Good. Anne Fletcher. Mariner Books. 2002.

You Can Free Yourself from Alcohol and Drugs: Work a Program That Keeps You in Charge. Doug Althauser. New Harbinger. 1998.

Sobriety Demystified: Getting Clean and Sober with NLP and CBT. Byron Lewis. Kelsey & Co. 1996.

The Thinking Person's Guide to Sobriety. Bert Pluymen. Bright Books. 1996.

"Warm Turkey: Other Routes to Abstinence." William Miller and A. C. Page. *Journal of Substance Abuse Treatment, 8*, 227–232. 1991.

How to Quit Drugs for Good. Jerry Dorsman. Prima Publishing. 1998.

How to Quit Drinking without AA (2nd ed.). Jerry Dorsman. Prima Publishing. 1997.

8 PRACTICING HARM REDUCTION

How to Take Care of Yourself While Still Using

By now you probably don't need to be reminded that we believe that you can make positive changes, even if you continue using alcohol and drugs. We'll remind you anyway because that belief goes against all of the conventional wisdom that says "get rid of the drugs and your other problems will vanish, or at least you'll be able to work on them." Harm reduction is about reducing harm in all areas of your life, not just in your drug use. You're probably already practicing harm reduction. Keeping household cleaners away from your children is harm reduction. You may not want to stop using bleach in the laundry; you just want the kids to be safe from it. Wearing your seat belt just about every time you get in your car and never ever drinking and driving is harm reduction, big time. So it's not unreasonable to assume that you can reduce other harmful effects if you want.

Of course, quitting all mind-altering substances *could* help ease problems in other areas of your life. If you've decided to quit, there are plenty of resources out there for you. For starters, this book has suggested that you look at your reasons for using and pay attention to your patterns, your stresses, and your strengths. The information on emotions and drugs can help you see what might be driving your use and how your brain chemistry is being altered. By developing a hierarchy of needs in the three major arenas of your life—drug, set, and setting—you should have a clearer idea about what else will need your attention if you decide to quit using altogether. We believe this kind of self-knowledge is essential to achieving and maintaining abstinence.

There are many self-help books and several different types of self-help or professionally facilitated groups in addition to the 12-Step meetings. Some of these alternative groups include SMART Recovery, Women for Sobriety, and Life Ring (all are listed in the Resources appendix). There are also many counselors and therapists who can help you. A counselor who is familiar with the harm reduction philosophy will help you keep *all* of your issues in focus, rather than just paying attention to your sobriety, or lack thereof.

If, however, you've decided not to be abstinent, or you've decided you want to get there gradually, you will be trying different patterns or methods of using and drinking, ones we suggested in the last chapter or ones you thought of yourself, before you cast out your drugs altogether. As you tackle your relationship with drugs, we recommend that you first take a good look at whether you're taking good enough care of yourself in other ways. It's a whole lot easier to change or give up something that's important to you if you feel you're getting fed in other ways, either literally with delicious food or emotionally through good relationships, intellectually by stimulating work, projects, or entertainment, or spiritually by a caring community or religion.

When faced with many problems that need your attention all at once, it will help if you've figured out your hierarchy of needs—perhaps you've already made a list of the areas you've decided are necessary to take care of. But, remember, just because something is necessary doesn't mean it's doable. You must also pick things that are *manageable* and *tolerable*.

What have you come up with as your hierarchy of needs? What did you decide was important to you? Conflicts in your family? Legal difficulties? Tired all the time? Lonely? Depressed? Anxious? Hate where you live? Worried about your kids? Working too hard? Need a job? Bored with your job? Can't perform sexually, or just not interested? Need to exercise? Need to lose or gain weight? House needs cleaning? Laundry piling up every week, or every month? Bills piled up for six months? Start with what seems most important to you or the area you're most panicked about. Or start with what someone else would like to see you change or with a very private matter. Or start with what you think might be easiest to deal with. Taking even a small step can feel good to you and make you more optimistic about your ability to confront larger problems.

The first part of this chapter provides suggestions about ways of taking care of yourself in different parts of your life, whether or not you continue to use. In the last part, we give an example of someone else's hierarchy of needs and show how using the structure of "Drug, Set, Setting" can help you pick out one area at a time. Leave aside your specific drug-related concerns for the moment.

Taking Care of Yourself:
Body, Mind, Emotions, and Soul

Have you ever taken one of those stress analysis tests? They measure events or changes in your life that are stressful. Happy changes as well as difficult events are considered stressful. For each type of stress, you get a certain number of points. The most points are given for the most serious stresses: the death of a child or a spouse, getting divorced, birth of a child, moving or losing your home, changing jobs, being promoted or getting fired. Fewer points are given for less dramatic stresses like graduating from school or breaking a leg. But stress is stress, and all kinds of stress can make you vulnerable to catching a cold, losing your hair, losing your keys, yelling at your partner or kids, falling down the stairs, etc. Stress lowers your resistance to illness and accidents. Literally, it compromises your immune system. While your body is coping with stress, it is too busy to ward off illness.

Stressful experiences, whether happy or sad, have one thing in common: they all involve loss or change. Whether it's losing someone, moving to another place, starting a job, or having a baby, change and the stress that comes with it are usually inseparable. Losing or changing your relationship with drugs is no different. *Having* a relationship with drugs is stressful too. The drugs themselves can be hard on your body and mind. Dancing all night on E instead of sleeping can stress your system. Copping on an unfamiliar street corner can be dangerous and stresses your system. Not knowing if where you're using is safe from the police can create stress because all the time you're looking over your shoulder, your stress hormones are active.

In our experience, people who use drugs in ways that they consider problematic, and people who are therefore quitting, cutting down, or making other changes in their drug use tend to be worried, anxious, panicked, bored, self-critical, depressed, frustrated, combative or withdrawn from others, sleepless, fatigued, desperate, lonely, or angry. If you're reading this book, you're probably among these people. To cope with all these difficult feelings, your body sends an army of physiological defenses to keep you functioning as your energy is sapped. So to keep your body and mind as healthy and comfortable as possible while you're making changes, consider ways to reduce some of the stress.

There are many formal and informal stress reduction techniques. Formal stress reduction techniques include things like meditation, massage, and breathing exercises for those who can sit still. For those who can't, yoga, martial arts, walking, or more strenuous physical exercise in which you break a sweat and discharge some of the toxins being built up by your tension or by your drugs might work well. Singing in the car or the shower is also good, as is standing under a noisy, well-trafficked bridge (to muffle the noise) and shouting out your frustrations.

We know that people use drugs for reasons. Alcohol and other drugs are relaxing, stimulating, pain relieving, and pleasurable. We're not stupid—we don't generally use drugs to be self-destructive. So, as you go about changing your relationship with drugs, or even if you have decided to change nothing about your use, we want to talk about how to take care of yourself so you don't catch cold (or worse), fall down the stairs (or worse), or lose your keys (or worse).

Taking Care of Your Body

There are a number of basic steps you can take to take care of your body while you're using and while you're changing. These steps coincide with Maslow's hierarchy of basic needs.

Drink Enough Water. Being dehydrated is a common problem for drug users. Dehydration, which comes from not drinking enough water or losing too much of your body's fluids, can sneak up on you when you're dancing all night and sweating or sitting around all night drinking beer but not water. It can also come from going on a speed run that absorbs so much of your attention you simply forget to drink water. You might not even have access to clean water. People who smoke cigarettes, drink alcohol, coffee, and tea, and who use drugs that make them sweat should drink more water than others. Being dehydrated is also a problem for people under stress, who may increase their use of caffeine to offset fatigue. Eight cups of water a day seems to be the standard that you see recommended these days. From nutritional journals to medical books to exercise manuals, eight glasses is the standard.

Don't Forget to Eat. First of all, eat. Just eat. Then worry about *what* you're eating. Meat, fish, chicken, eggs, milk, cheese, nuts, and beans are good sources of protein that will stick to your ribs for a while. Complex carbohydrates (pasta, dense whole wheat and nut breads, brown rice, oatmeal, and potatoes) are also good sources of energy. Both proteins and complex carbs take a while to digest, so you won't get a sugar rush and the energy will last longer. Simple carbohydrates (white bread, white rice) are OK but won't last as long. Natural sugars (fruits and fruit juices) are good for quick energy but also don't last long. Natural sugars also contain some vitamins, which make them a better choice than processed sugars (candy, doughnuts, and, of course, alcohol), which are also good for a quick blast, don't last long, and usually end with a sugar crash. If you eat candy, have something with nuts in it, such as almonds or peanuts (as long as you're not allergic to nuts, of course). If you have a bagel, have it with cream cheese or peanut butter instead of just butter.

It is better to eat a little throughout the day, even if you're not hungry, rather than get very hungry and then stuff yourself. Basically, you want to keep your blood sugar as even as possible so that whatever drugs you're using are being taken into a system that isn't wired from not eating or crashing from a sugar high.

Stay Warm. Warmth is good for the body and for the emotions. There's a reason the words *cold* and *lonely* often appear in the same sentence. Beware of exposure to harsh weather. Partying outside in the winter can lead to hypothermia, which makes you feel even higher—but you're actually crashing. Even in milder seasons, deciding not to take a sweater to the beach party, for example, because the cocktails you all had at home first made you feel warm, can cause you harm once the sun goes down and the wind is blowing off the ocean. Exposure is a particular risk if you are homeless and live in a cold climate. If you are sleeping in the park on a cold night, you risk everything from death to frostbite to illness. Alcohol feels like it warms you on a cold night because alcohol stimulates the blood vessels near the surface of your skin to expand. But it is actually pulling the heat from your inner body to your skin, making your skin feel warm but lowering your body temperature. So try to find heat and warm clothing. Then if you still choose to drink, go ahead. You'll be less at risk of hypothermia.

Stay Safe. We will leave it to your own personal exploration to determine what types of harm you need to address to ensure your own safety. We consider safety risks any person, place, or instrument that puts you in danger of physical abuse, rape, murder, overdose, accidents, or disease.

The greatest health risk for women who drink alcohol and use other drugs is becoming a victim of violence. Alcohol makes you not as aware of danger and not as able to respond to it quickly. Of course, men may become victims as well, especially if you leave work at midnight, stop at the bar for a few stiff drinks, then walk home in a bad neighborhood alone. Also, being around other drunk guys increases the chance that someone will start a fight and you could get caught up in it. And it is a huge problem for transgendered people, who are at high risk for both partner and stranger violence. Sometimes drinking or using alone is the best practice if you're likely to be taken advantage of by someone else. If you can't use alone, make sure you stay awake! Watch your drinks. Don't take drugs that you don't know about from others. Learn self-defense. Learn assertiveness skills. Work with a therapist who can help you improve your self-esteem and change your pattern of choosing abusive partners. Find people who think you're wonderful and treat you well. If you don't know any, decide to start looking.

Sometimes drugs that make you feel relaxed and contented can actually put you at greater risk. GHB is such a drug. It is often called a "date rape" drug because it can make you physically unable to resist assault and unable to remember afterward what happened to you. Alcohol can also sometimes produce the same effect.

Using GHB, alcohol, dissociative anesthetics, or virtually all of the other central nervous system depressants by yourself creates an overdose risk. Overdose also is a risk for people who use heroin alone. In addition to the overdose risk, alcohol, GHB, nitrous oxide, ketamine, PCP, and household solvents put people at risk of accidents. They all cause lack of coordination and poor judgment. The same is sometimes true of hallucinogens. It doesn't happen as often as the hype would have you believe, but the risk of a bad trip, during which you *feel* unsafe even if you aren't really, warrants having a "guide" around—someone who's not high. And most fatal overdoses could be prevented by having a friend around who can do "rescue breathing" or call 911.

This is a time to do a decisional balance. Figure out which of your risks is most dangerous. Are you more likely to fall prey to sexual aggression? Or are you more likely to down a whole handful of pills, *not* test the strength of your shot, or drink too fast and end up unconscious? The bottom line is: if you're going to get drunk or really high, have someone around to steer you out of harm's way, but not someone who will take advantage of your altered state.

Other health concerns include unwanted pregnancies, sexually transmitted diseases such as chlamydia, herpes, and HIV/AIDS, and blood-borne diseases like hepatitis B and C. All of these are transmitted either by sex or by blood-to-blood contact, usually through shared needles, sometimes through shared toothbrushes or exchange of blood or other bodily fluids through open wounds or sores. You probably know the drill here—don't share needles, have protected sex unless you *absolutely, without a doubt*, know the health status of your partner, and even then, use your own toothbrush. But this is a harm reduction book. Do your best, as often as you can.

You might also pay attention to whether you're at risk for diseases such as diabetes, alcohol-related liver disease, tobacco-related lung disease or cancer, and heart disease. Now this is getting *really* overwhelming. If abstinence is not for you, moderation is probably the best practice to avoid these diseases. And, remember, you can decide to be abstinent or moderate in your use of one drug but make no changes to others.

Finally, incarceration is a safety risk. Your quality of life suffers greatly if you are incarcerated. Besides the well-known dangers of gang violence and sexual assault associated with jails and prisons, poor sleep, inadequate access to natural light, lack of exercise, inadequate medical and mental health treatment, and very bad food can have a negative impact on your physical and mental health.

Sleep. Our bodies need sleep. There is no way around it. Some of us need less, some more, but no matter what our physical needs, sleep is part of health. Some drugs—alcohol, for example—disrupt sleep, which can cause a buildup of sleep deprivation. Sleep deprivation can cause everything from garden-variety exhaustion to difficulty thinking or concentrating to irritability or excess aggression at its most severe. If you go on a three-day speed run, the risks to your body as a result of sleep deprivation increase. If you are under stress, sleep is often the first thing disrupted. Not getting enough sleep can trigger depression and anxiety.

So sleep. Nap in the afternoon. Nap at your desk at lunchtime. Nap in the morning after you take the kids to school or after the early shift is over. Trouble sleeping can also be helped by antidepressants, which work for both depression and anxiety. Talk to your doctor if you're having trouble sleeping— too long without sleep is very bad for you. The less you sleep, the lower your resistance to other illnesses.

In addition to some of the stress reduction techniques we've mentioned, you might also try natural remedies such as chamomile tea, warm milk, bananas, or turkey to help you fall asleep. There are sleep remedies that you can find at natural food stores, but don't forget to check out how they interact with the drugs you're using. Go to a natural food store where there is an expert buyer who actually knows the products. You might even be able to mention your recreational drugs without getting judged too heavily!

Manage Pain. We have talked about the emotional pain that goes along with drug use. One of the most underrated phenomena that drug users experience is physical pain. The fact is, pain is undertreated, in general, in the United States—and we're not just talking about people who have been identified as "addicts." We are talking about postsurgical patients, accident victims, and, most of all, people in chronic pain. Pain is so undertreated that the American Medical Association has written policy guidelines on the appropriate treatment of pain, and the state of California has passed a bill of rights for pain patients.

People who use drugs "recreationally" experience pain, too. Half the time you may be using recreationally to manage that pain! If you've been labeled an "addict," however, you'll have an even harder time getting adequate help with pain management. The problem is, the best pain medications are narcotics (opiates), the very same class of drugs into which heroin falls. Of course, people become dependent on heroin, and some become chaotic users of it. But heroin and all of its narcotic cousins also work best for pain relief. The latest major drug panic to hit the nation is that of Oxycontin, a time-released synthetic opiate that has become the "poor man's heroin." It's cheaper, doesn't have to be imported from Mexico or Asia, and can be ground up and injected. Unfortunately, when ground up, it loses its time-release properties, so it is too strong for many people to inject, and overdoses have increased dramatically.

But most people who use prescribed opiates for pain relief do not get addicted, because most people take their medications as prescribed. And we would be willing to wager that some of those people who take more than they've been prescribed do so because they are, in fact, not prescribed enough to hold back their pain.

The problem isn't necessarily with the doctors who refuse to prescribe pain medications. Those doctors who do attempt to help their patients adequately by prescribing narcotics are at risk of being investigated by the federal Drug Enforcement Agency for abusing their prescription privileges. The best way to start the process of getting adequate care for pain is to find the nearest pain management clinic. Most will use at least some additional nonmedical treatments, such as meditation or acupuncture. Most will prescribe some medications. Some might prescribe enough to take care of all of your pain management needs.

Taking Care of Your Mind and Emotions

Persuading you to accept that people use drugs for reasons is the point of this book. We said plenty about it in Chapter 4 and in some of our examples. Drugs work to help us with intolerable emotions or with an inadequate ability to express ourselves, experience pleasure, and have fun. When you begin to make changes in your drug use, these areas will need your attention. There are many good self-help books on the market that cover all of the following areas. Some we have listed at the end of this chapter and in the Resources appendix. What follows is intended just to remind you that it's not all about drugs.

Build Emotional Muscle. Most people who have problems with alcohol or other drugs have gotten into the habit of acting on their feelings rather than just feeling them. When I feel bad, I have to *do* something. Your typical action is probably to get tipsy, drunk, or high—anything to avoid those feelings. Uncomfortable feelings are well known triggers of cravings to use (to *do* something) and can undermine your best intentions to change your relationship with drugs. In the long run you'll have to learn how to tolerate and even appreciate feelings that now overpower you. Getting used to having feelings is a major task in the process of changing your alcohol and drug use. If you've quit using entirely, you'll notice this almost immediately: all of a sudden you're drowning in anger, anxiety, or even elation. If you're cutting down—changing how, where, or when you use—your emotions might take longer to wake up. Don't be surprised if you cut down on your pot smoking for a month and all of a sudden, *wham*! You're feeling really sad, crying at the least little thing, and have no idea why.

There are several ways to get yourself used to feelings so that you don't have to *do* something immediately. Practice is at the heart of any method. Just as exercise builds physical muscle, using your feelings will also increase your tolerance, stamina, and "emotional muscle" so that you will be less vulnerable to the stresses of being human. One easy option is to count. Remember being told as a kid that you should count to ten when you're mad before you do or say anything, so that you don't hit somebody, say mean things, or have a tantrum? Well, it's the same idea now. Just count and stay as still as you can. We all forget that feelings, even the strongest ones, change, maybe even evaporate. Each time you feel yourself getting really sad or angry or whatever, *count*. If you get to three and then can't take it anymore, that's fine. Get yourself to three and then scream, fall apart, whatever. Next time, maybe you can get to five or ten. Keep increasing the time between your feeling and taking an action until you can sit with most feelings, either until they pass (most do) or until you can plan what you want to do.

The other easy option is to do something else, to distract yourself. Counting is about holding it in rather than exploding. Some drugs, like heroin or pot, help you hold things in. Others, like alcohol, help you let them out. Often you end up letting things out that you regret the next day. If you can't sit still, can't hold it in, go ahead and let it out. But try something besides alcohol or slamming a hit. Run, walk, slam a door, go under a noisy bridge and scream. But try not to yell at your partner, kick the dog, or slam your fist into a wall. All those things take a while to heal and can add to the laundry list of problems you're trying to solve. Eventually you'll find your way to tolerating emotions without getting loaded.

Notice Your Toxic Thoughts and Beliefs. There are several types of thoughts that can get in the way of progress. Three of the most common are catastrophizing, self-loathing, and hopeless thoughts. *Catastrophizing* thoughts tell you that the worst thing possible is likely to happen (a catastrophe). If you are drinking too much and are sure you're about to get liver cancer, you're probably catastrophizing. Liver cancer is not that common, even for heavy drinkers. These kinds of thoughts often lead to the other two toxic responses of self-loathing and hopelessness. You think that you're the worst person walking the earth and *deserve* to get liver cancer (self-loathing). Once you've gone this far into self-hatred, the next part comes fast (hopelessness). Your thought process goes something like this: "I'm drinking so much that I'll probably die of liver cancer. I'm such a loser that I can't quit drinking. There's nothing else I can do. The hell with it—might as well get drunk."

These thoughts, beliefs, and responses create enormous emotional stress, which is already probably a weak point for you. Give yourself a break, at least for the moment. Chances are good you are *not* the worst person around, and chances are good you are *not* doomed to failure. Talk it over with a therapist who specializes in cognitive-behavioral techniques to stop toxic thoughts and beliefs, or get one of the many self-help books on the market that deal with these kinds of issues.

Use Your Mind. Drugs and alcohol often isolate people who use them from the nondrug-using world and from the kind of mental stimulation offered by getting involved with people, political issues, reading, cultural developments in music, art, theater, or movies. For some people, working too hard is part of that isolation. For others, the isolation comes from being bored and having too little to do. One of the major contributions of 12-Step groups is that they get people out of the house and involved with others. If you don't like 12-Step programs, however, you won't get this benefit. If you don't want to join a group or program, it might be very useful to you—and to the world of which you are a citizen—to get involved in a cause that you can support. Read the paper, go to movies, read a book, go to rallies, write letters to Congress about something that is important to you, defend the rights of drug users to have equal access to health care, whatever suits you. The important point is to remember that you *do* belong in the world. Your drug use does *not* strip you of your membership in the human race, and we all need and will benefit from your involvement!

Be Soothed. Sometimes we just feel bad—cranky, lost, or upset—for vague reasons that we can't quite articulate. It's like being a baby who can't talk yet. What we need at such times is to be soothed, to be comforted. Many drugs are very soothing. Someone once called alcohol "an emotional warm blanket." But you're trying to break your wholehearted reliance on alcohol and drugs. It's often some kind of physical soothing that we want or need, someone to rub our back or stroke our head and say, "Shhhh, everything's going to be all right now." If you have someone around who loves you, being physically close like that might be good. If not, get a massage, take a long hot shower, wrap yourself up in your favorite sweatshirt, sit in bed reading the sports section, or eat some mashed potatoes or other "comfort food." Just find something that feels good and comforting to your body at these times, and your mood will probably improve.

Have Fun. If your alcohol or drug use has gotten out of hand, chances are you're not having as much fun as you used to. Using takes a lot of time, money, and worry and doesn't give back as much as it did at first. This leaves you without much fun in your life. Switching drugs is probably not the answer to this particular problem. Let's try another tack. Can you remember a time in your life when you enjoyed something? Watching *The Three Stooges,* walking on the beach, swimming in the river, sleeping in the sun, throwing a football or a baseball, digging in the garden, writing poetry? Now is a good time to pick up an enjoyable activity like that again. If you don't have fun, quitting or changing your drugs is going to be a grind. If you don't remember what you used to enjoy, you'll have to get creative. Ask someone who knows you to tell you what you used to do for fun—or even what he or she does for fun now. Pick up a local newspaper and flip to the entertainment section or get your city's special weekly entertainment paper. Read it. Go to a movie or a show or a free concert in the park. Or check out the bulletin board at the library, a cafe, or the supermarket and see what's going on. Pick something out and *go do it.* You may or may not end up enjoying that particular activity or event, but along the way you might remember something you always wanted to try. Dealing with a drug or alcohol problem is not fun, so it's important that you *not* be working at it all the time! That's sheer drudgery.

What about Your Soul?

For many people, religious faith, spiritual practice, and the communities that spring from them comprise a vital source of support and guidance. When relationships, work, health, and finances are all sputtering, spiritual guidance can be a final thread of hope for substance users, just as they are for anyone who feels lost or despairing. Our question is not *whether* spirituality has a place in harm reduction but *how* to integrate what seem like contradictory beliefs.

On the face of it, spirituality and harm reduction seem unable sit together in the same room. The fundamental issue that creates tension between spirituality and harm reduction is the issue of power. Many religions, particularly monotheistic (the belief in one god) traditions, rely heavily on the surrender of power and control to god. How can putting my faith in Jesus, surrendering my will to the will of Allah, or my Buddhist efforts to let go of attachments coexist with my harm reduction efforts, which rely on *me* to use *my* power to exercise control over *my* life and *my* relationship with drugs? If harm reduction invites me to be the expert and to be in control of my decisions, how can I retain a spiritual life that asks me to surrender my power to god? Ultimately, you may be left with the question: how can I be a spiritual or religious person and adhere to my faith while investing myself in something that seems to contradict my beliefs?

The answer to this difficult question, which by now shouldn't surprise you, is complex. Just as your relationships with drugs and alcohol as well as family and friends are complex, your relationship with spirituality also may be complex. If you've been selfish when you use or drink, and you claim to have a religious practice, how do you rationalize your selfishness? If you've hurt others, how do you assuage your guilt? If you've ruined your career or lost your family, where do you bury your shame? The spirituality of AA tells you to "turn it over." "Let go, let God." Accept your "powerlessness." "Surrender" and follow the 12 Steps and all will be well. A small percentage of people find the answer in these suggestions. But we work with people who don't find the spirituality of AA helpful. That doesn't mean, however, that it is impossible to craft your own sense of deep spirituality.

We have seen many survivors of trauma who feel their god has failed them. They work hard to reconstruct a fractured relationship with god as part of their recovery. It may mean having to give up their pretrauma faith in god as benevolent, work through the feeling that god is arbitrary and mean, and get to a realization that just because their trauma didn't make sense doesn't mean that god doesn't exist. This new relationship with god is often more mature, a partnership in which both parties are responsible for how things work. Using *harm reduction* to deal with your substance use and its consequences may also change your relationship with your god.

There are many aspects of religion that *do* resonate with harm reduction. Three are most important. First, *accepting* yourself as you are and receiving acceptance from others are essential to understanding why you use drugs, and knowing why you use drugs is essential to figuring out what to do about it. Second, although harm reduction doesn't express it like this, *forgiveness* is a fundamental value. Guilt is paralyzing, and you must forgive yourself, and ultimately be forgiven for, the damage you have done, in order to move forward in the matter of finding solutions. Third, there must be *love*. To be a harm reduction therapist means loving the people we work with *just as they are*. We find their creative solutions to their lives inspiring. We don't minimize the damage done, but we appreciate that they do their best, and we look for the strengths, the humor, and the cleverness in their efforts to survive. What better spiritual practices are there than those of acceptance, forgiveness, and love? In the words of someone who attended harm reduction training and has developed a harm reduction practice, "This is the most Christian work with addicts I've ever seen."*

Spiritual practice, whatever form it takes, inherently possesses cultural and social possibilities for connecting people to each other and to the rest of the world. People pray together, participate in rituals such as lighting candles on Shabbat, or dance to music that joins the spirit to community and cultural tradition. The fundamental principle here is that religious practice can mean a connectedness to others, a relationship. And here we are, back to relationships—between you and spirituality, between you and Chivas Regal, you and the crack pipe, you and weed, between you and your beleaguered wife, or between you and god.

Taking Care of Your Whole Self: Using Drug, Set, and Setting

Once you've picked a problem from your hierarchy of needs, you can take specific, practical steps to take care of it—perhaps using the formula we talked about in the last chapter: *drug*, *set*, and *setting*. When you address issues with your drug(s), consider all the substitutions and small but signifi-

*Thanks to Annie Fahy of Athens, Georgia, for her deep appreciation and heartfelt practice of harm reduction.

cant changes we talked about in the last chapter. When you turn your attention to yourself, you may find many things on your list to take care of. Careful, this part can be overwhelming! Most of us could think of a couple of hundred things we'd like to change about ourselves—our hair, body shape, height, weight, our anger or passivity, depression or psychosis, our flat feet, our love of chocolate, our allergy to cats, you name it. When it comes to environment, we could think of another couple of hundred things we'd like to change—how much money we make, our partner's snoring, the color of the house next door, the fact that one kid is gay, the other so pierced you can see the sky through her ears, tongue, and eyebrows, our parents' hatred of marijuana and love of gas guzzlers and Scotch, the president, the vice-president, tax laws, racism, sexism, the fact that our noses freeze off for six months of the year in Michigan and we melt onto the sidewalk for the other six months in Florida. Pick carefully or pick randomly, but pick just one or two things at a time that you would like to change. Now we'll use one person's story (a composite, actually) to help you get started with your own plan.

Terry is forty-five years old and in a committed relationship. She works hard at a job that she doesn't particularly like, but it's not very demanding, so she has a lot of free time. Lately, though, she hasn't been feeling good. She's overwhelmed by small things, not sleeping well, losing weight and doesn't know why, and she can't talk to anybody because she's "not that kind of person." Terry's hierarchy of needs looks like this:

1. Family: My partner and I aren't having sex much anymore and she's angry.
2. Legal: If I get another DUI, I'll lose my license or go to jail.
3. General and/or mental health: I'm not feeling very good lately. I get sick a lot. I'm not sleeping, and I'm losing weight. I can't concentrate at work, and it's making me nervous about my job performance.
4. Drug use: My partner says I drink too much.

Using the *Drug, Set, Setting* framework, Terry came up with some solutions to #1, her partner being angry about not having sex very often.

Drug: Terry drinks wine in the evenings, sometimes up to a bottle. The only other drug she uses is a little coffee in the morning. As we know, alcohol is often a social lubricant, helping people relax and enhancing sex, especially if they tend to be shy or anxious about it. But Terry is drinking *a lot* of wine. It could be that her lack of interest in sex is a result of being too "relaxed" at the end of an evening. She could try having sex with her partner in the mornings or before dinner. It might also be, though, that the amount of alcohol Terry has been drinking has depressed her sex drive over time. If so, trying to have sex at a different time of day probably won't work. (Cutting down or quitting drinking for a while would be a good test of this theory.)

Set: It might be that Terry just doesn't have a very strong sex drive. This pattern has happened to her before in relationships. After the first few months, she loses interest. It'll take some creativity on her part and her partner's part to get things going again. They could buy a book on sex and read it together, go on a vacation together, go to romantic movies. It could also be, though, that Terry is depressed. Many of her other concerns point to depression, as does her low sex drive. If this is the case, antidepressant medication could help, even though some of them also have sexual side effects. She could make an appointment with a psychiatrist and discuss the situation. Still another possibility is that Terry has shied away from sex since she was raped a few years ago. The trauma of a sexual assault can seriously interfere with sexual functioning. Seeing a therapist who is experienced at working with trauma, with or without her partner, should help.

Setting: The only socializing Terry does is stopping on the way home to have a couple of drinks with colleagues. Terry and her partner don't socialize with other people, so they spend most of their time at home or out to dinner, but never with other people. Maybe they need some outside interest to rekindle their interest in each other. They could join an organized social activity—biking, a class at church, bowling, travel slide shows or lectures, book club, tennis lessons—or get involved in the community—visit and play cards with people on Sundays at a senior center, serve meals at holidays, teach kids to read. Finally, Terry and her partner live in an apartment building with a lot of neighbors. Another possibility is that Terry, being shy anyway, could be embarrassed about being heard while they're having sex. She might be especially self-conscious because they're lesbians, and she isn't sure what her neighbors think about that. Find a room that's not adjacent to someone else's, or turn on some music!

Now let's look at #2, Terry's DUI.

Drug: Terry could figure out how many drinks it takes to get her over the legal limit (usually it's more than one per hour, but we're all different) and make sure she keeps count. She could buy a breath-analyzing machine and have it installed in her car. That way the car won't even start if she's had too much to drink! She could decide not to drink on her way home from work or have one drink and then a sparkling water if she wants to hang out with folks for a while. She could decide that her drinking's gotten out of hand and quit altogether for while, as was suggested in the DUI class.

Set: Maybe Terry is so embarrassed by her previous arrest that she hasn't talked to an attorney about steps she could take to clear her record. Or maybe she doesn't like asking people for favors, so she can't ask someone to drive her home if she's had too much to drink. Would they really mind, or does she need to be more assertive? There are classes and books and therapists that could help her become more assertive.

Setting: Terry sometimes starts out the evening at happy hour, where there are lots of people, lots of salty snacks, and she's tense after a day at work where her boss never seems satisfied with her performance. She could take a walk to unwind and then join people for the last hour. Skip out altogether and go home and have something to drink there. Or, if she's the type of person who drinks her last dollar, she might persuade her colleagues to pick a bar closer to her house so she can walk home. Otherwise, she could take enough money for a cab.

In the case of #3 (her general and mental health), here are some ideas:

Drug: Terry has recently started taking medication for high blood pressure. She's had to try a few different kinds because of side effects. It'll be important for her to tell her doctor about feeling sick. Her stomach is also upset more than it used to be. She should make sure to have food in her stomach before she drinks to cut down on stomach upset.

Set: Terry used to be able to motivate herself to do things, but can't anymore. She could be depressed. It is not uncommon, even years after a trauma like rape. It might help to see a therapist to evaluate whether her mood is causing some of her physical symptoms. Or maybe she just can't sleep as well as she could when she was younger. She hates the thought of getting older, and it may be hard for her to admit that. She might try talking to friends about how they're dealing with the ups and downs of aging.

Setting: Terry's company relocated recently, and now she's working in an office with a lot of other people who have kids who are always sick with some bug. Maybe she could move her desk to a spot out of traffic? Or she could ask her coworkers to take some cough syrup so they're not spreading germs around as much. Or maybe developing a better social life with her partner would help with her mood.

Terry was able to use her hierarchy of needs to make a list of concerns in her life, some of which had nothing to do with her drinking. If one of the most significant areas of concern on *your* hierarchy is alcohol or drug use, and you've decided you don't want to quit, then use the suggestions from Substance Use Management (SUM) as a practical guide to reduce harm and change your relationship with the drugs you use.

There are many different solutions to #4, drinking too much. It is possible that any of the changes above will resolve Terry's problematic relationship with alcohol. If not, here are a few other possibilities.

Drug: Terry could start by actually counting the number of drinks she has at any one time, then reduce that amount by one, or two, if she can. Or decide that she'll drink only on certain days and not on others. How much does she think is okay? Two glasses of wine? More or less? She has to know her standards before she can try to moderate her behavior. She should consider alternating alcoholic drinks with nonalcoholic ones. Or she might want to quit altogether for a while to get her tolerance down, then see if she can practice moderation.

Set: Terry needs to ask herself why she drinks. Does she really know, or does she do it now just because it's become a habit? Does Terry come from a culture of regular drinking? She may feel, on the one hand, like she is fitting in but that, on the other, things are getting out of control. Maybe she drinks the most—whether at the bar or at home or at dinner—when she thinks her partner is going to approach her to make love and she wants to *not* freak out.

Setting: If Terry is out after work with hard-drinking friends, it'll be harder to control herself. Learning how to say no ("drink refusal skills") would come in handy. If Terry and her girlfriend both drink a lot together, it would be good for them to talk it over and see if they both feel that the drinking is getting out of hand. They should then work together on any or all of the issues we've discussed.

This is a long list of possible steps to solve four problems. Where to start? If Terry doesn't want to start with cutting down on her drinking, then she will start somewhere else. The biggest bind is that many of the other solutions involve asking others for help. The list includes seeing a therapist to talk about the rape, getting a medical and a psychiatric evaluation for depression and antidepressant medication, asking for rides home, and seeing a lawyer. Since she is not assertive, this will be hard. What might be most helpful for Terry is to weigh a decisional balance about the pros and cons of asking for help before she tries to figure out where to go for what. In the meantime, she could try walking home from the bar. At least she would be changing *something*, which would increase her confidence. In Chapter 10, we'll see how Terry works all of this out.

If you feel overwhelmed by how complex your hierarchy of needs seems to be, go back to Chapter 6 and copy the chart again so you can see all the possibilities on one piece of paper. Then pick *anything* and focus on making a decisional balance. If you're stuck and can't figure out what to pick, consult with a therapist for at least a session or two to get some sense of direction. The next chapter focuses on how to find help that will work for you.

SOURCES AND SUGGESTED READINGS

Go back to the workbooks listed at the end of Chapter 5 for help with taking care of yourself.

Pain management is a difficult issue for a lot of people. This book is pretty technical, but worth a look:

> *Pain and Its Relief without Addiction: Clinical Issues in the Use of Opioids and Other Analgesics.* Barry Stimmel. Haworth Medical Press. 1997.

You can also get important information on pain control from this organization:

> The National Foundation for the Treatment of Pain; Joel Hochman, Executive Director. *www.paincare.org*

For spiritual inspiration, this book has a chapter on harm reduction:

> *The Soul of Recovery: Uncovering the Spiritual Dimension in the Treatment of Addictions.* Christopher Ringwald. Oxford University Press. 2002.

9 FINDING THE RIGHT HELP

You're the expert. Only you can control your life and your behavior. Only you can decide what you need, what to do, and what to change. Even if you're under the supervision of a judge or the watchful eyes of your husband, wife, partner, parents, children, or any number of other people who would like to stop you from using once and for all, you can defy their wishes till hell freezes over. Or until you do some time behind bars where, rumor has it, you can still use. Or you end up in a hospital bed or, heaven forbid, the morgue.

Although we have encouraged you to consult often and thoroughly with yourself, there are times when getting help that is beyond your own knowledge and wisdom is necessary. In fact, we fully expect that this book will be only one of many resources you will use. By *resources* we mean other books, people, pets, places—things that may bring you comfort, support, encouragement, wisdom, ideas, reassurance, perspective, or hope.

In a country that values independence and self-reliance, seeking help is viewed by many people as a sign of weakness. Try not to feel ashamed when you think about reaching out. Other people see things that we don't. Other people might even care about us more than we care about ourselves! That's very helpful if we're being neglectful or abusive of ourselves. Other people sometimes know more than we do, at least about *some* things. But help has to be *helpful*, not stressful. If the support you're being offered feels like it adds pressure instead of alleviating it, you need to reduce the harm of help. This chapter describes formal kinds of help—professional therapists or programs and nonprofessional self-help groups—that can provide what personal relationships may not be able to offer, or that can lend a hand when going it alone isn't working.

How do you know when it's time to seek help? Warning signs can be found in your body, your mind and emotions, and your surroundings. If, despite your efforts to make positive changes or at least hold steady, your body feels more pain, you're moving more slowly, your energy is waning, your skin and hair look less healthy, your hygiene is poorer rather than better, it's probably time to ask someone to help you check out what's going on. (A medical evaluation would be a good place to start.) If your mind is more disorganized, your mood more depressed or anxious, or your emotions angrier, sadder, or more labile (up and down), it's probably a good time to seek out a therapist or a psychiatrist. If your environment is crumbling around you— you're losing your job, your family, or your home, your friends are avoiding you, you are hanging around with people who take you further into harm's way—you might consider finding a place where you will be accepted as you are right now. A church, a 12-Step meeting (even if you don't want to quit), or a harm reduction program or group might be a place to look for support.

Help comes in all shapes and sizes. Choosing what kind of help *you* want can energize you or immobilize you. Beware, the help that will be most helpful is what feels good. This may be hard for some of you to believe. You think to yourself, "Working on my problems isn't supposed to feel good! I need a therapist who will be tough on me, call me on my shit, not let me get away with anything." Most of us in this country have bought the "tough love" philosophy, just like we've swallowed the "pull yourself up by your bootstraps" idea, hook, line, and sinker.

Working with a "tough" therapist may be your way of accepting the anger your loved ones feel toward you. It is also possible that working with a tough therapist will be just another way to feel beaten up, just in case you haven't beaten yourself up enough. It may even be a way to *avoid* strengthening the part of yourself that needs to take responsibility for making your own decisions. A tough therapist can keep you dependent because you end up relying on his or her judgments rather than your own. Although it is true that reducing harm is painful, difficult, and confusing at times, the overall feeling of your therapy need not be painful. In fact, the more painful it is, the less likely you will want to stick with it. And the more fun you have with your therapist, the more likely you will be to want to go back. Therapy is supposed to reduce harm, not recreate it for $90 an hour.

Your family and the people who are intimately involved in your life do not have to respect your decisions. After all, they are sometimes negatively affected or deeply hurt by your drinking or drug use. They have the right to their own feelings—to push you, make demands, issue ultimatums, and otherwise scream and shout. Although sometimes it would be more helpful if they didn't, they, too, have been taught that tough love is the only way, especially if they have attended "codependents" groups or Al Anon. But a therapist or counselor does not have the same right to be demanding. Therapy or any other form of help should be a partnership in which you and the helping person share your respective wisdom, both working to further your goals. Look for a therapist, a treatment program, or a self-help group with whom or where you feel accepted and respected.

Finally, make sure there is room for flexibility. Harm reduction is a process that's different for everyone. There is not one way to get better. The solution cannot be prescribed. It is in your best interests to find a therapist or counselor who doesn't lay somebody else's tried-and-true solutions on you and who doesn't push you down any roads you don't want to travel.

Therapy: What It Is and How to Get the Kind You Want

There are as many types of therapies as there are breakfast cereals. You can work on your problems individually, you can do it in a group, with your family, or as part of a couple. You can work with a therapist who sits quietly, offering few words, or you can work with someone who is very active and offers many suggestions. You can work with a therapist who adheres to a behavioral model—change your behavior and your habits and feelings will follow—or a therapist who works in an analytic model—understand the origins of your behavior, develop an honest and deep relationship with your therapist, and changes will follow. This description is a little oversimplified, and many therapists blend approaches. A therapist will tell you about what he or she does when you call for an appointment.

You can find a therapist who works privately in his or her own practice, or you can find a therapist who is affiliated with a nonprofit clinic or a community mental health clinic, where you are more likely to find flexible fees. **The most important factor in finding a therapist is to feel that there is a good fit between you and the therapist.** You have found a good fit if you feel understood, respected, or even neutral. You are in a poor fit with a therapist if you feel bossed around, misunderstood, or positively awful, either physically or emotionally. A certain degree of discomfort and anxiety is to be expected in a first session with a therapist. After all, you are talking about things that take years to reveal in other relationships. When you are talking about drug use, you may be revealing things that you have told no one else. Wanting to use after a particularly stressful therapy session is normal. However, if you feel so much discomfort that you feel like jumping out of your skin, it is either the wrong therapist for you or the wrong time to be in therapy. If you have that feeling and want to quit, talk about it with the therapist first, just to see what he or she thinks. If you feel too much pressure to continue, try talking to someone else before you give up. That will tell you if it's the person or the timing.

The purpose of therapy is to provide a context in which you can develop a relationship with a professional with whom you can talk about your experiences, build enough trust to be truthful, and begin to address the harm in your life. The depth and duration of therapy is different for everyone. Just because your friend shares the most intimate secrets of her sex life with her therapist, and you talk with yours about why your boss keeps giving you crappy assignments, doesn't mean your friend is doing therapy "better" than you. Just because another friend saw someone only six times and is better doesn't mean you have to rush through your therapy. And just because some people spend many years in therapy doesn't mean yours will take forever. Your therapy is as unique as your fingerprint, and it should have your fingerprints all over it!

When you're looking for a therapist or counselor, we recommend interviewing several on the phone and making an appointment to see one or two of them. This is called *shopping* and is perfectly well accepted in the therapy profession. Try to remember the following: when in doubt, *don't*. If you speak with a therapist on the phone and just don't feel right about the conversation, or don't feel terribly drawn to him or her, trust the instinct and move on. There are thousands of us, although admittedly the choices are more limited if you live in a rural area. In that case, consider training your therapist to work well with you by insisting that the two of you focus on what *you* think you need and perhaps by requesting that the therapist do some nontraditional reading about drugs and drug use.

What if your instinct is to find a tough, "no bullshit" therapist? Pay attention to all instincts, but keep in mind that toughness that feels hurtful is not the same thing as firmness, and rigidity is not the same thing as consistency. Try to steer clear of a therapist who makes you feel like a hopeless jerk or presumes to know what's best for you.

Some of the questions you might want to ask a therapist in a phone interview are covered in the following material.

• *What are your credentials?* See a therapist who is licensed by a professional organization. A professional's license binds her to the ethical standards of her licensing board. Someone with an MSW (a master's degree in social work), should be licensed in the state in which he is practicing. Similarly, an MFT (marriage and family therapist) or a CADAC (certified alcohol and drug abuse counselor) should be licensed. A CADAC does not need to have master's level education and is trained to provide drug counseling but not psychotherapy on other psychological issues, although she might be helpful in other areas. A psychologist has a PhD or PsyD degree and is licensed at that level. Some therapists have doctoral degrees, but are licensed at a master's level (either as a social worker or a marriage and family therapist) and go by the name of their license. Still others have a master's degree and the corresponding license (social work or MFT). An MD (medical doctor) is someone who has been through medical school, internship, and possibly residency, and should be board certified in psychiatry. A psychiatrist can prescribe medications but may not have had training as a psychotherapist. A psychoanalyst is someone who has one of the other degrees and then has had many years of advanced training to practice therapy or psychoanalysis. He doesn't have a license as a psychoanalyst, but he should have graduated from a psychoanalytic institute. There are many institutes that train professionals in many different styles of working with people.

• *What about interns or trainees?* Many clinics and some private therapists employ people who have acquired their academic degree, who are not yet licensed by the state, and who are in training to become therapists. Everybody needs to learn his or her trade, and therapists must spend a lot of time studying and practicing. An intern may actually have quite a bit of experience, even before acquiring a license. The main point to consider if you hook up with a therapist-in-training is *the person supervising your therapist: what formal training is your therapist receiving while you work with him or her.* You should check out the credentials of the supervisor, because that's the person who will guide your therapist through *your* treatment.

• *Do you have any special training?* Most professionals are required to receive ongoing training to maintain their license. You will want to know if the therapist has any specific training in harm reduction, addiction, psychopharmacology (the biology of the brain, medications, etc.), trauma, or depression, to name the most relevant.

• *What's your fee?* Can you pay for therapy, or does your insurance cover it? Does the therapist offer a sliding scale based on income? Many therapists may point out that you are, after all, spending money on drugs, and they may be more reluctant to negotiate a lower fee. On the one hand, they need to understand that you can't turn over your drug money to therapy all at once. On the other, they have a point. If you are of limited means, you may be faced with a tough decision. Try doing a decisional balance in which you weigh the pros and cons of your drugs versus paying for therapy. See if you can negotiate a lower fee at first and agree to increase the fee as you are able to relinquish some of your drugs, once you have a stronger relationship with your therapist.

- *How long is a session?* The norm here is anywhere from forty-five minutes to an hour. Flexibility is one thing, but be wary of a therapist who says "We'll go as long as we need. Some days you may need more time than others." This is a therapist who probably struggles with keeping good boundaries and being consistent. Besides, would you want to be the person with the 2:00 appointment, tapping your fingers at 2:30 while you wait for the 1:00 appointment to finish up?

- *Who are you?* The answer to this question may or may not help you. If it's important for you to have a therapist who is similar to you, or has spent a lot of time working with people similar to you (typical characteristics that people find important are race, gender, sexual orientation, and age), the answer may help you. Some therapists concentrate on working with a group of people with whom they feel particularly helpful or comfortable. Remember, it's all about how you and the therapist fit together.

- *How often would I need to come in?* Once a week is the most common frequency for therapy sessions. You may want less or more. This is about what's necessary, manageable, and tolerable. Being in therapy is a little like peeling off layers of dead skin. Peeling dead skin is necessary for your health, but the skin underneath is soft and delicate. Any therapist should help keep the peeling to tolerable levels—not so many layers at a time that you feel raw. If you are in a particularly delicate state, slowing down the process by meeting less often can help. On the other hand, meeting more often gives you more support, sort of like putting up scaffolding around a building that's being stripped and repainted. Then there's the issue of what's manageable. Usually this means what you can afford, either money-wise or time-wise. If a therapist is firm about the frequency that she recommends, find out why. She's either noticed something in your work together that she feels strongly about (for example, a pattern in your life whereby you dismiss or underrate the help you need) or she's rigid about how she practices.

- *What do you think about working with someone who's not sure he [or she] wants to be "clean and sober"?* Is the therapist a die-hard abstinence-only therapist, or does he have a harm reduction philosophy? Even if he isn't specifically trained in harm reduction psychotherapy, he might intuitively be flexible and understanding with drug users.

- *How do you feel about people starting and stopping therapy?* From a harm reduction perspective, you should be able to take a break if you feel ambivalent or overwhelmed. You should be able to move (in the stages of change) from preparation to action to contemplation and back again—a hundred times, if necessary—without your therapist questioning your ability to be in therapy or labeling you "resistant" or "in denial."

• *What would make you fire a patient?* Some therapists don't feel equipped to work with a client who is drinking heavily or using and has no plan to quit. Some therapists don't feel equipped to work with a client who has relapses; they see it as a "treatment failure" and will send you off to an inpatient treatment program until you are "ready" for outpatient therapy. This is not a harm-reduction-friendly therapist. Keep looking.

• *Would you need to talk with my husband [wife, parole officer, former therapist, parents, employer, etc.]?* The right answer here is that communication with other people is entirely up to you. Anyone, regardless of age, has a right to confidential psychotherapy. Confidentiality can be broken only under extreme circumstances—if you are an imminent danger to yourself or others. The most common "others" to be concerned about are children or elderly people, usually ones in your care. Therapists are entitled to establish their own standards and must inform you of them. For example, a therapist might ask you to sign a form saying it's OK for her to consult with your spouse. You aren't under legal obligation to sign, but the therapist might refuse to treat you if you don't sign. If that troubles you, find another therapist. The welfare of people under your care may be of particular concern for a therapist working with drug users. For example, are you using at a time and in a place that doesn't compromise your responsibilities? Don't be surprised or offended if the therapist checks in with you about this from time to time. It's reasonable and probably practical for you to be specific about how you take care of your kids or your elderly father. But if a therapist *assumes* that you are neglectful or abusive just because you're a user, that's time to wonder about that therapist's credentials as a harm reductionist.

• *What about emergencies?* All therapists should be set up to handle out-of-office-hours emergencies. If you know yourself to be someone who needs a good deal of support beyond your regular sessions, talk this over with the therapist and be sure he is able to offer that support.

If the answers to these questions satisfy you, make an appointment to see the therapist. In that first session, here are some things to look for:

• *Does the therapist seem interested in your ideas?* Being interested in your ideas suggests that the therapist is willing to collaborate with you. Remember: *you* are the boss of your life. Your therapist is there to help you, not rule you. Also remember who's paying whom.

- *Does the therapist insist that the therapy go a certain way?* Flexibility is important. If the therapist is too rigid in the way she runs a therapy session (insisting, for example, that you do exercises such as guided imagery, "empty chair" work, or talk about your history of abuse), she may not have the flexibility to deal with your many ups and downs. Techniques, or tools, that a therapist uses should feel helpful to you, not required.

- *Does the therapist seem focused or distracted?* Depending on whether you are seeing someone privately, through a hospital, community clinic, or other organization, the therapist might have distractions during the session—phone calls that he answers, a pile of papers up to the ceiling that keep grabbing his attention, knocks at the door. You have a right to be the center of your therapist's attention while you're with him.

- *Does the therapist give you homework? If so, does the homework feel doable?* Some people want the structure of homework; others feel it's too controlling. Homework often means writing. If you're in couple therapy, it usually means practicing communication between sessions. Some people get the shakes just thinking about their days in school and freak at the very word *homework*. The decisional balance is a classic homework assignment. It's very helpful, but we find that people often don't sit down with pen and paper and make their lists. It's OK for you to learn the concept of the decisional balance and then loosely apply it to the various ideas and feelings, wishes and impulses that float through your head during the week. You can always talk about them in therapy. No law says it works better if you write it down. This is where we encourage you to trust what seems right to you (not the people who have been encouraging/nagging you to find a therapist!).

- *Who provides backup for the therapist in an emergency when she's away?* Murphy's law of therapy is that something unusual will arise while your therapist is on vacation. Make sure you feel comfortable (or at least informed) about who you will be speaking with if your therapist is away.

- *Do you feel comfortable being with the therapist?* This is the litmus test. If you don't feel comfortable today, you probably won't next week either. A certain degree of anxiety is normal—this is a new person, possibly a new experience. But trust your instincts. If the whole thing feels creepy or depressing or so stressful you want to get drunk while you're sitting there, either find a different therapist or slow down—you may not be ready to dive into therapy.

The therapist may have a few questions to ask you, either on the phone or if you meet with her or him in person. Here are some questions therapists are likely to ask.

241

• *Have you been in therapy before?* Most therapists will want to know if you've been in any kind of treatment. If you have, they will want to know why you left or how it ended. Some, especially if they're in a clinic, might want to contact your previous therapist. You have the right to grant or deny permission. Don't give permission unless you feel it would be helpful.

• *How was your previous experience of therapy?* Therapists usually want to know how you have experienced other forms of therapy. If you've had a good experience, you can let your new therapist know what worked. If it was a bad experience, he or she needs to know what not to do with you.

• *What are you hoping to get out of therapy?* You may or may not be able to respond to this question, and the answer may change over time. That's OK. The question is intended mostly to get you thinking about what you want. It's good your therapist wants to know.

• *How will you pay for therapy?* Nobody likes to talk about money, but this is a reasonable question. Talk about insurance options, self-pay, and sliding scale (flexible fees). If you know that your cash flow is frequently disrupted by your using, talk this over with the therapist and establish some ground rules with which you are both comfortable.

Drug Treatment: What to Expect

Drug treatment is offered at varying levels of intensity. It is always focused on keeping you abstinent. Some require that you be drug-free before you start; others allow you a few days to get there and help you with detox.

Regular outpatient programs allow you live at home, go to work, and continue your usual (nondrug-using) life. You attend process (talking) groups, educational groups, and/or individual counseling for one or a few hours a week. Programs last for several months to two years. There also are Intensive Outpatient Programs (IOP), which run for about three hours a day, three to five days a week for several weeks or months. The next level of intensity is usually "day treatment," programs that last for perhaps two to four weeks and have all of the activities of an inpatient program except that you don't sleep there. Still another level of treatment available, residential programs take up part or all of your day with treatment activities. Some allow you to work, and you stay at the facility. Some of these programs are referred to as *therapeutic communities,* a term that dates from the 1950s. People can stay in some therapeutic communities for two years or more. Finally, the most intensive form of treatment is an inpatient setting, where you are in program activities all day, often part of the evening, and you stay at the facility, usually for either two to four weeks, or at least for a few days of detoxification. How long you stay at these facilities often depends on what your insurance company will pay for and what you can afford. They can be very expensive.

In both residential and inpatient treatment programs, your contact with the outside world may be limited, forbidden, or supervised. Research indicates that for most people, there is no more benefit gained from inpatient programs than from outpatient programs. If you feel, though, that you want to quit *right now* and just can't do it in your regular life, one of these programs will help get you started. Research shows that people who stay in residential treatment for a year or more tend to have better outcomes. Some of these programs will allow you to keep in contact with your regular therapist, but some discourage it, feeling that you need to focus exclusively on your addiction. This, of course, is not our point of view and may cause you some conflicts, but if you feel that you need to be separated from your everyday life, these programs can help you.

An outpatient program considered an entity unto itself is outpatient methadone treatment. These programs administer methadone, a synthetic opiate, as a substitute for heroin or other opiates. Methadone is administered only in strictly controlled, federally supervised clinics. Counseling, vocational skills development, and case management to help patients access support services are used to gradually stabilize people. Some patients stay on methadone for many years, some forever, whereas others eventually move from methadone to abstinence. Unfortunately, it is burdensome to be on methadone. You have to show up at the clinic every day and submit to random urine tests. Clinics vary widely in how respectfully they treat patients. Only when you demonstrate reliability over months or years are you allowed "take home" doses—a week's worth of doses, or the exact number of doses to account for each of the days of a vacation—in a locked box. There is a move afoot to allow certified physicians to prescribe methadone in their regular office or clinic practices. Since, as we said earlier, methadone or other opiates are essential medication for people whose endorphin systems may have been damaged by early trauma, this will go a long way to destigmatize methadone and to normalize the whole process of receiving treatment.

Outcomes of Drug Treatment

Outcomes of drug treatment have always been measured in terms of abstinence rates. They are not impressive. They usually hover around 25 percent, according to estimates. The only scientifically designed survey of drug treatment in the United States, conducted by the federal Substance Abuse and Mental Health Services Administration and completed in 1998, found abstinence rates of 21 percent several years after the completion of treatment. It is much more difficult to find out how many people *never complete* the treatment programs they enter, but it is the majority. The same study, interestingly, found much more impressive results when it measured *harm reduction* outcomes. These included *reduction* in drug use, criminal activity, unemployment, loss of children to the child welfare system, medical crises, and other quality-of-life issues. Improvement rates ranged from 23 to 43 percent in these areas. We can only imagine how much better treatment attendance and reduction in various harms would be if people got to *pick* their goals. Research in Europe, where there are real alternatives between abstinence and controlled use, indicate positive results. Furthermore, most people, given a choice, choose to work toward abstinence!

Shopping for Drug Treatment

Shopping for drug treatment is similar to shopping for a therapist. You have a right to ask questions in a phone conversation and, if you are satisfied with the answers, proceed to an in-person visit. Abstinence will always be the goal of treatment and often a prerequisite. This is less true for inpatient treatment programs that offer detoxification. (To require that you be abstinent before you show up could be dangerous!) Unfortunately, accusing clients of "denial" is often the method of choice. You might not be able to tell how strenuous this confrontational approach will be from a phone conversation. In most places, any drug use during the program will get you kicked out.

Ninety-three percent of programs—inpatient, residential, or outpatient—are based on the 12-Step philosophy of Alcoholics Anonymous. When that is the case, you will be required to attend 12-Step meetings as a condition of your participation in the program. Some treatment programs, especially some of the older "therapeutic communities," use confrontation, punishment, and humiliation to get you to go along with the program and to transform your "addictive personality" (there's no such thing, by the way). This is the ultimate in tough love. Since we believe that many drug users have already been traumatized and badly shamed, we find the idea of breaking someone's spirit in this way to be horrifying. Certain people do benefit from such an extreme approach: they overcome serious addictions and even criminal behavior patterns. By now you know that this is not an approach we endorse, especially for people who have been oppressed or traumatized.

Drug treatment programs tend to undertreat other problems, such as depression and anxiety. Some think that if you get too comfortable, you won't remember why you're there and you'll relapse. Some programs don't allow the use of prescribed psychiatric medications, but nicotine and caffeine are usually used freely! Many don't allow you to be on methadone either, despite the fact that using methadone could be very helpful to your efforts to stop using heroin or other opiates, to say the least. It seems odd to us that being comfortable is seen as dangerous. We think that being comfortable is not the same as being "in denial." Because there is growing pressure to treat people who have "dual diagnoses," however, it is possible that any program you call might allow use of psychiatric medications and might even have a physician available to prescribe them.

Since most programs tend to think that anyone who is abusing alcohol or other drugs can't make good decisions, you may find yourself pressured to take a view of yourself and your relationship with drugs that doesn't really fit with your true beliefs. All of these programs work by trying to help you become part of a community ("the fellowship," in the case of AA). You are encouraged to fully immerse yourself in the group experience. You are also told to pay attention to what others in recovery say and to distrust your own instincts. You end up going along with "the program." This kind of compliance, against your own judgment, often leads to relapse or "treatment failure." If you are going to use traditional treatment and/or self-help programs, you must either decide that you believe what they are saying and entrust yourself to the program, the counselors, and the other participants, or find other skeptics like yourself who can help you deal with the conflicts that will arise. A good harm reduction therapist should be able to help you manage these conflicts.

It might be impossible for you to use harm reduction techniques (other than abstinence) if you enter a traditional drug treatment program. A few outpatient treatment programs, however, are now including a harm reduction option. Some call it *pretreatment.* In other words, they are preparing you for the *real* treatment, which means abstinence and all the activities that go along with it. In San Francisco, thanks to the Department of Public Health, in all its wisdom, harm reduction is becoming a required option in drug treatment. If a program can't incorporate harm reduction into its philosophy, it must give you an alternative referral. We look forward to the day when all communities offer harm reduction treatment as an option.

If you are interested in exploring drug treatment, here are some of the questions you might want to ask:

- *What is your organization's philosophy?* You'll want to know if absti- nence is required to be in the program, and if it is, how relapses are han- dled. You'll also want to find out if counselors work from a disease model (you are powerless over your disease) or a behavioral model (you have the capacity to learn to control your behavior). This simple distinction will give you some sense of whether your philosophy jibes with theirs.

- *What is the intake process?* Some programs have you interviewed by several people, which can be exhausting. Some also make you wait, all the while getting or staying "clean and sober." This waiting is often seen as a test of your motivation.

- *How much do I get to be involved in my treatment planning?* This is a vital piece of information. You should be as involved as possible with your own treatment planning. Remember, you are the expert about your use. You alone have access to the best information about what will work and what won't work to help you. If a counselor tells you that all addicts are the same and they use a preset treatment plan, look elsewhere.

- *Who are some of the other people who might be in treatment with me?* If you are an alcohol user, will you be comfortable with needle users? Are there more men than women, and is this OK with you?

- *What is a typical day like?* Knowing the basic schedule can alleviate a good deal of your anxiety, and it will also help you see if there is enough, or too much, "program time."

- *How much time is spent in individual, group, family, or marital treat- ment?* If you don't want to involve your family, and the program focuses on family treatment, it won't be a good fit for you. Similarly, if you feel your spouse is an integral part of your efforts to reduce the harm in your life and the program does not involve spouses, you may not get what you need there.

- *What are the credentials of the counselors or staff?* You have a better chance of getting competent treatment in a professional environment where staff receive regular training. This does not, however, guarantee *good,* cut- ting-edge treatment. First, even if staff members are professionals, they might adhere to a philosophy that doesn't work for you. Second, there are very helpful unlicensed staff out there, just like there are incompetent pro- fessionals.

- *Do you employ people who are "in recovery"?* It may or may not be important to you to be helped by people who share your experiences.

- *What's your program's philosophy about psychiatric medications?* Some programs regard any and all drugs, including antidepressants and antipsychotics, as off-limits. We recommend you look for a program whose philosophy supports the idea that psychiatric medication can be helpful in your struggle with drugs or alcohol.

• *What happens after I leave your program? Is there ongoing support?* Ongoing support is important, as is the philosophy of the "aftercare" program. You will want to know what the continuing care providers think about relapse and how it is handled. If they kick you out of aftercare or force you to start over, we would suggest you look elsewhere.

• *How does your program define success, and what is your program's success rate?* These answers will tell you a lot about an abstinence-based philosophy versus a harm reduction-based philosophy. If success is defined as absolute and total abstinence and you want a program that uses a harm reduction model, this program will not be helpful to you. You will also want to know how many of the people in the program are successful. Remind the person with whom you are speaking that you do not want an "advertisement" but rather some information to help you gauge whether you will be successful and for how long.

• *Can I talk with some people who have been through your program?* There's nothing like the horse's mouth to give you an inside look. Be wary of places that don't want you to speak with former customers. Be wary of places that offer up a list of names without stating that the people they are offering have agreed to waive their confidentiality.

These questions are very assertive and, unfortunately, many alcohol and drug treatment program staff might become defensive when faced with your wish to talk about the details of their program. For sixty years, the 12 Steps of AA and the confrontational style of programs, not to mention the assumption that abstinence is the gold standard, have reigned unchallenged. You may be labeled as "difficult" or "resistant" rather than seen as an equal partner. If that's the feeling you get, run!

Self-Help Options

By definition, self-help programs are not professionally led. They are supportive groups of peers, all of whom have suffered from alcohol and other drug problems, who come together to help each other stay abstinent (except in the case of Moderation Management, which helps group members manage their drinking). Alcoholics Anonymous and its sister programs are, by far, the most available of all the self-help groups. AA is a spiritual program of support, based on the disease model of addiction. It teaches the 12

Steps, which involve accepting one's powerlessness and undertaking a number of exercises in surrender, self-examination, and making amends, followed by a life of giving back. A number of other programs that offer alternatives to the spiritual approach of AA have sprung up in recent years. Except for Moderation Management, they all expect their members to have abstinence as their goal, although most do not reject people who have not achieved it. All of these alternative programs are listed, with descriptions, in the Resources appendix.

Harm Reduction Treatment: Training Your Therapist or Counselor

No drug treatment programs, except the Harm Reduction Therapy Center, with offices in San Francisco and Oakland, California, and a few other programs and therapists in private practices, exclusively use a comprehensive harm reduction model. The Resources appendix gives you some places to start, and The Harm Reduction Therapy Center's website has links to other harm reduction programs and specialists around the country (*www.harmreductiontherapy.org*). The Internet has become a storehouse of information about addiction, with thousands of references to harm reduction sites, and if you search, you may find something that fits your needs. If you know of any people to add to our list, please contact us. The more people who get involved, the easier it will be for other people who need help.

There are some programs and many individuals who use harm reduction principles but may not call themselves harm reductionists. If you are specifically looking for a harm reduction psychotherapist, you will probably have to say so when you are shopping. Since harm reduction is relatively new in this country, and still very controversial, your search will not be easy. You will have to explain what you mean. You might then be surprised that therapists are willing to work with you once they understand the idea. Many therapists who call themselves cognitive–behavioral or life skills therapists use harm reduction approaches intuitively or as part of some other training and practice. The principles are not unique to harm reduction. In fact, they are the basis of any good therapy. It's just that therapists have been told to refer people who use drugs to "drug treatment," that it is not their business to address drug issues. Still other people have an incomplete view of what harm reduction is, so they may deny that they use it but actually do! Some people think harm reduction is only about needle exchange, or is not in favor of abstinence at all, or think it is about drug legalization. *Tell them this is not true!*

The interview questions in this chapter are meant to help you find out how closely a therapist's values and methods conform to harm reduction principles. These questions can also be the start of a conversation with a therapist you like but who thinks he or she doesn't want to get involved in harm reduction.

Finally, many therapists are willing to read something that you suggest in order for them to understand your needs. Show them this book. Talk about it with them. Give them the professional reading list from the Resources appendix or the Harm Reduction Therapy Center website. Patt has written a very readable book for professionals on this topic: *Practicing Harm Reduction Psychotherapy*, published in 2000 by The Guilford Press.

Finally, some drug and alcohol treatment programs have introduced harm reduction principles in parts of their programs. Sometimes these are referred to as *pretreatment groups* or as *decision groups.* They are helpful if you want to examine the harmful effects of your alcohol or other drug use but aren't sure if you want to quit. Most of these programs will not accept you into their "regular" treatment program, though, until you decide to become abstinent. From our point of view, of course, there is no such thing as pretreatment. Once you begin a process of self-examination, you are in treatment, on the journey called *recovery.* The next chapter describes what this journey looks like for people who are practicing harm reduction.

SOURCES AND SUGGESTED READINGS

Here are some references that can tell you what you can expect from different types of help and that provide analyses of what works and what doesn't:

Handbook of Alcoholism Treatment Approaches: Effective Alternatives (3rd ed.). Reid Hester and William Miller, Eds. Allyn & Bacon. 2003.

Harm Reduction Psychotherapy: A New Treatment for Drug and Alcohol Problems. Andrew Tatarsky, Ed. Aronson. 2002.

Hooked: Five Addicts Challenge Our Misguided Drug Rehab System. Lonny Shavelson. New Press. 2001.

"Matching Alcoholism Treatments to Client Heterogeneity: Project MATCH Posttreatment Drinking Outcomes." *Journal of Studies on Alcohol, 58*, 7–29, 1997. (You can look at all of the results of this major study by doing a web search with the keyword *Project MATCH*.)

Practicing Harm Reduction Psychotherapy: An Alternative Approach to Addictions. Patt Denning. Guilford Press. 2000.

Recovery Options: The Complete Guide. Joseph Volpicelli and Maia Szalavitz. Wiley. 2000.

Treating Substance Abuse: Theory and Technique (2nd ed.). Frederick Rotgers, Jon Morgenstern, and Scott T. Walters, Eds. Guilford Press. 2003.

The Truth about Addiction and Recovery. Stanton Peele. Simon & Schuster. 1991.

And for your therapist:

Practicing Harm Reduction Psychotherapy: An Alternative Approach to Addictions. Patt Denning. Guilford Press. 2000.

Harm Reduction: Pragmatic Strategies for Managing High Risk Behaviors. G. Alan Marlatt, Ed. Guilford Press. 1998.

Motivational Interviewing: Preparing People for Change (2nd ed.). William R. Miller and Stephen Rollnick. Guilford Press. 2003.

"Warm Turkey: Other Routes to Abstinence." William Miller and A. C. Page. *Journal of Substance Abuse Treatment, 8,* 227–232. 1991.

"Strategies for Implementation of Harm Reduction in Treatment Settings." Patt Denning. *Journal of Psychoactive Drugs, 33*(1), 23–26. 2001.

And any other readings your therapist might choose from the treatment or research sections of the Sources and Suggested Readings in the appendix.

10 IS HARM
REDUCTION WORKING?

We can't think of a more reasonable question to ask yourself than "Is harm reduction working for me?" Everybody wants to know this answer. People also usually want to know whether harm reduction or abstinence is best for them (or, even more often, for someone else!). You have shaken loose some old ways of doing things. Maybe you've shifted from the contemplation stage of change to the action stage. Or you've shifted from the precontemplation stage to contemplation. You've made a single positive change or many. Research on the stages of change indicates that thoroughly negotiating each stage before moving on to the next leads to better success at meeting your goals. But simply having "done some work" may not tell you if harm reduction is working for you.

Sylvia, the woman in the Introduction whose husband left her and took the kids, had a bad time for many months. She lost her job, and she and her father became dependent on his Social Security. While she and her husband were separated, they went into counseling, and she did make one final stab at AA, but she hated it. She realized this approach was not what she needed, feeling it was too preachy and judgmental. She had grown up in a fundamentalist Christian community, which she always thought of as hypocritical because the supposed Christians were very racist. She came across SMART recovery (see the Resources section in the appendix), found a good therapist, and was able to slowly taper herself down to one or two cocktails on Saturdays. Sylvia's husband is still not satisfied and believes she will be OK only if she is abstinent forever. Sylvia would like to quit drinking altogether, partly as a role model for her kids, partly for her health, but for now she thinks of her one or two drinks as a reasonable protest against her husband's rigidity and control. Nevertheless, they got back together and agreed to continue couple therapy.

Sylvia has since gotten another job and is working full time now that the kids are teenagers, which gets her through the 2:00 to 6:00 P.M. stretch without drinking. Even though she feels guilty about seeing less of her kids, and her evenings are really crazy with chores, working has eased their money trouble and given Sylvia a feeling of greater independence and control. The whole process took about two years. She doesn't attend any support meetings, which still makes her husband uneasy, but she has made some friends at work who don't drink and who have helped her discover other fun things to do. They either play cards or go to a movie every Friday night.

There could have been many points along the way when Sylvia might have said, "This just isn't working." Like when her kids asked her why she was still drinking and keeping the family apart. Or when her husband left for one night during an argument. But she was able to remember that progress forward almost always includes some stops along the way and even some steps back to make sure of the direction. She kept coming back to the idea that *any positive change* meant she was still doing the right thing, at least the most right thing she could handle at that moment.

For some of you, the successes of harm reduction have come in days or weeks. For others it may take months or years, so you feel it isn't working, or it's too soon to tell, and for sure it's taking way too long. Some of you have struggled to make changes and have not succeeded at all. Or you may have set out to reduce your drinking or smoking with some success, but trouble still surfaces (or new troubles emerge) from your newfound infatuation with another substance. Maybe you've been on methadone for six months and you've used heroin only twice, but you're not sure you should be smoking so much pot. Then again, for many of you harm reduction may be virtually indistinguishable from just another day. How will you know what's working?

First let's define what *working* means. Harm reduction works for different people in different ways. It comes in every size and shape you can imagine. It works in very small ways, like changing the color or brand of your rolling paper, to very big ways, like quitting pot altogether. Every person trying to use harm reduction should be generous but realistic about measuring improvement. This means that if you're thinking of giving up because you don't see any improvements at all, be generous with yourself: Have you made things worse, or are you maintaining, hanging on? Have you killed anyone, or are the people close to you all still alive and kicking? Are you still alive? If your life was going downhill, and you stopped the downhill slide, maybe that's progress. Stabilizing your use, leveling off before you lose everything, might just have saved your life or someone else's.

On the other hand, if learning about harm reduction has made you so relaxed that you write off everybody's worries about you as drug hysteria, check again. Be realistic. Was there anything that *you* were worried about that needs attention? The likelihood is that, since you are still reading this book, you are taking your relationship with drugs seriously, have an appropriate level of concern, have not climbed into that hole we mentioned earlier in the book, and are waiting out the storm with your favorite drug.

We haven't put it this way before, but harm reduction has steps, too. There are really only four steps to practicing harm reduction. They are the stages of change—contemplation, preparation, action, and maintenance. They take each of us very different lengths of time to travel. There are many curves and switchbacks, which most people call *relapse.* If you are at any one of these stages, harm reduction *is* working. Once you reach the termination stage, you are "over it" and no longer need to practice harm reduction consciously. Now you are taking good enough care of yourself out of habit.

In other words, if you are at any of these stages, you are in the process of "recovery." *Recovery* is another word people in harm reduction don't talk about much. It is a word that is too closely associated with AA's 12 Steps. But all it means is that you're getting healthier. You're being as honest as you can. You're putting effort into doing less harm to yourself and others. You don't have to be all finished. You don't have to quit using. You can take breaks. You get to decide how much work is the right amount. And you get to choose which harmful effects you want to work on based on their impact on your life. If you're doing any of these things, particularly if you're doing them consciously, you're making progress. The motto of the Chicago Recovery Alliance—"any positive change"—is all we humans can expect of ourselves.

You can measure positive changes by following the sequence of this book. You will know harm reduction is working if you . . .

   . . . **are thinking about your relationship with drugs.**
   . . . **are setting some goals, knowing what you want and what you need.**
   . . . **are on the way to making changes that you like.**
   . . . **have achieved your goals.**

Thinking about Your Relationship with Drugs

If you're still reading this book, it's likely that you're evaluating your relationship with drugs. You can't change until you've made some decisions. You can't make decisions until you've studied yourself and your drugs. You can't easily study yourself and your drugs if you're locked into labels such as *addict* or *alcoholic*. When you lock yourself into one of these definitions, your use of drugs is explained by your label. If you've managed to leave the label aside and stick cotton in your ears when others call you names, you're on the harm reduction road.

Here are reminders of some key points to consider when evaluating your relationship with drugs and examples of how some of the people in this book handled this first step.

Be flexible about labeling yourself (or someone else) an addict.

Remember Daryl, the man in the Introduction who had been smoking pot every day for fifteen years and feeling OK about it but was now wondering what to do with his life? His friends had always told him that he had inherited the disease of addiction from his alcoholic parents, and that he should beware any drugs, especially alcohol. He was never convinced, but when his dad died of lung cancer last year, he got scared enough to quit smoking. Within a month he was drinking every weekend and still no happier with his job. He had also gotten a DUI—his first ever—and was beginning to wonder if he *had* inherited a disease. Something still didn't seem right to him, though.

Daryl came across harm reduction while searching the websites on addiction, and it clicked. He got himself into therapy and discovered that although smoking pot (and playing basketball) had helped him be able to tolerate his parents' drinking, it had also deprived him of the ability to be a good student. At his therapist's suggestion, he started taking a couple of courses at the community college. It wasn't until he bombed a midterm exam that he started scrutinizing his weekend drinking binges. He realized that his *motivation* for smoking or drinking was the problem. He didn't care enough about himself, had gotten into a bad habit of wanting to get "out of it," and the result was self-destructive and self-defeating. He had never really taken himself seriously or thought about what kind of adult life he wanted to live. His pot smoking and, later, drinking weren't about being an addict. They served to prevent him from being a well-developed person—from making adult choices and being responsible for living his life to the fullest.

Kendra, the woman in Chapter 1 who had lost her job and was smoking pot and snorting heroin with friends, moved along almost effortlessly—so effortlessly that when things started getting better for her, her brother put more and more pressure on her to go to NA. He would tell her she couldn't possibly be getting better—that heroin was too addictive a drug, she must be on a "pink cloud" (in a honeymoon period) and in denial about her addiction. She would be back to it as soon as there was a problem at work, and it wouldn't be long before she would be shooting it again. Every time she told him that things were better—that she had gotten another job and had less time for heroin or that she was just depressed about being poor—he would focus on the fact that she was depressed and tell her she was a drunk waiting to drink. For a while she stopped talking to him altogether, because she felt so misunderstood by him.

Things fell apart for her when she started to get nervous and, at her brother's urging, agreed to see a counselor at a drug treatment clinic. The counselor confirmed her brother's worries and educated Kendra about how denial works.

Kendra decided she must be practically delusional, her denial was so deep. She didn't feel *any* of the things her counselor or her brother said she did. Was she really so out of touch with her own feelings? For a while she felt crazy, trying to reconcile her feelings and the feedback she was getting from her counselor. She got very anxious, started having trouble sleeping, and lost weight as she searched inside herself to see if she really wanted to snort. Her counselor referred her for a psychiatric evaluation, and she was prescribed an antianxiety medication and an antidepressant.

To her surprise the medications made her feel like a new person. But to her counselor's and brother's surprise, she found a pretty independent voice inside and told them both to lay off. She quit seeing her counselor, stayed on the antianxiety medication for about two weeks, and still takes the antidepressants. She hasn't touched heroin, still smokes a little pot every few days, and feels satisfied with her job. She's been thinking about learning some more about how to budget her money so she won't have to be poor forever.

Be realistic about the harm you are, and are not, doing. Don't panic, but don't underestimate. Measure your level of use with an objective eye.

Remember Hillary from Chapter 1, who worked in a café for about three years and used speed with her coworkers to get through her shift? At first she was using only once a day, just before the dinner rush, but then she was using at the beginning of her 4:00 P.M. shift and maybe a couple of times before she closed up at midnight. She began having trouble sleeping and started to notice her short temper with her child and her waxy skin. She wondered if she was now an "addict" but decided it was just job stress that was making her feel so bad and function so poorly.

Know why you use.

Terry is the woman who was having sexual, legal, and maybe drinking problems in Chapter 8. Her drinking had increased after she was raped a few years ago. Her drinking also seemed to be related to her symptoms of depression, and to her attendance at the after-work happy hours, where she liked to unwind and hang out with folks in a situation where she didn't feel so shy. She got a little overwhelmed and confused by trying to figure out what was causing what, or if all these things were just coincidental. She decided to see a therapist for help in evaluating the seriousness of each of her issues. Together they decided that the first issue to tackle was the rape a few years ago, since it might be at the root of her sexual inhibition, her depressive symptoms, and her drinking too much. It seemed the most likely cause, if there was a cause, of her other problems. This made sense to Terry and felt like it would relieve her of an enormous burden of fear she had been carrying ever since. They decided that if she didn't notice any improvements in her other issues within a few months, they would look for other things that might be driving Terry's drinking.

Setting Goals and Knowing What You Want and Need

If you've studied your relationship with drugs enough to start making some decisions, you're well into the contemplation stage and heading toward the second step, the preparation stage. Setting goals comes after you say, "All right, all right, I'll *do* something about shooting speed." You don't know what yet, you don't have to be happy about it, but you're ready to commit to making some change. To negotiate this step, here are the tasks involved and how other folks have accomplished them.

Know how you feel about change.

Despite the sensible plan she made with her therapist, and her relief in talking about her rape, her nightmares, and her fears, Terry wasn't thrilled at the thought of changing her drinking habits. She liked her after-work routine. She didn't want to lose it. She also couldn't really imagine developing a richer life with her partner. They had always had a stay-at-home kind of life. She skipped several therapy sessions. She drank a little more on the way home. At least she wasn't driving—*that* was a change she could live with! Finally, her therapist suggested that they talk about what it might mean to her to change her drinking habits but not worry about making any actual progress.

Determine your hierarchy of needs. Listen to your own voice about what you need and want.

Danny, the young man struggling with schizophrenia who is intermittently homeless, got angrier and angrier about being pushed around. He felt controlled when he lived in residences for the mentally ill or drug treatment programs. He felt ashamed and young when he stayed with his parents. And he certainly didn't enjoy being homeless. He liked drinking and smoking crack sometimes, and he didn't like being so restricted that he had to sneak around until he got busted. "What the hell do I *want*?" he said over and over. "OK, number one, a roof over my head where nobody gets in my business. Number two, some money in my pocket. Number three, control over what drugs I take and when."

That seemed clear enough to Danny. It took him a couple of years to achieve his goals. He had to put his name on a waiting list for subsidized housing where they don't do anything to you if you use drugs as long as you don't cause trouble for other people in the building. (They have those kind of places in San Francisco.) They do have counselors, and they have money managers who help you pay your rent at the beginning of the month. Then the rest is yours. When he finally moved into his small studio apartment in a supportive housing program, he was in heaven. For months, he got loaded right after rent day, then had no money for the rest of the month and had to eat at the free lunch places around the city. That was a big drag. Also, the counselors would see him looking pretty bad, agitated at times and losing weight, and try to get him to talk to them. But what the hell did he move here for if he was going to have counselors in his business? Wasn't this his own home, for goodness sake?

He did finally decide that control was not exactly what he had achieved by blowing all his money by the fifth of the month. He hadn't achieved having money in his pocket either. So he got his money manager to give him a weekly stipend. That helped him space out his alcohol and crack use.

Danny had decided what he needed and wanted and had taken care of these things one at a time. A few years later he had built relationships with the other residents and the counselors. Some would ask him what he got out of smoking crack. "Don't you get crazier, man?" So what? he thought. But the questions got to him, so he went back to the drawing board to think about whether he might want something different in terms of the drugs he was putting into his body. For as long as we have known him, he has tinkered with his medications and other drugs. He went to school to get training as a computer tech, has girlfriends from time to time, and lives a reasonable life.

Work a decisional balance, about one, two, or all of your identified needs.

Stella is the woman who was mourning the death of her husband with help from Xanax and alcohol. With the increased pressure from her kids, her boss, and her EAP counselor, she knew she had to make some changes but didn't know where to begin. Her job and her grief and loneliness were the issues needing attention, with a decision about what to do with her alcohol and pills the goal. She put them all together in a complicated decisional balance.

On the one hand, alcohol blotted her out at night so she didn't have to think or feel. And Xanax eased the hangover she woke up to the next morning, which helped her face the day. On the other hand, she still felt awful at work and was irritable, sloppy, and in trouble. She certainly couldn't go along with the recommendations of the alcohol treatment counselor whose group she ended up in, but she did learn an interesting piece of information: Xanax has a particularly nasty crash when it wears off. On the one hand, it was the only drug her doctor had given her, and on the other hand, it might actually be causing her trouble at work more than alcohol. She thought about other ways to handle loneliness besides drinking. She couldn't imagine, however, going to any of the familiar places she and Victor used to go to—the restaurants, movie theaters, parks, even the grocery stores. Therapy didn't seem to be an option, since she had already been told that no one would help her talk about her loss until she quit drinking. And she couldn't quit drinking. . . . Nothing was coming clear—she was well and truly stuck. So she decided to keep going to the support group to keep herself out of trouble and just experiment with various ideas to see how they would feel. We'll visit her again later.

There was just one last safety measure. Her job was vital to her wellbeing. It was financially important, was the only connection she was able to maintain with people on a consistent basis, and even though she was not doing her job very well, she knew it was something she was good at. In preparation for making changes that would ease the pressure at work, she set herself one basic goal: be honest with her boss on the bad days.

Distinguish between what's the drug, what's you, and what's your environment.

Masa is the young man who was cycling between extremes of depression and psychotic episodes and using ecstasy and speed at dance clubs. With the help of a counselor at the student counseling center of his college, he was able to start untangling the various factors that were contributing not only to his attraction to ecstasy and speed but also to the way the drugs were interacting with his depression and psychotic experiences. He figured that he had been depressed on and off since his teens, so he and his therapist made a close study of the different things he felt in a "post E depression" and his memories of the "pure depression" he had felt in his teens. Ultimately he determined that underneath the E depression, he was still pretty depressed most of the time. He and his therapist wanted to figure out how his intermittent psychotic experiences figured in before considering antidepressants. The more they talked, the less it seemed that Masa had bipolar disorder. His very high highs only happened with speed but didn't seem to have come up before he had started using it. Finally, they determined that he did have depression, which was exacerbated by ecstasy and lifted by speed.

This first clarification led Masa and his therapist to discuss *where* he was using. It wasn't only the fun of the drugs; it was being with lots of people who felt just fine about his being gay, who encouraged him to explore his wild side and break out of some of the traditions he had grown up with. And the excitement he felt when he was out with these accepting people made him less aware of the harm he was experiencing. He usually didn't drink enough water, but that had never gotten him in trouble. He got really overexcited. He used a lot of speed with guys he met, not knowing at first that speed can make you psychotic.

It seemed that the culture he had grown up in and its attitudes about his being gay and the culture he was currently drawn to were the key ingredients here. He probably needed to be treated for depression, because he'd had symptoms for several years. The depression might very well disappear once he has accepted himself and gotten his parents' and relatives' voices out of his head. Come to think of it, maybe *that* would get rid of the psychotic voices first. Untangling clubbing, sex, and drugs would prove more problematic. Nothing could beat the excitement. It seemed he first needed to find a friend or lover or two who weren't into that scene to give him an alternative place to feel at home. Then he would see if he could become less reliant on the drugs for connection.

Get an idea of what stage of change you're in for each issue, or at least the first few.

Cheryl is the woman who was sexually abused as a child and now finds that drinking loosens her up enough to have sexual relationships with men, but that it also unleashes much of the anger that destroys those relationships. She identified several issues she wanted to deal with: her relationships with men, her abuse history, the anger that seemed to connect her current relationships to her past abuse, the aftereffects of drinking (fatigue and irritability), and the attitudes of her friends. She was at a different stage regarding each of these issues.

Although she felt certain that her abuse history was at the core of much of her troubles, she felt overwhelmed by its magnitude and remained unable to think about it for the first year of therapy. Discovering that she was in the *precontemplation* stage on this topic meant that she should move on to something else for now. Every now and again, her therapist would gently remind her that she might consider telling her what had happened. Cheryl finally accepted an eight-session referral for EMDR (eye movement desensitization and reprocessing—a technique that has proven successful in helping some people manage and/or let go of traumatic memories). This EMDR experience helped her develop a sense of safety when remembering her history and moved her closer to agreeing to talk to her therapist about it.

In the meantime, Cheryl considered (*contemplated*) changing something about her drinking to cut down on how tired and irritable she felt so much of the time. She weighed the downside of evenings alone without drinking versus the upside of days at work not biting people's heads off. She weighed the upside of not drinking and fighting with boyfriends against the downside of being tense when a man touched her.

She decided she was definitely ready for *action*—to swear off relationships for a while, which was the easiest way for her to reduce the pressure to drink. The only *preparation* required was to rehearse what she would say when men called her for a date. She knew she wouldn't "relapse" and go out with a guy because she was truly sick of her terrible relationship pattern. All she needed to do was to *maintain* that new action—saying no—and eventually deal with her lack of trust—which, of course, brought her back to her childhood abuse.

Pick the issue that you're finished contemplating, the one that's closest to the preparation stage, and make a plan or try out a few ideas.

Stella had decided that excruciating loneliness was the most important issue to take care of first. Since she felt loneliest at home, and since alcohol is easier to obtain, she thought about stopping the Xanax in the mornings and still allowing herself a few drinks at night. She knew her job would be even more challenging without Xanax helping her through her hangovers. And, anyway, she didn't like the feeling alcohol gave her at night, especially knowing she wouldn't have her hangover pill in the morning. She backtracked and decided to reverse her plan. She gave up the alcohol on weeknights and stuck with the Xanax. She worked hard to find things to do out of the house most nights so that she would be home alone less. Those nights were still awful, but knowing she could rely on Xanax in the morning eased her anxiety both at night and when she woke up. She was still left with the problem of being almost impossible to work with when withdrawal set in, but because she was mentally clearer, colleagues were not suspicious about "addiction." They assumed she was moody because she was finally feeling her feelings about losing Victor.

All of this attention to the details of how she felt taught her something about herself, and the experience of having insight into herself was refreshing. Since she had been with Victor for most of her life, she had been dependent on him for her sense of self every waking moment. She had had no practice figuring out what would make her feel fulfilled. She enjoyed the feeling of paying attention to herself. It made her feel less lonely. She continued to think about Victor a lot, but it began to have some distance. She also began to notice that using the Xanax make her feel dependent, indeed in some of the ways she had depended on Victor. She challenged herself to develop the same independence she had discovered in paying attention to her feelings about alcohol, and soon she was taking great pride in the mornings she got to work without taking Xanax.

Making Changes That *You* Like

You've set certain goals for yourself, and some or all of these goals are being met. Your goal last month was to drink on Fridays instead of Saturdays. You are now drinking on Fridays and only rarely on Saturdays. Or, your goal might have been to quit everything. What you've done so far is to restrict your pot use to evenings, your speed use to once a month, and to study your impulses and reactions closely when you use. Or you've quit alcohol and heroin but still use pot. Harm reduction is working.

Manage your drug use better.

George had tried ecstasy a few times and loved it. After seeing someone get really sick at a club and end up in the hospital, however, George didn't know whether or not to do ecstasy again. No one else he knew had ever had any trouble with it, and he was reluctant to ask anyone about it. He found harm reduction through a party drug site on the Internet and got some excellent information about how to use ecstasy safely. Not using as often is recommended. It's also good to take vitamin C. He has developed a sort of before-hours ritual with his friends, where they play music and drink water. They never drink alcohol. They also pick a "designated driver" to keep tabs on how much they've used, who they're buying from, how long they've been dancing, and whether they're drinking water.

Do less harm.

Hillary took a look at what she liked about her job—everything from the money to the good friends she had at the restaurant. When she thought about everything in terms of a decisional balance, she realized that the best times she had with her friends occurred when she was high, but that the person she liked most at work was a college student who *didn't* get high. She was worried that even if she changed jobs, she'd have trouble quitting.

She also realized she didn't have to stick with dinner shifts, so she got a different waitress job doing lunches and an occasional dinner. She gets high with her old friends now and then but doesn't feel like it rules her schedule or that she depends on it.

Her parents and her friend from her old job still put pressure on her to quit altogether, but Hillary doesn't want to give it up. She plans to at some point, but not until she figures out what she wants to do with her life. She's thinking about taking a class so she can finish college. Hillary is using harm reduction in just the right way, to make changes in her life, as she needs to.

Develop new goals as you go along.

Now you're sober all weekend, but you feel agitated and jumpy. Harm reduction is still working; it's just that now your goal has changed. You don't have to address drinking on the weekends; you may need to work on finding interesting things to do with your family on Sundays to help ease the jumpiness, or staying busy on Saturday to keep away from the bottle. As life shifts and successes are accumulated, your goals will shift as well. Harm reduction is working.

Mike was the attorney, married for fifteen years. With two teenage kids and a new baby in the family, Mike's drinking was increasing steadily, as were fights with his wife, sleep deprivation, and drunk driving. He went to AA meetings for a few weeks, but he couldn't relate to the program and refused to go back. The older kids were getting very upset by his drinking, and his son had begun having trouble in school. Mike had wondered if he was an alcoholic or just suffering from stress.

The snowballing problems eventually led to a marital separation, and Mike discovered that without his family around every day, he drank even more. He and his wife went into therapy. It was that therapist who suggested that Mike try managing his drinking instead of trying to quit. His wife was very negative about such a compromise and wanted to focus on getting Mike to stop completely. Mike's first plan was to record every drink he took. His goal was to go to bed when he couldn't keep his handwriting within the lines on the page.

It took three weeks of talking about it before Mike began working on this goal. He and his wife and their therapist talked a lot about what his wife could do when she was frustrated that he wasn't abstinent. She still wasn't prepared to let him come home until he quit, and she was angry to have all the responsibility of the kids. Mike talked about his fear that he wouldn't be able to do his simple writing task. It made him feel foolish. Being able to voice their fears helped establish their first sense of partnership in years. Mike was able to stick with his assignment for two months before he and his wife decided to add another goal: to go outside for five minutes to get fresh air after every drink.

Step by step, he decreased his drinking (and increased his sleep) through these and other creative methods. He moved back home after nine months of steady progress. One night the baby woke up, and he ended up trying to get her to go back to sleep for about two hours, all the while not drinking. He realized he could be up in the night and not drink. Then he decided to try not drinking at all at least one night a week. The less he drank, the more he slept. The more he slept, the better he and his wife got along. The better they got along, the better he felt—and the less drawn to drinking he felt.

Take in positive comments from others.

The success of harm reduction isn't necessarily measured by whether you're feeling better. Sometimes you may still feel terrible, but others around you are commenting on your improved attitude and behavior, your clearer eyes, increased energy, and better outlook or mood. Actually *feeling* better may take some time. Sure, you're drinking on Fridays and not usually on Saturdays, but your family is noticing how much nicer you are to be around on Sundays. Harm reduction is working.

A year and a half after the whole process in therapy began, Mike is still drinking on weekends but stops when he feels tired. He still worries about where his drinking might lead, but now his wife is the big harm reduction advocate. She keeps telling him to look at the positive changes he's made and reminds him that as long as they're talking to each other and he continues in therapy and being a good father, she's got no complaints. Mike likes hearing that. He started thinking about getting some more support and decided to check out an AA meeting. To his surprise, he found it helpful, even though when he went a couple of years ago he had hated it. Now that he doesn't feel coerced, the meetings give him a way to hear how other people have quit drinking entirely. He thinks he'll try that himself someday.

Move through your hierarchy of needs — take care of things besides your drug use.

Cheryl, like Stella, knew that her job was an anchor to her well-being. But it was her overarching feeling of being unsafe that haunted her. Besides with men, she often felt nervous at work, at home, or driving. Making a list of all the things she needed to make her feel protected became a number-one priority. Comfortable clothes, walking with friends rather than alone at night, hot showers, women's self-defense classes were some ideas she came up with. What most people do intuitively had to be planned consciously. Next on her list was gaining the support of her friends. She knew she needed to feel a sense of belonging in both social and professional settings. She began to make an effort to identify people who made her feel comfortable. She thought about how people make, or don't make eye contact with her, whether they seemed to notice she was working hard, whether they reminded her of her brother, whether they interrupted her when she was talking, and so on. This not only increased her feeling of intimacy with her friends but made her feel alive, interested, and engaged.

Get help if you need it.

If things aren't going well and you've been trying to do this on your own, you might decide to get professional help. You might decide to add a traditional treatment modality to these harm reduction methods if you haven't done that already. Perhaps going to some AA or NA meetings, even though you're not particularly in favor of that approach, would be a kind of "booster shot" to help you move more quickly. Some people decide to go into a residential program if they want to be clean and sober, because the structure and support are much more intense than regular life. If you're having trouble staying off the booze, you could try a drug that prevents you from enjoying its effects or one that makes you sick if you drink. These extra things, even if you do them for just a little while, might get you jump-started when you feel like you're stuck.

After four years on the muscle relaxant Soma, which Gloria had originally taken for her neck injury following a car accident, her primary care physician discovered she was getting prescriptions from other doctors. Fortunately, instead of discontinuing her medications, he first prescribed therapeutic massage. After she had stabilized her use, he sent her to a pain clinic to learn various techniques for pain management. Not only did pain management help with the discomfort in her neck, it also helped her tolerate the gradual reduction to a lower dose of Soma. Her doctor also suggested that Gloria look into EMDR (eye movement desensitization and reprocessing), which, as noted, can be helpful for people who have experienced a traumatic event. She has another two months of decreasing her medication before she expects to be off it completely. Although Gloria was physically dependent on Soma, she felt her success in getting down to a lower dose came because her doctor never treated her like an "addict."

You Have Achieved Your Goals

Maintain your desired changes.

Jorge, the man in Chapter 5 who was trying to break from his routine of drinking at Sunday dinners with his family, made a plan to leave early a few times and see how that went. It did help him cut down on his drinking significantly, which made Monday mornings much easier. He drinks with friends on the weekends and has lost about ten pounds. He now goes to his parents' house every other week and stays for no more than two hours. After he dropped that first ten pounds so easily, he started looking at how much he was eating when he smoked pot. It wasn't that it was so much, but he was definitely lazier when he was stoned. After he got his brother to join a basketball team with him, he found that he wasn't as interested in smoking pot. He likes the feeling after basketball with his brother better than the feeling of being stoned and alone.

Feel confident in yourself.

Daryl is still in school, studying his butt off and working weekends instead of drinking, so that he can finish school and become a basketball coach. He drinks with friends some Friday nights. He occasionally smokes a joint, which he enjoys a lot, but he is keeping his eyes fixed on having a job doing something he loves.

Mature out of your relationship with drugs. Get "over it."

Remember Yolanda from Chapter 2? She had gone from smoking heroin to shooting it with her boyfriend. Her new independence after moving out of her parents' house was stressful, and heroin helped relax her. Since she had always been a good student, kind of nerdy and never considered cool, she was excited to have a boyfriend who was a little on the edge. When he encouraged her to shoot heroin, it was irresistible at first. She could feel herself sinking into it, losing track of her goals, not to mention her other friends. After about a month, feeling terrible and scared about where she might be headed, she broke off the relationship and started smoking pot.

Yolanda continued to smoke until her senior year in college, when she was invited to join a singing group. Smoking had definitely impaired her vocal range, but she still sounded good. Eventually she got interested in sounding better, made friends with two of the other members of the group, and was drifting away from the friends who smoked a lot. By the time she graduated from college, she was just smoking every few days to unwind. This remained her pattern.

Continue to grow. Keep working on whatever took you to your relationship with drugs and on whatever challenges come next.

Richard, the newly married man from Chapter 4, was dealing with his serious drinking problem for the first time in therapy. This focus opened the door to awful childhood memories of listening to his father beat his mother and sister. Even though he is building a good life, with a wife who supports him, the memories follow him and he has concerns about repeating the violence in his own life that he witnessed as a child. In therapy he talks about emptying his pockets of all his pain and anger, only to round the corner and discover there's more stuff in his pockets. Now that he and his therapist are communicating well about how much, when, and why he drinks, he's begun wondering if the positive changes will add pressure to have children soon. He wonders if he'll be a good parent. If they don't have children, he worries about whether the marriage will be a happy one. "It never ends," he says, exasperated.

It doesn't end. The challenges come whether we welcome them or not. But we have choices about how much harm we do and how much suffering we endure.

SOURCES AND SUGGESTED READINGS

"How Drug Users Measure Success in a Harm Reduction Setting." Terry Ruefli and Susan Rogers. *Harm Reduction*. Ernie Drucker, Ed. On-line journal. 2003.

11 HOW TO TALK TO FAMILY AND FRIENDS ABOUT HARM REDUCTION

The questions people ask and the things they say to you usually reflect the worries they have about your drinking or drug use and their hope that you'll stop. Sometimes these questions or comments are confrontational, or at least they sure sound that way. Ideas that are intended to be helpful can indicate either a poor understanding of your relationship with drugs or the fear, anger, and frustration people feel about how you're managing your life.

This chapter aims to translate the ideas of this book into user-friendly, put-'em-in-your-pocket and bring-'em-out-when-you-need-'em answers to people's concerns. Its purpose is to equip you with brief statements about harm reduction that respond to (1) the myths people have about drugs and drug use, (2) questions people ask you about the harm reduction approach, and (3) questions *you* have about this harm reduction stuff. We offer some possible "translations" of the common questions and statements people make about using and quitting, as well as some thoughts about why these questions get asked. Finally, to demonstrate that harm reduction is not completely beyond the scope of our sound bite society, we offer a few harm reduction sound bites.

Myths

You Have to Hit Bottom to Get Better

Why people think this:

Some people think change is possible only when you feel so bad you can't stand it anymore. The pain must become greater than the pleasure to precipitate change. The idea that hitting bottom is a requirement for getting better reflects a hope that you'll get desperate enough to *do something right now*. It also voices an angry wish that you will experience some *real* suffering as punishment for your drug-related transgressions. For some, this comes close to a puritanical or other strict religious belief that you must be punished to cleanse your sins and purify your soul.

What you can say:

Getting better is different for everyone, and not everyone "hits bottom" before learning how to get better. Besides, if I keep waiting to hit bottom before making any changes, I might be dead before I get there. Or somebody else might be! If you're talking about a "wake-up call," a punch in the face like losing my job or my wife, the phone has been ringing off the hook for years. I'm *awake* to most of the trouble I've caused. In fact, sometimes I get high to stop all the noise. Harm reduction *is* helping me. It's helping me decide what to do. It's also breaking down the changes I want to make into manageable steps, so I might actually *get* somewhere.

If You Think You Don't Have to Quit, You're in Denial

Why people think this:

People want results, and the only result we've talked about in this country for the last seventy years is *total abstinence*. Anything short of that has implied avoidance, denial, and continual drug-related crises. People just aren't familiar with alternatives to abstinence that also reduce very real harm.

What you can say:

Denial would mean I was pretending things aren't so bad. I know they're bad, I'm just trying to make them better more gradually than you might like. I'm dealing with my relationship with drugs all the time. I'm feeling pain, shame, and self-hatred. I'm looking as hard as I can as fast as I can at when, why, and how I use. Once I understand all that, I will decide what I can change about my use. Change can mean using less. It can mean using more safely. It can also mean using nothing. I'll figure it out, and I'll do it at the right pace and in the right order so I stand a chance of maintaining what I've done.

People quit drugs all the time. Most of them start again, too. How many times have you heard the joke "I can quit smoking—I do it every day"? It refers to the fact that people who think they can just quit are often in denial of their real and complicated relationship with drugs. But look at the statistics on methadone treatment or needle exchange. Many, many people have avoided HIV by substituting their opiate for methadone or by visiting a needle exchange program. Other changes are often more effective than quitting, because they actually succeed.

It's All or Nothing

Why people think this:

People think that quitting drugs or alcohol is an "all-or-nothing" matter mostly for two reasons. First, we have a "black-and-white" culture that does not tolerate shades of gray particularly well. It's in our language of drug treatment and AA: You're either "clean" or "dirty"; you're "in the program" or "out there." These concepts aren't much different from the religious idea of "saved" or "sinner." Remember, AA grew from religious roots. Second, to draw the line that distinguishes success from failure, and because AA was started by a man who could foresee only two alternatives—drunk or sober—because that's what *he* could imagine, people see *using* as failure and *not using* as success.

What you can say:

The idea that using is an all-or-nothing matter comes from the experiences of the handful of people who developed the idea and for whom this happened to be true. But the all-or-nothing model is not true for everyone. It's my life, drugs and all. My drugs have helped me at the same time as they've caused problems. I've figured out I don't want to suffer so much, and I don't want to hurt you anymore, but if I stop now, I won't know how to cope, so I'm learning how to cope with feelings at the same time as I'm cutting down gradually. You see, I can do two things at once, or I'm learning to.

Once an Addict, Always an Addict

Why people think this:

Some people think that using drugs is a slippery slope that always ends in addiction—which always means catastrophe. Because the (small) minority of people who join AA and the (small) minority of people who go to drug treatment haven't managed to control their use yet, a stereotype has emerged that says this is the way it is for everyone.

What you can say:

Seeing *all* drinkers and users as evolving the way Bill Wilson did is like living in Europe five hundred years ago and believing that the world was flat simply because the political and religious leaders said so. Or, it would be like living in this country two hundred years ago and thinking women shouldn't vote because they're the property of men. Today we know that the world is round and that women aren't property. Do we have to wait another two hundred years to redefine drug use? The fact is, most people who use or have used drugs *don't* get addicted. Moreover, just like we get over other bad habits, many people have controlled their drinking or using, even after having a problem. We don't hear from these people, either because they're using illegal drugs that they don't want to publicize or because they just don't make a fuss. C'mon, everybody knows *someone* who stopped abusing drugs or alcohol. Some of them quit, some drink or use moderately. If they can learn moderation, why can't I?

Addiction Is a Disease with No Cure

Why people think this:

Profound hopelessness, anger, and frustration are at the top of the list of feelings people have about your using. It helps them believe you are a victim of an incurable disease rather than a person making, at times, lousy choices. In the absence of other "cures" for alcoholism, AA persuaded a whole generation of people, including doctors, that the experience of its members defined the experience of all alcohol abusers. Thus the disease idea got professionalized and integrated with the "once an addict" idea. These "facts" have been absorbed into our culture as "the truth." But they are no more "true" than the "fact" that women used to be the property of men.

What you can say:

Bill Wilson wasn't necessarily wrong; he just didn't speak for me. I know that the idea of having a disease is comforting to people who tend to be judged or punished or who blame themselves for everything. They don't have to feel like a bad person if they have a disease. And that's good, because feeling like a bad person is often more harmful than anything—using drugs in a destructive manner is a great way to keep punishing yourself and anyone else who makes you feel shitty. For me, I'd prefer to be thought of as a person who has been making problematic choices for a reason. I don't need to feel diseased. I can take responsibility for my choices, and I'd appreciate it if you don't bad-mouth me while I'm working on changing those choices.

Addiction Is a Disease over Which You Are Powerless

Why people think this:

The disease model represents a significant advance over the moral model, in which addiction was seen as a moral failure. The disease model let us stop judging people and start seeing them as suffering. Although on the surface it has a ring of sympathy (it's not that you're a jerk; it's the disease), it is also patronizing to condemn a drug user to unending powerlessness. The problem is, powerlessness is akin to weakness, and in this country, weakness is still a moral flaw.

What you can say:

I've learned that I have control over a whole lot of my life, including my drug use. I've also learned that there are situations in which I am *actually* powerless. I can't control the weather. I can't get out of a traffic jam. I can't stop the street wars in my neighborhood. I'd love to control other people, but I usually fail. I can't stop racism. I vote, but I seem to be powerless to stop the redistribution of income in this country from the poor to the rich, so people like me will never feel like I have enough to take care of myself. I actually have much more power over myself than I have over the world around me. And I don't want to give away that power by joining something like AA.

Your Life Won't Get Better until You're Sober

Why people think this:

Again, in a society that views things in all-or-nothing terms, most people don't see that there are degrees of "better," some of which have nothing to do with drinking and drugs.

What you can say:

I'm already better. Even though using still affects many parts of my life, they're not all affected the same way and to the same degree. I can make some things better simply by changing some of my using patterns. Since I stopped drinking at Sunday dinner, the number of arguments with my wife went way down. I'd call that better. Anyway, are sober people "better," or are they just sober?

How to Answer Questions about Harm Reduction

Say, you and a friend get on the elevator at the twenty-fifth floor. You have until the elevator reaches the lobby to describe harm reduction.

What is harm reduction, anyway?

Harm reduction is a new way of dealing with drug and alcohol problems.

What's new about it?

For the last seventy years, our goal for drug use and problem drinking in this country has been total abstinence, and the first step is . . . *total abstinence*! Harm reduction's goal is to *reduce* the harm done by drugs or alcohol. The first step is to evaluate how you can do that—figuring out what the harm is and then what the solution is to each problem. Abstinence usually isn't the first step. In fact, some people never quit altogether.

Whoa. I thought addicts had to quit.

First of all, not everyone with a problem is an addict. Second, most people who drink or use don't even get into trouble. But if you do, there are lots of ways out of trouble, and different people have different methods and take different amounts of time.

How long does it take?

Just like it takes months or years to develop a habit, it can take months or years to unlearn it. It depends on a lot of things, like how much harm

273

you're doing in the first place, why you use, how much you want to change, and how quickly you can work through your ambivalence about your drugs. It's different with each person, since we're all unique.

Why is working through ambivalence important?

Because feeling ambivalent about changing usually keeps you stuck on the fence. To make positive changes in your drug habits, you need to get off the fence. That takes a lot of "on the one hand . . . on the other hand" thinking before you know which hand wins.

So then what?

So then you do whatever you can. You don't smoke before work. You get help for your depression. You stop sharing needles. You get couple counseling. You stop borrowing money, which means you have to make do with less speed. Then you get more sleep. You do whatever seems healthier, whenever you can. There are a million choices. You do your best.

Hmmm. Sounds a little wishy-washy.

It isn't wishy-washy. It's human and it's *realistic*.

How to Respond to Some Challenges about Harm Reduction

You're just making excuses.

I know it sounds like excuses. I know it sounds like I'll think up any ridiculous thing that would justify using. What I'm actually telling you is that there are reasons I use, and those reasons are real. Drugs are like my medicine. I know I've gotten into a little trouble lately. I'm not blind. But what I'm *trying* to do is make changes that I'm really ready to make. I'd rather change a small thing that sticks than make a total transformation that lasts only a day.

So what are you doing about it?

I'm using harm reduction. In the harm reduction approach, learn what my drinking is all about, what harm it creates in my life and yours. Then

I'll figure out what I can change about my drinking to make it less problematic. If it turns out that quitting is the only way to take better care of you and me, so be it. We'll see.

You really just want to keep using.

Well, sure, I'd like to keep my pot, my drinks, my cocaine, my ecstasy, and my poppers. You enjoy your coffee and your cocktails, if nothing else. Why shouldn't I? But what I really want is to feel OK. As I study my drugs, my relationships, my self-esteem, and everything else, if I find that my drugs aren't what's causing my problems, then they'll stay and I'll move on to some other solution. The problems in my life may be that I don't really like my job, or I really want children but haven't met the right guy yet. Not having a glass of wine or a line or a hit isn't going to change those things. Changing jobs or getting out to meet more people might.

If you think you can drink while you're trying to stop using speed, you're nuts.

I'm not nuts. I've tried to stop using everything at once, and that was nuts because it didn't work. You know what they say at AA: "Insanity is doing the same thing over and over again and expecting different results." I started to feel insane the tenth time I tried to quit and failed. Now I'm trying something different. Now that I'm not totally paranoid from using speed, I'm getting more sleep, and I'm not overwhelmed by life because I can still chill out with a drink when I need to.

Your Own Questions

Sometimes it doesn't take a skeptical friend, relative, or coworker to start us questioning the value or practicality of using harm reduction. We have questions in our own heads that gnaw at us. We are, after all, part of the same world as all those other questioners. We've learned the same "lessons" about alcohol and other drugs. Here are some of the questions that might come up for you in an internal conversation, and our answers to them.

Will harm reduction work for me?

It really will. The beauty of harm reduction is that it is tailor-made for each person. There are thousands of things to try in your efforts to reduce harm, including abstinence. You can be a harm reductionist and go to AA. Or you can try other people's methods of quitting, either gradually or all at once. There is no right way and no wrong way. That means that there *is* absolutely a way for you.

Will I ever be OK?

Of course. For starters, there are already many things that are OK about you, and we haven't even met. It's just not humanly possible to be all bad. Second, you will be what you believe you are. So get working on your self-esteem if you don't like yourself. Finally, nothing stays the same. But if there's a risk that you could do yourself more damage or get out of control or more out of control, you will have to be careful. If you can stop yourself from a downslide, chances are you will get better.

How realistic is it to think about getting better without going through rehab?

It's actually better to make changes in your drug use in a "real-life" setting. Being in rehab definitely immerses you in a certain kind of culture that helps you quit immediately and stay off drugs as long as you're there. But being immersed in something like rehab, even when it's helpful, can be too artificial. Lots of people attain abstinence in rehab but can't maintain it on the outside It's much better to weave progress into your everyday life, because that's where you'll learn what works or which parts of your plan work best.

How realistic is harm reduction, in general?

Actually, more people who have completed *traditional* drug treatment achieve harm reduction goals than abstinence. The harm reduction approach is new, so not many programs have been studied formally. Needle exchange, the most extensively studied harm reduction program, has been overwhelmingly successful at meeting its goal of reducing the spread of infectious diseases (without increasing drug use). It is also a good entry point for people involved in, or contemplating, abstinence-based treatments. Methadone maintenance, now considered part of the harm reduction arsenal, consistently nets the best results of any drug treatment program in the United States.

The most comprehensive study of drug treatment graduates found fairly low abstinence rates after a few years (21 percent) but better improvement (23 to 43 percent) for things like staying out of jail, staying employed, avoiding depression, and *reducting* drug consumption. An older study by the RAND Corporation found that a few years after graduating from treatment, 25 percent of the people were out of control, 25 percent were abstinent, and 50 percent were moderating their drinking. We all know that any significant change takes time and we get better at it the more we practice. Treatment works best when people stick around—and, in our experience, more people stick around longer for harm reduction treatment than for traditional treatment. Not only is harm reduction realistic, it's real, and it's what we really do.

Will I be sick my whole life?

You're not sick now. You're trying as best you can to manage your life. It's just that some of your methods might be problematic.

Some Sound Bites

We couldn't resist compiling this brief list of sound bites. The list is not complete, by any stretch. Make up your own. Let us know what works. These sound bites can become your everyday mantras, a way of reminding yourself of the principles of harm reduction and how you are working to improve your life. Put them on stickers, put them on a T-shirt, say them quietly while you're counting to ten, waiting for a bad feeling to pass.

Just Say Know

Change Sucks

Harm Is Relative

Reasons Are Reasons

Excuses Are Reasons

A Little Less High, a Lot Less Harm

Any Positive Change

A LETTER TO FAMILY
AND FRIENDS

You've picked up this book for one reason. Someone you care about is drinking or using drugs, and you're worried. In ten seconds you can think of fifty ways he is creating problems in his life. And in another five seconds you can think of a hundred ways she is creating harm in yours. Whether your spouse or partner, your child, a parent, or a friend, you have stood by this person as he or she has tried or refused therapy. You have stood by him as he has tried or refused AA or NA or rehab. You have left, kicked her out, or considered it, believing that if you didn't, you would only enable her to continue using. You've returned because you love this person, fear for him, feel sorry for him, or all of the above. But you returned feeling defeated and weak. Nothing you do seems to help.

Being the loved one of a person with an alcohol or other drug problem can be excruciating. You weather profound helplessness, frustration, anger, and fear. Today's optimism, induced by fervent promises of "Never again," is replaced by tomorrow's disappointment when those promises are broken. You end up struggling with extraordinary questions about loyalty, love, support, and limits. How much help is too much? How long should you put up with it? How many times should you cover for him and pick up the pieces? How many times do you open the door to let her come back and sleep it off again before you lock the deadbolt and say "Not this time"? Should you give up hope of her ever changing, preferring to keep some peace in the family instead of continuing to fight for improvement?

Much is available to you in the way of Al-Anon, Al-Ateen, or Nar-Anon, ACOA (adult children of alcoholics), and support groups. In all of these groups you continue to hear that the only *real* help you can offer an "addict," while protecting yourself and your integrity at the same time, is to lovingly detach and get out of harm's way. You're told you need to stop "enabling" and practice "tough love." (The toughest part of this love is that's it's so hard to practice.) You keep hoping he'll recognize how he is hurting himself, the devastation he's causing his children, or that he's inches from losing another good job. But the truth is that people can see only what they're ready to see, and sometimes all you can do is sit back and wait. Now *that's* tough.

Along with the rest of us, you've learned that addiction is a disease and that immediate and total abstinence from all mind-altering substances, along with the support of the 12 Steps, is the treatment. You've come to believe that surely he must *want* to continue using, or else all the trouble he's had would have convinced him to give up his cocaine, heroin, alcohol, or other substance. It must be true that her denial is so thick that only "hitting bottom" will motivate her to get sober. You've been told to stop bailing her out, stop cleaning up the mess, and let her face the consequences of her choices. Eventually, you're told, she'll hit bottom. If she lives through it, maybe then sobriety will be possible. And only with sobriety will come a life.

Having believed in this, you've urged her into treatment. But in spite of the universal acceptance and popularity of abstinence-based treatment models in the United States, the person you're trying to help has not gotten better. The advice to detach from the person you love has felt too harsh. You've loved your daughter since before she was born, and it is unthinkable to abandon her to her addiction in the hope that she will hit bottom and get better before it kills her. A person may never fully recover from the death of a child, so every ounce of your parental soul seeks a way to help her.

As a spouse, you do not really believe that your life will be better if you leave your husband, even though his drinking is out of control, he's left the care and feeding of the family to you, and he's intermittently abusive. On the other hand, you've had it with the promises and disappointments. You're exhausted by fear and by the suffering that drugs and alcohol have caused. Maybe you're also ashamed or feel terrible for others he's hurt. You're tired of being patient, loving, and *passive* in the face of all this. You're about to take the advice to get tough. Quit or get out.

The problem is, though, tough love doesn't work. And it feels awful to everyone involved. It's unrealistic to expect people to change complicated behaviors *just like that*. Any approach that limits you to an all-or-nothing choice ignores the reality of how people change. People change in incremental steps, practicing new behaviors and new ways of coping with life and with feelings over time. The crucial ingredients to making lasting change are *understanding* and *support*. When we expect immediate change and refuse to be with a person during this process, we undermine the very goal we're trying to accomplish. Banishment seldom leads to reconciliation.

Understanding does not mean, however, that you do not *set limits*. You set limits with a two-year-old, and you set limits with an adult. But you are setting limits on *behavior*. Limits keep a child from running into traffic, touching a hot stove, and eating poison. Adults need somewhat different limits. "You can't yell at me" and "I won't let you take all of our money and spend it on drugs" are some of the limits you might need to set. The point is, it is more useful to separate a person from his or her behavior: we are not the sum total of our behaviors, although we can come pretty close sometimes! Running into traffic, touching a hot stove, or eating poison doesn't mean a child is stupid. Spending all of our money on drugs doesn't mean we are stupid adults. We may just be ignorant of the consequences, curious, or overcome by need.

Behaviors can be changed. Aspects of our personality can change. But *all* of us first must have a basic sense of being valued to make it worth our while to take care of our bodies, minds, and emotions. We get that sense of worth early in our lives from those around us—our parents and siblings, our extended family, our peers, and our teachers. You are probably concerned about someone who is no longer at an early point in his or her life. The older we get, the less we can expect the unconditional love that should exist between parent and child. Relationships become equal partnerships in which we have to earn the love and respect of others, even our parents. Once we reach late adolescence or adulthood, the only place to get unconditional love—more commonly called "unconditional positive regard"—is from a therapist, a person who specializes in understanding emotions and building self-esteem, a person we do not have to take care of beyond paying the agreed-upon fee. You are not your partner's therapist. You are not your child's therapist. And you are not your boss's or employee's therapist. You're limited by the fact that you're in a mutual relationship where you, too, have needs that you're obligated to honor, especially if others are dependent on you. You don't have to provide unconditional love to an adult, as much as he or she might need it.

Even if you've endured someone's drinking and drug use for twenty years, even if you now feel crushed by guilt for having let harmful consequences occur, for giving tacit permission to be terrorized, abused, or worried sick, **it's OK to change your mind now.** On the one hand, you're partly responsible for the marriage you've been in all this time, even if it's just because you didn't complain. On the other hand, you now know that you don't have to live like that anymore. You have a right to alleviate your own suffering. You might even have an obligation to others, particularly to children who are in harm's way and who have no power to change their environment.

Tough love, however, is often a reaction to years of anger at yourself for having endured for so long. Reactions can sometimes produce more trouble than the problems you are trying to solve, however. This is how we come to have relationships that cycle wildly from anger to remorse to reconciliation and back again.

The harm reduction approach suggests that you undertake the same kind of balanced evaluation of different options for taking care of yourself that we have encouraged drug users to undertake: to weigh the pros and cons carefully so that whatever action you take or don't take reflects the complexity of your relationship with your son, daughter, partner, husband, wife, girlfriend, boyfriend, best friend, or colleague. Just as the drug user needs to respect the complexity of his or her relationship with drugs before making decisions that will actually *work* and that can be *maintained,* you need to respect the complexity of your relationship with the drug user.

Harm reduction does not believe that you have to end a relationship to improve it. Nor is abstinence necessarily seen as the basis for an improved life. Nor does an "addict" have to "hit bottom" to become motivated to make positive changes. Instead, harm reduction suggests that making incremental changes in drug-using behavior, along with incremental improvements in emotional coping skills, are realistic and reasonable goals. Abstinence may come at some point, but for most of the people with drug or alcohol problems, it is not a first step.

We know that this new perspective is a lot to swallow. It goes against everything you've learned about what addiction is and how it should be treated. How can someone who is still drinking or using the very drugs that make everything worse get better? We're asking you to develop an entirely new set of ideas about this person you love and his or her relationship with drugs and alcohol. Your ability to be helpful to this person, and to take care of yourself, will be enhanced by a change of perspective.

Understanding the User and the Difficulties of Change

Think about yourself for a moment. You may never have had a problem with drugs or alcohol. But maybe you've had a health problem such as high blood pressure. Your doctor gave you strict instructions about what to do to prevent stroke or heart attack. Get more exercise. Cut way back on your salt intake. Take the medications prescribed. You might respond to this medical advice in a couple of different ways. At first you are afraid, and you quickly form a determination to control this disease. You might go home and throw away all the peanuts and potato chips and dust off the exercise bike. You exercise every day. You take your pills. Then you go to a barbecue, and the ribs smell *so* good. A little salt won't make *that big* a difference, you say. Or your feet start to hurt, and the bike pedals feel so hard. Better not work out for a while. Or you don't have the energy that you used to and your sex life isn't so good. Must be the damn pills. You may fight the urge to slack off and win for a while, but more likely you will wage many battles over a long time until you make changes you can stick with. Sometimes these changes are a less-than-ideal compromise between doctor's orders and your not-so-perfect self. Your friends will understand, because they do the same thing. One friend has diabetes and never checks her blood sugar, relying instead on some intuitive sense of when the levels are too high, at which point she cuts back on carbohydrates. She says that life is too short to worry all the time. Another friend spends more than he earns and has a huge credit card debt. He vows to leave the card at home when he goes out, but if there is a sale on . . . well, that's different, right?

This is how life works. You identify a problem and try to deal with it in your own way, without hard and fast rules. You make compromises with reality. You are sometimes more and sometimes less honest with yourself about how you're doing. You are more likely to make a positive change if you have some control over how you do it and if the way you do it tends to be a way that's manageable for you. That's harm reduction. It's the same for problems with alcohol and other drugs as it is for any other problem that necessitates a behavior change.

Naturally, this puts you in a difficult position. On the one hand, how can you allow the person you are concerned about to be in charge of his or her life when things are clearly out of control? On the other hand, you're not really in charge of anyone but yourself anyway. There are a few things about drug use that you might want to consider while you're trying to address the harm that's being produced in *your* life. Understanding the perspective of the person with the drug problem can help you formulate your own plans.

It's Normal to Want to Alter Your Consciousness

Most people have tried to alter their consciousness at some point. Some of us like to listen to a certain kind of music and feel "swept away" by it. Children twirl around in circles to make themselves dizzy and then fall to the ground giggling. Many of us fix huge amounts of food for holidays and celebrations and eat until we're groggy. Some people fast and meditate to have visions. And people try illegal drugs and legal ones (alcohol and cigarettes and caffeine) for the same reasons: they want to see how it feels to feel different, to alter their usual state of mind. This is normal behavior. And it has become an adolescent rite of passage for the majority of kids in America. Most of them come through this experimental phase just fine. Some suffer serious harm along the way. A few die. It's important to keep in mind, especially for young people, that drug *use* is not the same as drug *abuse*. And when we try to understand the internal workings of a person with an addiction, it's useful to remember that at least some of what's driving their behavior is the same thing that moves all of us—curiosity.

People use drugs for reasons. Sometimes those reasons are the desire to participate in a rite of passage. Sometimes it's to dull the pain of the past or deal with the stress of the present.

Let us also not forget the heavy reliance in America on medication to treat all manner of ailments. Antihistamines, cough suppressants, antibiotics, diet supplements, and stimulants for weight loss, weight gain, or performance enhancement are used liberally. We no longer want to *endure* simple colds, flu, allergies, or sore muscles. Goodness knows, we don't want to *tolerate* them or ride them out. We want to *eradicate* them. Some of us take antidepressants and sleeping pills at the first sign of a bad mood or a bad night's sleep (whereas others' serious depression and anxiety disorders often remain untreated). We take all manner of medications to change our moods and our feelings. And it's all socially sanctioned. In fact, it's increasingly expected. But we think that someone who smokes marijuana or drinks wine to calm down is somehow different from the rest of us.

Denial and Ambivalence

The concept from the disease model that speaks most clearly to families is that of denial. If the user does not stop using as a result of all the trouble he or she gets into, denial must be the reason. Denial is being misused here. The real definition of denial is as a psychological defense (in the form of a true lack of memory) against some fact or event that is too painful or troublesome to tolerate consciously. We believe that drug users use the defense of denial no more frequently than anyone else.

Let's say you have a personal limitation that, although not life threatening, feels like a "fatal flaw." Your fatal flaw is that you are a terrible cook. In your heart of hearts, you know that the only thing that stands between you and bland spaghetti, blackened meat loaf, and runny eggs is the Chinese restaurant on the corner. But when your friends at the office organize a potluck, you want to show off, so you consider making your special mashed potatoes. You decide instead to bring a few quarts of kung pao from the Chinese restaurant. A few of your colleagues jokingly ask if you even know how to cook! You tell them you're a fine cook, but you didn't have time to make anything.

Are you in denial? Of course not. You know that lumpy, watery mashed potatoes are disgusting, that no one will eat them and you will be humiliated. But you're torn. You want to join in and be part of the office event. You also want to hide your fatal flaw. You aren't in denial. You lied!

Maybe you're in a relationship that isn't going so well. You've put a lot of energy into trying to work things out, but your partner still gets really angry and yells at you, sometimes even threatens you. Some of your friends have noticed and are worried. They keep telling you that you should either insist on going to couple counseling or leave the relationship. You've suggested counseling, but that makes him or her even angrier. So now you tell your friends that it's not really that bad, that you've been telling them only the bad stuff, and they don't get to see how wonderful your partner can be most of the time. You tell them that you also bear some responsibility for how things are going. You tell them that the two of you are talking more now, and you're sure things will get better soon.

Are you in denial? Probably not. You could simply be expressing hope and optimism. You're fully aware of the problems in the relationship and may even realize that you're not the cause of your partner's anger. But you love, and don't want to lose, this person. This is the first relationship you've had in two years. You're ambivalent about doing anything that might rock the boat. So you *minimize* the problems and focus on more positive aspects. In this way you're expressing your hopefulness that the relationship will work out and blocking out your friends' more pessimistic assessment. It's all in the eye of the beholder.

There is surprisingly little actual denial on the part of people who use alcohol and other drugs. Every time a drinker is confronted about her use of alcohol, she feels it. She may be lying, minimizing the problem, ambivalent, hopeful that she can make it better, hopeless about doing anything different, or fearful about losing that warm blanket that alcohol wraps around her each evening, but she's not in denial. Layers upon layers of defenses have been built up around her drug problem, and when confrontation cuts through all of that, what comes back at you sounds a lot like denial. It's not denial; it's the wall built up to protect herself from the onslaught of your confrontation. Confrontation breeds armor, not awareness or thoughtfulness.

Powerlessness

We all like to feel that we can have an effect in our lives, that we have the power to accomplish things. We like to believe that we have some degree of power over people as well. We send back the cold food at a restaurant, believing it'll come back hot. We explain the dangers of smoking cigarettes to our children in the hopeful certainty they won't smoke. We exercise and eat right, believing we'll live a long, healthy life by doing so. When things aren't going well, we have to believe that we can *do* something about it. Have you ever coached a kids' baseball or soccer team? You tell them all the time that *they can do it*. You try to instill a sense of confidence in their power to be better than the other team. We all need to feel a sense of power in our lives to get out of bed in the morning and go about our work. It's hard for a person to feel powerful when he has a drug or alcohol problem that seems to be running his life. But just like you, he needs to believe that he *can* take control, to use his power to solve this problem. Believing that you *can do it* is called *self-efficacy*. Studies of self-efficacy show that it's one of the major factors that make positive behavior change possible: the more self-efficacy one has, the more one can make positive changes. And positive change is one of the cornerstones of harm reduction.

The first step of Alcoholics Anonymous, however, is to admit that you're *powerless* over drugs and alcohol. This first step is used as the entry point into almost all treatment programs in the United States. It's an idea that puts a lot of people off. Most people, including those with alcohol and other drug problems, tend to bristle or wince at the idea of being powerless. It makes us feel weak and frightened. In a larger context, we live in a society in which power is regarded as essential to taking one's place in the world. The idea of proclaiming powerlessness goes against how things work in this country. Moreover, there are many, many people—here and all over the world—who already experience so much powerlessness, so little say in the quality of their lives, that recommending that they voluntarily embrace powerlessness as some kind of beacon is an insult of the highest order. The lasting effect of racism, sexism, and other forms of discrimination is to withhold power from the targeted people, the power to control their own destiny and to take part in the goods of society. The lasting effect of child abuse is to deprive people of their god-given power to control their own bodies. People rightfully fight against any attempt to deprive them of power. And yet we see this resistance to the mantle of powerlessness as bad in the case of people who have a drug or alcohol problem, many of whom also have a history of trauma. The fact is, a person who doesn't have confidence in his or her power to change *never will*.

The Harsh Self

When a toddler sees a toy she wants, she grabs it. She hasn't yet learned to say to herself, "That's someone else's toy; I need to ask if I can borrow it." She has little awareness of others' feelings. But, more important, she has no *guilt* about doing exactly what she wants. She hasn't learned to be ashamed or to hide her true wishes. Somewhere between toddlerhood and adulthood, she develops the capacity to think about others, to contain her impulses, and to impose some controls on her behavior. She also learns about shame and guilt. She learns that, if she really shows off her unedited self and her unfettered desires, someone is very likely to make her feel bad about it. It's important, of course, to have rules to live by and to consider the rights and feelings of others. Too often, though, we are taught by harshness and ridicule to feel ashamed when we make a mistake.

The average adult, although usually not conscious of it, has internalized an "observer" who determines right from wrong, makes moral and ethical judgments, and imposes punishment for bad behavior. Punishment imposed from within is felt as either shame or guilt. Roughly speaking, guilt is the feeling that your *behavior* is bad; shame is the feeling that *you* are bad. It is commonly believed that people who abuse alcohol and other drugs have not developed this internal observer. Since they drink to excess or use drugs that are illegal—and seemingly without regard to consequences—it is assumed that they have an "anything goes" attitude. It often seems as if they don't care that others are hurt by their actions, worried, or ashamed. People think they have an internal observer that is lax and indulgent. Quite the opposite is true. The typical observer inside a heavy user or abuser of alcohol or other drugs is likely to be very active in its punitive and harsh judgments.

Someone with a harsh internal observer can't please himself or anyone else. In his own eyes, he doesn't look right, dress right, say the right things at the right time, ever get an A on a test, or get a date. She's too fat, too flat-chested, too slow, too clingy, too pushy, too quiet, too loud, or too sensitive. He feels old and stupid and weak and ashamed and guilty. The self-recrimination goes on and on, and it's constant. Only drugs can mute this strict internal voice for a while. So even at a time when it makes no sense to use cocaine—like immediately after you tell your girlfriend that she's really obnoxious when she's had too much—she goes ahead and uses some more. She (probably) doesn't do this because she doesn't care what you think, but rather because she feels ashamed by your criticism and needs to escape that feeling. Coke will make her feel better fast. It'll get her away from your voice—which matches her internal voice. This is not a great way for her to deal with your feelings and wishes. It just explains her actions.

When you're disappointed in yourself—you screwed up a task at work, scolded your kids because you were in a bad mood, were dumped by your boyfriend—you usually have some type of internal conversation with your observer. It goes something like this:

"Hey–you really messed up there."

"Jeez, I know it."

"Well, what are you gonna do about it?"

"Talk to my friends. Try to fix it. Maybe I'll go to the movies and get my mind off it."

When a person who has developed a drug problem is disappointed in something he's done, the conversation goes something like this:

"Hey–you really messed up there."

"Jeez, I know it. I always do that. I'm the biggest asshole on the planet. Everyone says so."

"Well, what are you gonna do about it?"

"Do what assholes do—I'm gonna drink and avoid anybody who could possibly remind me of what an asshole I am."

So the person drowns out her harsh observer. Then family members or friends often unwittingly take on the role of the supposedly absent observer. A spouse will become the voice of reason, punishment, judgment, or morality. Or a parent will scold an adult child as if she were a toddler again. As the loved one or friend of a drug abuser or drinker, you find yourself angry and frustrated, feeling the weight of responsibility but none of the authority you need to make things different.

Understanding Yourself: How Harm Reduction Can Help You

"Promises, Promises": The Reality of Failures and Relapses

For those of you who have been dealing with a drug-abusing loved one for a while, you may be feeling cynical about his or her promises to quit, or stay in treatment, or pay back money he or she took from you. How can you hope that it'll be any different this time? You don't want to get your hopes up, yet you can see the hurt in his or her eyes when you express skepticism about the latest batch of promises. The reality is that most people with significant alcohol or drug problems try many times and many different ways to help themselves before they manage to make lasting changes. It's important not to ask for promises. This usually just results in lying and secrecy. And it's the lying and secrecy, as much as it is the broken promises, that strain your relationship.

What harm reduction asks of you is to hold the paradox of no longer putting up with behavior that hurts you—you can, and should, express your feelings, state your needs and expectations, and make demands—even as you realize that your demands and pleas don't usually result in lasting change. You have your own *decisional balance* to work. (For a more detailed discussion of the decisional balance, please see Chapter 5.) Deciding to take one action or another first requires you to weigh the pros and cons of each. Holding the paradox, then, means that you can be at the end of your rope and still know that change will happen, albeit slowly and with many setbacks along the way. You can feel as if you were going to burst with impatience and still understand that change takes time. You can fully expect a person to change his or her behavior and at the same time openly discuss the lack of progress.

People who become interested in harm reduction sometimes bring with them a pervasive sense of failure and self-reproach. The harsh internal observer finds fuel at their failure to "get with the program" or "face the problem." The isolation and hopelessness that grow from this sense of failure often drive continued use. As a family member or a friend, **it is vital that you grab any opportunity *not* to reinforce the user's internal observer.** When drug users beat themselves up for relapsing, it's not an invitation for you to join in!

Of course, it's no time for simple optimism either. You certainly don't have to act like a cardboard cutout Mary Poppins, merrily singing that the glass is half full. It is just a matter of remembering the person inside the drug use who is struggling in the only way she knows how to survive both the distress caused by drug use and the pain of the things that brought her to use in the first place. Dishing out harsh criticism or extracting promises won't help her, and blaming yourself won't help you (or her) either.

There Are No Rules Except the Rules You Make

So what *are* you supposed to do? Just let him destroy his life and yours? Refuse to continue the relationship? How are you supposed to know what's best? Now is the time you will be invited to take a new approach. And the first rule is, there are no rules except the ones you make.

This may not be exactly what you wanted to hear, but the fact is, no one knows what you should do. All the advice about not "enabling" drinking or using, all the talk about not being "codependent," can push you into making up rules that you might not really want to enforce or that you don't even have the power to enforce. People might tell you to do things that violate your own values about loyalty and family. If you don't abide by their advice, then you get labeled as someone who is supporting another's addiction. Harm reduction principles can help guide you while you're figuring out what might be best for you and for your loved ones.

Identify the Harm You Are Suffering. Make a detailed list of the harm that another person's drug problem is causing you. Are you losing sleep? Are you paying his bills, leaving you without enough money to buy your medicine or food? Is he bringing people home who might endanger you or your children? Is he acting up in public when you're out together? Is he stashing illegal drugs at your house, putting you at risk of arrest or losing your home?

Next, try to be objective about this list. Which things are actually related directly to drug or alcohol use? Try to make distinctions between the actual activity of drug using and the behaviors that might go along with it. Is the harm really that your cousin smokes weed or that he smokes in your car when you are going somewhere together? *He* may have a marijuana problem, but the harm to *you* is that he's smoking an illegal drug in your car. Or how about your boyfriend, who is using a lot of speed and staying up all night, you can't get to sleep either? While *he* may have a drug problem, *your* problem is that you're not getting enough sleep. If your son keeps asking you to pay the rent because he's snorted his money up in cocaine, *your* problem is that you can't pay your mortgage and his rent at the same time, even if *his* problem is cocaine (and homelessness).

By looking at the problems in this way—by separating out which problems are directly connected to the drug or alcohol use, per se, and which ones involve behavior associated with it—you can plan your decisions and responses in such a way that you are more likely to reduce the harm to *yourself*, even if the other person doesn't change his or her drug use.

Distinguish between Being Harmed and Feeling Hurt. It might be hard to make this distinction, but it's a necessary one for a lot of people. Commonly, what's happening is not that you are suffering actual harm because of a loved one's drug or alcohol problem but that you feel hurt, disappointed, anxious, and maybe angry as well. We are not dismissing these feelings.

Hurt feelings are sometimes as harmful to your well-being as a wrecked living room, a drug bust, or going without food. Your feelings are important and serve as a guide to your decisions. And too much hurt and anger are harmful to your peace of mind and perhaps even your health. What we're suggesting is that you try to figure out the difference between your emotional reactions to your loved one's drug use (which may range from anger to disappointment to worry to hopelessness, etc.) and actual destruction. Are you losing money, sleep, your job? Are your other family members being victimized? Or are you suffering from the disappointment of failed expectations and hopes, from watching a good person spiral down?

Affirm Your Values and Needs, but Beware of Tough Love. You have your own hierarchy of needs, just as we talked about in Chapter 6. Do you need peace and quiet to function at your best? Or do you like excitement and challenge? Are you basically a loner who just wants family around sometimes? Or are you a social person who enjoys interacting with lots of different kinds of people?

If there are many things you might like to change about the person whose drug or alcohol use is affecting you, you may quickly feel overwhelmed when you start making the list. Too often people just give up. Nothing changes, at least not for the better. One place to start is by thinking about your values and your beliefs about how things "ought to be" in a family or between friends. You probably have some values about loyalty. Maybe you believe that you're supposed to stick with a person through hard times. Marriage vows say just that: "for better or worse." What's important to you? Your hierarchy of needs might look something like this:

I want to be able to worry less about my parent/child/partner.
I want to feel pride in my family.
I want my friends to be able to come to me when they're in trouble.
I don't want a lot of excitement—I like things to be predictable.
I want my children to be able to count on me.
I want my neighbors to respect me.
I want to give back to my community, not create problems.

Now think about how you came to be involved with this person who has a drug or alcohol problem. What did you enjoy and admire about her before the drug or alcohol problem emerged? Have those qualities all gone away or just some of them? Does she depend on you for support, emotional and/or financial? Has this support been given freely by you? Ideas of loyalty and self-sacrifice are too often criticized in modern American society when it comes to people with alcohol and other drug problems. The stigma of mental illness or physical disability is changing, and the role of the caretakers of these people is now a valued one. Not so for people with drug and alcohol problems. Why is it that we're not supposed to help them in the same way we help other people with serious problems? Is it because their behaviors seem so voluntary, or so much about seeking pleasure? Is it because we're uncomfortable with people who seem out of control?

Consider how we treat people with other problems that are called diseases. Both diabetes and schizophrenia are chronic disorders that have a course that is often deteriorating. There are certain things patients with diabetes or schizophrenia can do to prevent or slow down the progressive course of these diseases. For example, they can be encouraged to monitor their food intake, exercise regularly, take their medicine, avoid stress, etc. When they (inevitably) don't always follow medical advice, we as caretakers may feel frustrated or worried, but we don't usually throw them out of the house! We try to protect them from serious consequences and motivate them to take better care of themselves. Drug and alcohol abuse have been included in the list of mental disorders by the medical establishment as a way of destigmatizing people, but society hasn't really come to terms with what that means. Just look at how differently we feel about insulin and drugs that treat schizophrenia versus methadone to treat heroin dependence! On the one hand, addiction is considered a disease, and people who have it need help. On the other hand, we shouldn't "enable addicts" by helping them when they most need it—when they are out of control and suffering the worst consequences. While we don't subscribe to the idea that addiction is a disease, we wonder why the people who do are so inconsistent.

What harm reduction suggests is that you adopt the same attitude toward people with alcohol and drug problems that you do toward people with other chronic problems, such as asthma, diabetes, or schizophrenia. Even though you may get frustrated or feel afraid, you don't usually cut them out of your life if they don't follow medical advice or common sense. Even though their behavior may put not only themselves at risk, but you as well, you usually try to work things out to preserve the relationship. You might try to save money so that if your partner dies of untreated diabetes, you won't lose the house. You might make sure that your partner has enough sick leave on the books to cover her absences due to episodes of illness that have been increased by her harmful or neglectful behaviors. But we don't tend to use "tough love" on people with these types of problems.

"Tough love" hasn't helped most people overcome a drug or alcohol problem, either. It has caused a lot of pain on both sides and has separated people from those who are most important to them. You may have to separate yourself from your drug-using parent, friend, partner, or child. Hopefully, you will not have to do this until you have tried other, less dramatic limits. The harm reduction approach suggests that you balance your own needs and values with your attachment to your drug user and then allow yourself to take care of yourself *and* to be compassionate when you set limits.

Establish Your Bottom Line. Trying to figure out what you *do* want to do about someone's alcohol or other drug problem is similar to the process that the drug user is going through. Each of you is coming at the problem from a different perspective, but the guidelines are pretty much the same. What is your bottom line? What is necessary, what can you manage, how much can you tolerate, and what has got to change? First of all, you do not have to do *anything* differently, if you don't want to. You do not have to do anything someone else tells you to do. It's up to you, and there are no right answers.

Start with your hierarchy of needs, your values, and the list of harmful effects that you've come up with. There is probably at least one thing that's "non-negotiable"—something that you just can't put up with or that must change *now*. Maybe you will no longer allow illegal drugs in your house. Ever. Or maybe you will not tolerate being around your friend when he or she's been drinking. You don't need to rationalize or explain your limits. You can just make the rule. Sometimes trying to explain your limits just leads to an argument. "I don't *always* drink too much, so why can't you come over?" or "Where am I *supposed* to leave my drugs, out on the street?" So don't explain, if you don't want to. Just say, this is the way it is.

You will have to establish some methods of enforcement and some consequences for breaches when you lay down your bottom line. If you make a rule that your friends can't bring illegal drugs into your house, are you going to do a strip search before you let them in? Are you going to ask other people to find out and tell you? And then what? Will you really tell them to leave? Will you call the police? It's important for you to think these matters through before issuing your rules. If you're not clear and committed, you and the person you're trying to influence will be in the same position you are now—having to negotiate tricky situations in the heat of the moment.

It's possible that you are at the point where you aren't interested in small changes. You want her to quit! Maybe you've decided to demand that she get into treatment. One point to consider if treatment is your bottom line:

how will you respond to a relapse? Are you unwilling (or unable, at this point) to tolerate a relapse? What if she relapses but stays in treatment? And what kind of treatment are you saying she has to take part in? What if she quits using but also quits treatment? What if she has, say, just one drink, then quits again immediately? Will you allow her any negotiating room? Any second chances? The stricter your limits, the more likely you are to make it impossible for your loved one to stay connected to you, at least in the short run. Is disconnection something you can live with? Are you really at the end of your rope? If so, stand your ground. If not, think carefully about how you want to state your demands.

The main point to remember is that your limits are about *you*. They are not necessarily the only solutions, and they may not even be the *right* ones for your using friend. You are setting limits to help resolve *your* problems; those will be the *right* limits for *you*. The person with a drug or alcohol problem will figure out what works for her. She will go through her own process of change, no matter what you dictate or how involved you are with her. These limits, rules, and boundaries are about YOU.

Now What Do You Do?

Let's go back to your cousin who smokes marijuana when the two of you are out driving in your car. You really think he has a problem with pot. And you get nervous having the drug in your car. What if you get stopped and the police smell it? You could go to jail, and you would certainly pay a hefty fine. You've been asking him why he smokes so much, but he just tells you that you're trying to stop his fun. He doesn't think he has a problem. He just likes to use it to relax after a hard day at work. The two of you are at a stalemate in terms of *defining* the problem, let alone solving it. You aren't getting anywhere trying to convince him that he has a problem. And, in fact, *your* biggest problem is that he smokes in your car and puts you at risk. Stop talking to him about smoking pot. Save your energy. Just set a limit about smoking in your car: "Put it out or get out. Now." You might also decide not to let him smoke in your presence or around your parents and kids. In this way, you reduce the harm to you and those around you without spending your energy trying to get *him* to change.

Now about your boyfriend who uses speed and keeps you up so late you're too tired to work the next day. You're really worried about his speed habit and would like for him to stop or, at least, party only on weekends. But he doesn't see it that way, and you just end up in an argument. There are other solutions that will probably work better than demanding that he stop using speed now and forever. Being willing to end the relationship over this issue is one way. But let's assume you value the relationship and don't want to end it. You could make it clear that if he's using, you want him to spend the night with friends. Or you could stay somewhere else. The point is to generate a number of solutions by separating drug or alcohol use from problem behaviors associated with it. That way you don't have to get frustrated if he doesn't want to deal with his drug use. It's also possible that the "natural consequences" your boyfriend now has to face (sleeping on the floor at a friend's house) will become part of his decisional balance. He might one day decide he'd rather sleep in bed with you than do speed at night.

Each possible action on your part probably has risks and benefits associated with it, just like a person's drug or alcohol use has both risks and benefits. Writing out a decisional balance will help you decide what you want to do. Beware the unintended consequences of pressure. Tracy spent her lifetime feeling pressured by her mother to lose weight. Her mother tried guilt, criticism, bribery, persuasion. Tracy ate more in the presence of her mother than anywhere else. When her mother died, well into Tracy's middle age, she joined a gym and started to exercise. Pressure, especially from someone close to you, can backfire.

Let's say your daughter, a crack user, comes by your house while you're at work and steals your TV. By the time you discover it, she has pawned the TV for cash and is already high, maybe even crashing by now. You consider your options. Have her arrested. Demand that she go retrieve the TV. Offer her cash to get it. Bargain with her that you won't turn her in if she goes into rehab. Kick her out of the house. Do nothing.

Let's look at what harm or help might be embedded in each of these alternatives.

Option	Harm	Help
Have her arrested	Jail is dangerous and doesn't teach people anything. Creates animosity between you and her. Having a criminal record creates employment problems and stigma.	Wake-up call. Teach her a lesson. Get her away from you and your stuff. *(cont.)*

Option	Harm	Help
Demand that she get the TV back	She'll fail, because she doesn't have the money or doesn't know where it is.	Force her to deal with you and work to get your forgiveness.
Offer cash	Uses it to buy more drugs.	You get your TV back.
Bargain	She might call your bluff.	Maintains relationship.
Kick her out of the house	She'll be homeless and a target for other sources of harm (violence, poor nutrition, prostitution, etc.).	Forces her to make a choice.
Do nothing	You'll lose more of your stuff.	She'll eventually feel bad and stop stealing from you. Maybe stop using, too.

Still another option: On the other hand, you could decide to pay for therapy for your daughter. Obviously, she's used all *her* money to buy drugs, and if she can't afford both drugs and therapy, she's not going to go to therapy now. *Paying for therapy is not enabling her drug habit; it's enabling her to enter treatment.* You have no other power to affect, one way or another, her choice to use crack right now. She might discover that she uses more after she feels criticized by her husband about their lack of money and that, in fact, their marital relationship is an area in which she feels empty and sad. She might discover she is able to limit her drug use to weekends and start marital therapy. If her husband gets a more regular job, their finances improve, and she feels less pressure to be the perfect provider, she might even quit entirely. You might make a huge difference in the eventual resolution of her drug problem by helping her sort out her marital and work problems.

The most painful situation for families is when someone is both drug dependent and mentally ill. Many people with schizophrenia, for example, use alcohol as a way of quieting the voices in their heads. Some use marijuana because it makes them feel less agitated. Some smoke crack as a way of making them feel more alive, a feeling they've lost since becoming ill and taking their medications. The majority of people with schizophrenia also smoke cigarettes. This mixture of drugs can often cause disturbing symptoms and pose danger in the house, such as fire. Using their money for alcohol and drugs often means they don't pay their rent and end up homeless.

If you have financial resources, you could consider a number of interventions. Don't demand that your son quit using all drugs. Folks with mental illness have a harder time quitting than anyone—they have more problems to medicate. You might consider paying your son's rent for him (directly to the landlord) to prevent homelessness. You might put up good smoke detectors so that if he passes out with a cigarette burning, he won't burn down the house. You might arrange to drive him to his doctor's appointments and give him money to fill his medication prescriptions. You can thereby reduce the harmful effects both to yourself and to your son.

The major principle of harm reduction is to strive for *any change in a positive direction*. At first, the change made may not directly affect a person's use of alcohol or other drugs. You don't have to pretend to like your decisions or the problems that this person is causing you. You don't have to keep quiet about your worries. Nagging is a way of showing concern. It just isn't a very effective change strategy. You don't have to avoid talking about his or her drug or alcohol use and how you feel about it. You just have to stop making empty threats. Demand what you must and tolerate what you can while your friend or loved one struggles to find his or her way.

You may not know this, but **abstinence** is **a harm reduction strategy**. Don't be afraid to ask for it, but remember: he or she might not be able or willing to quit right now. Even for people who *have* decided to quit, it takes time, relapse is the rule, and they stop and start numerous times before achieving lasting abstinence. How you respond to these natural "slips" is important. Anything that suggests to the person that he or she'd better not tell you when he or she's used will set up the possibility of secrecy and broken communication.

Finally, don't give up. Everything changes. And harm reduction actually allows for change better than more dramatic interventions. Focus on strengths, not weaknesses. Look for any positive change. Praise progress. And ask, "Is there any way I can help you?"

SOURCES AND SUGGESTED READINGS

For more on change, the decisional balance, and responsible drinking and drug use:

Changing for Good. James Prochaska, Carlo DiClemente, and John Norcross. Avon Books. 1994.

Responsible Drinking: A Moderation Management Approach for Problem Drinkers. Fred Rotgers, Marc Kern, and Rudy Hoeltzel. New Harbinger. 2002.

Safety First: A Reality-Based Approach to Teens, Drugs and Drug Education [brochure]. Marsha Rosenbaum. Drug Policy Alliance. 2002.

The Australian National Council on Drugs sponsors the Family Drug Support Project, run by Tony Trimingham, who has advocated for safer injection sites and works with families and drug-using members all over Australia. *andc.org.au/about/members/trimingham*

For critiques about the existing drug treatment system and drug policy:

Drug Crazy: How We Got into This Mess and How We Can Get Out. Mike Gray. Routledge. 1998.

Hooked: Five Addicts Challenge Our Misguided Drug Rehab System. Lonny Shavelson. New Press. 2001.

Recovery Options: The Complete Guide. Joseph Volpicelli and Maia Szalavitz. Wiley. 2000.

The Truth about Addiction and Recovery. Stanton Peele. Simon & Schuster. 1991.

RESOURCES

Professional Harm Reduction Alcohol and Drug Treatment

Harm Reduction Therapy Center (HRTC) (formerly, Addiction Treatment Alternatives)
Patt Denning, PhD, and Jeannie Little, LCSW
423 Gough Street
San Francisco, CA 94102
415-863-4282
www.harmreductiontherapy.org
pdenning@harmreductiontherapy.org
jlittle@harmreductiontherapy.org
    HRTC also specializes in training other therapists and treatment providers in harm reduction therapy.

Frederick Rotgers, PsyD, ABPP, Associate Professor of Psychology
Assistant Director of Training and Internship Coordinator
Department of Psychology
Philadelphia College of Osteopathic Medicine
4190 City Avenue
Philadelphia, PA 19131-1693
Phone: 215-871-6457
Fax: 215-871-6458

Andrew Tatarsky, PhD
Harm Reduction Psychotherapy and Training Associates
31 West 11th Street, 6-D
New York, NY 10011
212-633-8157
www.harmreductioncounseling.com
info@harmreductioncounseling.com

Addiction Alternatives, Marc Kern, PhD
A division of Life Management Skills, Inc.
Beverly Hills Medical Tower
1125 South Beverly Drive
Los Angeles, CA 90035
310-275-5433
www.addictionalternatives.com
habitdoc@addictionalternatives.com

Guided Self-Change Clinic
Nova Southeastern University
Community Mental Health Center
Maltz Psychology Building
3301 College Avenue
Fort Lauderdale, FL 33314
954-262-5968
www.cps.nova.edu/~gsc/
gsc@cps.nova.edu

Practical Recovery Services
A. Thomas Horvath, PhD
8950 Villa La Jolla Drive, Suite B112
La Jolla, CA 92037-1704
858-453-4777
www.practicalrecovery.com
info@practicalrecovery.com

Harm Reduction Organizations

The Harm Reduction Coalition (HRC)

The Harm Reduction Coalition is the primary representative of active drug users and their issues in the United States and has many active users as members. It was one of the driving forces in creating needle exchange programs around the country which it continues to support. Needle exchanges are excellent places to get support from other users. Some communities also have needle exchange sites for youth. HRC is more up-to-date than most organizations about the risks and benefits of drugs. They have a lot of printed educational materials, very inexpensive and very understandable, about many of the drugs people use and about safe injection techniques. HRC's every-other-year conferences are a great place to get educated and to meet other users (and ex- or non-users), professionals, street outreach workers, and family members of users, who can become a support network.

Harm Reduction Coalition (HRC)
22 West 27th Street, 5th Floor
New York, NY 10001
212-213-6376
www.harmreduction.org
hrc@harmreduction.org

1440 Broadway, Suite 510
Oakland, CA 94612
510-444-6969
hrcwest@harmreduction.org

Drug Policy Alliance (DPA)

A new name for two classic drug policy organizations: The Lindesmith Center and the Drug Policy Foundation. DPA sponsors important legislation to counter the effects of the War on Drugs, fights for the rights of people incarcerated under current drug policies, and maintains an excellent library of scholarly and practical resources about drug policy and public health harm reduction interventions.

Drug Policy Alliance
70 West 36th Street, 16th Floor
New York, NY 10018
212-613-8020
www.drugpolicy.org
nyc@drugpolicy.org

Legal Affairs
717 Washington Street
Oakland, CA 94607
510-208-7711
legalaffairs@drugpolicy.org

1227 Paseo de Peralta
Santa Fe, NM 87501
505-983-3277
nm@drugpolicy.org

1225 8th Street, Suite 570
Sacramento, CA 95814
916/444-3751
sacto@drugpolicy.org

925 15th Street NW, 2nd Floor
Washington, DC 20005
202-216-0035
dc@drugpolicy.org

2233 Lombard Street
San Francisco, CA 94123
415-921-4987
sf@drugpolicy.org

119 South Warren Street, 1st Floor
Trenton, NJ 08608
609-396-8613
nj@drugpolicy.org

The San Francisco office of the Drug Policy Alliance (under the direction of Marsha Rosenbaum) has created a special project, Safety First, that responds to requests from parents about teenage drug use by providing honest educational information.

415-921-4987
www.safety1st.org

DanceSafe

DanceSafe's unique characteristic is that the staff and volunteers show up where the drugs are. They are available to educate you about drugs, safe use, and drug interactions. They also have testing kits to test your pills, especially ecstasy, and tell you if you are about to take what you thought you bought. DanceSafe provides a wonderful and pragmatic service. They are sort of like Rock Medicine, the medical staff and drug experts that the Haight Ashbury Free Clinic sent to rock concerts decades ago.

Most unfortunately, since the prospect of the federal RAVE Act (Reducing American's Vulnerability to Ecstasy)—which was not passed but which would have made club owners and party organizers responsible for the drug use of their patrons—many such business owners have banned DanceSafe from their premises, for fear of implicitly acknowledging the reality of drug use and thus taking responsibility for the drug use of their patrons. On New Year's Eve 2002 two young people died at a dance party in San Francisco and several more were hospitalized. DanceSafe was on the premises, but they were allowed only to distribute condoms, not provide any safer drug use education or pill testing. Although the RAVE Act was not passed in 2002, it has been reintroduced to Congress, this time called the "Crack House Statute Amendments" as part of the larger "Illegal Drug Anti-Proliferation Act."

DanceSafe has a lot of very useful information about ecstasy on its website, an E-zine, health tips, up-to-date pill testing results, regional contacts, and lifesaving information about safer drug use and safer raving.

DanceSafe
c/o HRC
22 West 27th Street, 5th Floor
New York, NY 10001
510-834-7500
www.dancesafe.org

The Chicago Recovery Alliance (CRA)

CRA offers a great deal of support to drug users in the Chicago area, with very educated needle exchange and street outreach workers who represent many using communities, including youth and gay and transgendered people. CRA is hoping to open a youth-oriented drop-in center in Chicago. Its director, Dan Bigg, is one of the leading experts on substance use management in the United States.

Chicago Recovery Alliance
Dan Bigg
PO Box 368069
Chicago, IL 60636-8069
773-471-0999
www.anypositivechange.org
cra@attglobal.net

Self-Help Programs: Abstinence-Based

Women for Sobriety (WFS)

The philosophy of WFS is to support women in achieving and maintaining abstinence from alcohol. Introductions are first name only but do not include the "I'm an alcoholic" tag. The groups are abstinence-based, and the focus is more future- than past-oriented. Groups are small—about six women. Moderators are women who have achieved at least one year of sobriety, know about the WFS program and philosophy, may have read some literature about addiction, but have no formal training.

Women for Sobriety, Inc.
PO Box 618
Quakertown, PA 18951-0618
215-536-8026
www.womenforsobriety.org
NewLife@nni.com

Secular Organizations for Sobriety (SOS)

SOS has three basic characteristics: it is secular (nonreligious), abstinence is the goal, and self-help is the way it works. Meetings generally open with a statement about SOS, but the structure varies from group to group. Any time away from alcohol is considered sober time. If a person is abstinent for a year then relapses, he or she is considered abstinent for a year with a relapse, unlike in AA, where your sober time is counted only *since* your last relapse.

SOS International Clearinghouse
The Center for Inquiry-West
4773 Hollywood Boulevard
Hollywood, CA 90027
323-666-4295
www.cfiwest.org/sos
sos@cfiwest.org

Resources

LifeRing Secular Recovery

LifeRing is a self-help group based on a philosophy of secular (nonreligious) mutual support and discussion of all life issues, including work, relationships, the law, drugs, or anything else deemed important to the members. It subscribes to the traditional abstinence model and views any use as relapse. Meetings are unstructured and informal. At a typical meeting a "convener" calls the group together and reads a statement about LifeRing, indicating there are no steps and no sponsors and that discussion is open and intended for mutual help. The convener is not a professional but rather a participant charged only with calling the group to order and reading this statement. Members of the group go around and introduce themselves on a first-name-only basis. Discussion is then open, and participants talk about how the week has gone. Others respond, and there is open and free discourse with the intention of providing mutual support. Meetings last about an hour.

LifeRing Service Center
1440 Broadway Suite 312
Oakland CA 94612-2023
510/763-0779
www.unhooked.com
service@lifering.org

SMART Recovery

The goal of SMART Recovery is to build skills to maintain abstinence. Introductions are informal, and meetings are led by "coordinators" who may or may not have had a drinking problem but have been sober at least a year and adhere to SMART principles. No formal training is required to be a moderator, but training sessions are offered and coordinators are encouraged to attend. Since SMART is recognized by the courts as an alternative to AA meetings, you might run into some folks who are required to be there and may be somewhat resistant to working on their drug or alcohol problems. Participants do not have sponsors. Confidentiality is strictly enforced— you could be removed from the program for talking about others in the group outside of the group meetings. SMART is for people who like a do-it-yourself approach with very little structure. Group membership shifts, and there is a good deal of turnover— people get what they need and then leave.

7537 Mentor Avenue, Suite #306
Mentor, Ohio 44060
440-951-5357
www.smartrecovery.org
srmail1@aol.com

Rational Recovery (RR)

Rational Recovery employs a method called Addictive Voice Recognition Technique, a behavioral program that can be self-administered through a variety of different media, including self-help groups, books, and seminars. The technique teaches how to recognize the irrational "voice" that drives one to relapse and offers specific strategies to resist this impulse. Rational Recovery is vehemently anti-AA, and most recently tend not to hold formal groups meetings, but give people the information to work this program on their own.

Rational Recovery
Box 800
Lotus CA 95651
530-621-2667
www.rational.org
rr@rational.org

Self-Help Programs: Non-Abstinence-Based

Moderation Management (MM)

The goal of participants in MM is moderate drinking. Only if moderation fails do people revisit their decision and consider abstinence. MM was developed for problem drinkers rather than for other drug users. There is no inherent reason why the principles could not be applied to other drug use. The maximum levels of drinking recommended were based on studies of people's optimal success when trying to moderate, so users of other drugs would need to determine their own optimal levels for moderating their use. As we recommended in the chapter on Substance Use Management (which is really a drug user's MM), the right levels of other drugs are dependent on the nature of the drug and the physical and mental health and circumstances of each user.

MM groups are process oriented and incorporate a good deal of education. MM is approved by the state of California for DUI sentencing. Groups can be very diverse, including those with problematic early-stage drinking and those in advanced stages of alcoholism. Although participants are generally not interested in abstinence, guidelines set out by the World Health Organization for safe drinking are offered. The philosophy of MM is not to be alone with the experience of drinking and to be accountable to peers who share similar goals regarding alcohol use.

Groups meet in person in some communities. There are also online groups. All information about meetings can be found on their website. In New York, they share office space with the Harm Reduction Coalition.

Moderation Management Network, Inc.
c/o HRC
22 West 27th Street, 5th Floor
New York, NY 10001
212-213-6582
www.moderation.org
mm@moderation.org

Here is a comparative chart of several self-help programs, developed by Marc Kern of Addiction Alternatives in Los Angeles:

SELF-HELP GROUPS

	Rational Recovery	Self-Management and Recovery Training	Secular Organizations for Sobriety	Alcoholics Anonymous, NA, CA, MA	Women for Sobriety	Moderation Management
Goal	Abstinence	Abstinence	Abstinence	Abstinence	Abstinence	Moderation
Main Technique	Addictive Voice Recognition	Identifying and changing destructive thinking	"Priority One" is not drinking	The 12 Steps	Spirituality and self-empowerment	Self-monitoring and life balancing
Habit or Disease?	Habit	Habit	Disease	Disease	Disease	Habit
Suggested Length of Program	Brief	6–24 months, or until the skills are mastered	Until the pleasures of sobriety are greater than the pleasures of using	A lifetime	As needed	6–18 months, or until you decide that this goal is not for you

Emphasis on Social Support	None	Moderate	Strong	Essential	Strong	Moderate
Spiritual/Religious Emphasis	None	Optional	None	Essential	Strong	Optional
Suggested No. of Meetings per Week	None	1–3	2–3	Daily	1–3	1–2
Group Size	0	5–15	5–15	2–100s	5–15	5–15
Drugs/Alcohol	Both	Both	Mainly alcohol	Both	Mainly alcohol	Only alcohol
Cost	Books and trainings	Donations	Donations	Donations	Donations	Donations
Effectiveness	Has not been scientifically tested	Techniques proven to be effective	Has not been scientifically tested	Effective for 5–15 percent of abusers	Has not been scientifically tested	Proven effective for early stage problem drinkers
Availability	0 groups	250 groups nationally	300 groups nationally	Very available	250 groups nationally	15 groups nationally

Online Guided Self-Change Programs

Behavioral Self-Control Program for Windows

This is an interactive software program for alcohol moderation training that consists of eight computer-assisted sessions. It gives you individualized feedback and helps you assess your chances of succeeding at moderation, shows you how to set up rewards for yourself, deal with triggers, etc. The single-user version (there is also one for therapists) is listed at $45 plus $10 s/h within the United States, $20 outside the United States.

Drinker's Check-Up (also works with drugs)

Another interactive software program for assessment, feedback, and decision making about your alcohol use, as well as secondary information about drug use. (Download program from *rhester@behaviortherapy.com*)

Reid Hester, PhD
Behavior Therapy Associates
3810 Osuna Road NE, Suite 1
Albuquerque, NM 87109
505-345-6100

Informational Websites

Treatment

- *www.habitsmart.com*—Alternative resources and theory, plus links to relevant sites.
- *www.killthecraving.com*—Information about ERP (Exposure Response Prevention).
- *www.peele.net*—Stanton Peele's alternative approach to addiction. His site has articles, a question-and-answer section, as well as information on books by Peele and other authors.

Needle Exchange

- *www.nasen.org*—Supports needle exchange as a valid way to stop the transmission of blood-borne pathogens in IV drug-using communities. Also has links to people all over the country doing practical public health, and provides information about their NEX (Needle EXchange) conference (which has been canceled for 2003).
- *www.needleexchange.com*—Santa Cruz County Needle Exchange Program with information on youth-related harm reduction approaches and drop-in sites.

Pain

- *www.paincare.org*—The National Foundation for the Treatment of Pain; Joel Hochman, Executive Director.

This organization is dedicated to improving the treatment of pain, a condition that often causes people to abuse medications.

HIV

- *www.thebody.com* and *www.projectinform.com*—Information about interactions between HIV, HIV medications, and recreational drug use.

Youth

- *www.fraize.org/ufostudy*—Based in San Francisco, has information on the UFO project, a study of the risk factors and needle exchange use associated with hepatitis B and C and HIV in injection drug users under the age of thirty. Also has comprehensive referral information.
- *www.harmreduction.org/YOUTH1.html*—National list of organizations that provide harm reduction-based youth services from the Needle Exchange Youth Caucus, a work in progress.
- *www.hify.org*—Health Initiatives for Youth, good information with resources for sale (health-related youth zines, among other information), as well as youth-health education workshops and links to other youth-specific sites.
- *www.safety1st.org*—Information for parents who want to be educated about how to talk to their kids regarding drug and alcohol use.

Family Support

- *www.fds.org.au*—The Australian National Council on Drugs sponsors the Family Drug Support Project, run by Tony Trimingham, who advocates for safer injection sites and works with families with drug-using members all over Australia.

Drugs and Safer Use

- *www.dancesafe.org*—E-zine, health tips, up-to-date pill testing results, regional contacts, lifesaving information about safer drug use and safer raving.
- *www.erowid.org*—Otherwise known as The Vaults of EROWID, contains comprehensive information on just about any drug you can think of, with stories from users about their experiences of various drugs.
- *www.drugpolicy.org/library/bibliography/driving/index.cfm*—Information about marijuana and driving; search the main site for more information about drugs.
- *www.ravesafe.org*—South African site, very big, with lots of information, such as specific drug information, safety tips, and a question-and-answer section.
- *www.partysafe.org*—Health advisory information, hepatitis A and B vaccine information, and ecstasy testing kits for purchase.

Policy and Criminal Justice

- *www.sentencingproject.org*—Statistics and reports on the impact of criminal justice policies in the United States, with special sections on drug policy and racial inequities.
- *www.drugpolicy.org*—In addition to information and publications on drug policy, the Drug Policy Alliance has a large library and online "bookstore."

SOURCES AND SUGGESTED READINGS IN HARM REDUCTION

Self-Help Books

(*Highly recommended.)

The Addiction Workbook: A Step-by-Step Guide to Quitting Alcohol and Drugs. Patrick Fanning and John O'Neill. New Harbinger. 1996.

The Angry Book. Theodore Rubin. Simon & Schuster. 1998.

The Anxiety & Phobia Workbook. Edmund Bourne. New Harbinger. 1995

Changing for Good. James Prochaska, Carlo DiClemente, and John Norcross. Avon Books. 1994

Getting Off Right: A Safety Manual for Injection Drug Users. Rod Sorge and Sara Kershnar. Harm Reduction Coalition. 1998.

Getting Real about Teens and Drugs: A Practical Guide [brochure]. Rodney Skager and Marsha Rosenbaum. Drug Policy Alliance.

How To Quit Drinking without AA. Jerry Dorsman. New Dawn. 1991.

Kill the Craving: How to Control the Impulse to Use Drugs and Alcohol. Joseph Santaro, Robert Deletis, and Alfred Bergman. New Harbinger. 2001.

The Miracle Method: A Radically New Approach to Problem Drinking. Scott Miller and Insoo Kim Berg. Norton. 1995.

Problem Drinking. Nick Heather and Ian Robertson. Oxford University Press. 1997.

Resisting 12-Step Coercion: How to Fight Forced Participation in AA, NA, or 12-Step Treatment. Stanton Peele, Charles Bufe, and Archie Brodsky. SeeSharp Press. 2000.

Responsible Drinking: A Moderation Management Approach for Problem Drinkers. Fred Rotgers, Marc Kern, and Rudy Hoeltzel. New Harbinger. 2002.

Safety First: A Reality-Based Approach to Teens, Drugs and Drug Education [brochure]. Marsha Rosenbaum. Drug Policy Alliance. 2002.

7 Weeks to Safe Social Drinking: How to Effectively Moderate Your Alcohol Intake. D. J. Cornett. Universe. 2001.

The Small Book (rev.). Jack Trimpey. Dell. 1992.

Sober for Good: New Solutions for Drinking Problems—Advice from Those Who Have Succeeded. Anne Fletcher. Houghton Mifflin. 2002.

Sobriety Demystified: Getting Clean and Sober with NLP and CBT. Byron Lewis. Kelsey & Co. 1996.

The Soul of Recovery: Uncovering the Spiritual Dimension in the Treatment of Addictions. Christopher Ringwald. Oxford University Press. 2002. (There is a chapter about harm reduction.)

*The Straight Dope Education Series [brochures]. Harm Reduction Coalition. 2001.

Take Control Now! A Do It Yourself Blueprint for Positive Lifestyle Success. Marc Frederick Kern. Life Skills Management Publishing. 1994.

The Thinking Person's Guide to Sobriety. Bert Pluymen. Bright Books. 1996.

*The Truth about Addiction and Recovery. Stanton Peele. Simon & Schuster. 1991.

You Can Free Yourself from Alcohol and Drugs: Work a Program That Keeps You in Charge. Doug Althauser. New Harbinger. 1998.

Alcohol, Drugs, and Pharmacology

(*Highly recommended.)

Benzodiazepine Dependence, Toxicity, and Abuse. A Task Force Report of the American Psychiatric Association. 1990. (technical)

"Benzodiazepine Treatment of Anxiety or Insomnia in Substance Abuse Patients." Domenic Ciraulo and Edgar Nace. *American Journal on Addictions, 9*(4), 276–284, 2000. (technical)

*Buzzed: The Straight Facts about the Most Used and Abused Drugs from Alcohol to Ecstasy. Cynthia Kuhn, Scott Swartzwelder, and Wilkie Wilson. Norton. 1998.

Clinical Handbook of Psychotropic Drugs (12th ed.). Kalyna Bezchlibnyk-Butler and J. Joel Jeffries. Seattle. Hogrefe & Huber. 2002. (technical)

Clinical Pharmacology Made Ridiculously Simple. James Olson. MedMaster. 1994. (technical)

Drugs, Behavior, and Modern Society. Charles Levinthal. Allyn & Bacon. 2002.

Drugs and the Brain. Solomon Snyder. Scientific American Library. 1996. (somewhat technical)

Essential Psychopharmacology: Neuroscientific Basis and Practical Applications (2nd ed.). Stephen M. Stahl. Cambridge University Press. 2000. (technical)

*From Chocolate to Morphine. Andrew Weil and Winifred Rosen. Houghton Mifflin. 1993.

A General Theory of Love. Thomas Lewis, Fari Amini, and Richard Lannon. Random House. 2000.

How to Stop Time: Heroin from A to Z. Ann Marlowe. New York: Basic Books. 1999.

*Marijuana Myths, Marijuana Facts: A Review of Scientific Evidence. Lynn Zimmer and John Morgan. The Lindesmith Center (now the Drug Policy Alliance). 1997.

Molecules of Emotion: The Science Behind Mind–Body Medicine. Candace Pert. Touchstone. 1997.

Naltrexone and Alcoholism Treatment. SAMHSA Center for Substance Abuse Treatment. Treatment Improvement Protocol #28. 2002. (technical)

Nicotine. Joy Schmitz, Murray Jarvik, and Nina Schneider. In Joyce Lowinson, Pedro Ruiz, Robert Millman, and John Langrod, Eds. Substance Abuse: A Comprehensive Textbook (3rd ed.). Williams & Wilkens. 1997.

Pain and Its Relief without Addiction: Clinical Issues in the Use of Opioids and Other Analgesics. Barry Stimmel. Haworth Medical Press. 1997. (technical)

Pharmacotheon: Entheogenic Drugs, Their Plant Sources and History. Jonathan Ott. Natural Products. 1996.

*A Primer of Drug Action: A Concise, Nontechnical Guide to the Actions, Uses, and Side Effects of Psychoactive Drugs (rev.). Robert Julian. Holt. 2001.

*The Pursuit of Oblivion: A Global History of Narcotics. Richard Davenport-Hines. Norton. 2002.

*Sisters of the Extreme: Women Writing on the Drug Experience. Cynthia Palmer and Michael Horowitz, Eds. Park Street Press. 2000.

Uppers, Downers, All Arounders (3rd ed.). Darryl Inaba, William Cohen, and Michael Holstein. CNS Publications. 1997.

The User's Voice, published by The John Mordaunt Trust, c/o Drugscope, 32–36 Loman St. London, SE1 OEE. Or e-mail them at usersvoice.jmt@drugscope.org (This is a newsletter that gives specific information on drug use, policy, and drug safety; see the March–April 2002 issue for marijuana tips.)

Harm Reduction and Other Treatment Resources

(*Highly recommended.)

"Diana: The Fear of Feelings and the Love of Wine." Patt Denning. In Andrew Tatarsky, Ed. Harm Reduction Psychotherapy: A New Treatment for Alcohol and Drug Problems. Aronson. 2002.

"Effective AIDS Prevention with Active Drug Users: The Harm Reduction Model." Edith Springer. In Michael Shernoff, Guest Ed. Counseling Chemically Dependent People with HIV Illness. Journal of Chemical Dependency Treatment, 4, 141–157, 1991.

Handbook of Alcoholism Treatment Approaches: Effective Alternatives (3rd ed.). Reid Hester and William Miller, Eds. Allyn & Bacon. 2003.

"Harm Reduction Group Therapy: The Sobriety Support Group." Jeannie Little. In Andrew Tatarsky, Ed. Harm Reduction Psychotherapy: A New Treatment for Drug and Alcohol Problems. Aronson. 2002.

*"Harm Reduction in Mental Health: The Emerging Work of Harm Reduction Psycho-

therapy." In Patt Denning and Jeannie Little, Eds. *Harm Reduction Communication*. Harm Reduction Coalition. Spring 2001.

Harm Reduction: Pragmatic Strategies for Managing High-Risk Behaviors. G. Alan Marlatt, Ed. Guilford Press. 1998.

Harm Reduction Psychotherapy: A New Treatment for Drug and Alcohol Problems. Andrew Tatarsky, Ed. Jason Aronson. 2002.

"Harm Reduction Psychotherapy Makes Clinical Intervention More Effective." Patt Denning. *The National Psychologist*—Special section on addictions, *9*(4), 4–5B, 2000.

"Harm Reduction: Reducing the Risks of Addictive Behaviors." G. Alan Marlatt and Susan F. Tapert. In John S. Baer, G. Alan Marlatt, and Robert J. McMahon, Eds. *Addictive Behaviors across the Lifespan: Prevention, Treatment and Policy Issues*. Sage. 1993.

Motivational Interviewing: Preparing People for Change (2nd ed.). William R. Miller and Stephen Rollnick. Guilford Press. 2003.

Practicing Harm Reduction Psychotherapy: An Alternative Approach to Addictions. Patt Denning. Guilford Press. 2000.

Recovery Options: The Complete Guide. Joseph Volpicelli and Maia Szalavitz. Wiley. 2000.

"Strategies for Implementation of Harm Reduction in Treatment Settings." Patt Denning. *Journal of Psychoactive Drugs, 33*(1), 23–26, 2001.

"Therapeutic Interventions for Individuals with Substance Use, HIV, and Personality Disorders: Harm Reduction as a Unifying Approach." Patt Denning. *In Session: Psychotherapy in Practice, 4*(1), 37–52. 1998.

Treating Substance Abuse: Theory and Technique (2nd ed.). Frederick Rotgers, Daniel S. Keller, and Jon Morgenstern, Eds. Guilford Press. 2003.

"Warm Turkey: Other Routes to Abstinence." William Miller and A. C. Page. *Journal of Substance Abuse Treatment, 8*, 227–232. 1991.

Theory and Research about Drug Use, Abuse, Treatment, and Related Issues

(*Highly recommended.)

"Acupuncture as an Adjunct to Methadone Treatment Services." Elizabeth Wells, Ron Jackson, O. Rachel Diaz, et al. *American Journal on Addictions, 4*(3), 98–214. 1995.

Affect Regulation and the Origin of the Self. Allan Schore. Erlbaum. 1994. (technical)

"The Codependency Movement: Issues of Context and Differentiation." Judith R. Gordon and Kimberly Barrett. In John S Baer, G. Alan Marlatt, and Robert J. McMahon, Eds. *Addictive Behaviors Across the Lifespan: Prevention, Treatment, and Policy Issues*. Sage. 1993.

"Contemporary Psychoanalytic Theories of Substance Abuse: A Disorder in Search of a Paradigm." Jon Morgenstern and Jeremy Leeds. *Psychotherapy*, 30, 194–206. 1993. (technical)

Creating the Capacity for Attachment: Treating Addictions and the Alienated Self. Karen Walant. Aronson. 1995. (technical)

Decision Making. I. Janis and L. Mann. Free Press. 1977. (technical)

Drug, Set, and Setting: The Basis for Controlled Intoxicant Use. Norman E. Zinberg. Yale University Press. 1984.

Evidence Based Research on the Efficacy of Needle Exchange Programs: An Overview. Eric P. Goosby, Special Assistant to the Director, National AIDS Policy Office, White House. San Francisco Department of Public Health. 2001.

Harm Reduction: A New Direction for Drug Policies and Programs. Patricia G. Erickson, Diane M. Riley, Yuet W. Cheung, and Patrick O'Hare, Eds. University of Toronto Press. 1997.

"How Drug Users Measure Success in a Harm Reduction Setting." Terry Ruefli and Susan Rogers. In Ernie Drucker, Ed. *Harm Reduction* (on-line journal). 2003.

"Matching Alcoholism Treatments to Client Heterogeneity: Project MATCH Posttreatment Drinking Outcomes." Project MATCH Research Group. *Journal of Studies on Alcohol, 58*, 7–29. 1997. (You can look at all of the results of this major study by doing a web search with keyword Project MATCH; technical.)

The National Household Survey on Drug Abuse. The U.S. Substance Abuse and Mental Health Services Administration (SAMHSA), *www.samhsa.gov/oas/nhsda.*

"The Natural History of Drug Use from Adolescence to the Mid-Thirties in a General Population Sample." L. Chen and D. Kandal. *American Journal of Public Health, 85*, 41–47, 1995. (technical)

One Hundred Years of Heroin. David Musto, Ed. Auburn House. 2002.

Relapse Prevention. G. Alan Marlatt and Judith R. Gordon, Eds. Guilford Press. 1985. (See, especially, the section on the abstinence violation effect, or the "what the hell" effect, pp. 41–43, and the section on alcohol expectancies, the tendency to experience different effects because of expectation rather than the biological effects of alcohol, pp. 137–150; technical.)

"Roles of Drinking Pattern and Type of Alcohol Consumed in Coronary Heart Disease in Men." Kenneth Mukamal et. al. *The New England Journal of Medicine, 348*, 109–118. Jan. 9, 2003. (technical)

The Self-Medication Hypothesis of Substance Use Disorders: A Reconsideration and Recent Applications. Edward Khantzian. *Harvard Review of Psychiatry, 4*, 231–244. 1997. (technical)

*"A Life-Span Perspective on Natural Recovery (Self-Change) from Alcohol Problems." L. C. Sobell, J. A. Cunningham, M. B. Sobell, and T. Toneatto (pp. 34–68). In John S. Baer, G. Alan Marlatt, and Robert J. McMahon, Eds. *Addictive Behaviors across the Lifespan: Prevention, Treatment and Policy Issues.* Sage. 1993. (technical)

RAND Corporation Drug Research Policy Center. There are many studies about drugs and alcohol and their social impact available on this website: *www.rand.org/ centers/dprc/DPRCpubindex.html*.

Services Research Outcome Study (1998) and other treatment outcome data sources. Substance Abuse and Mental Health Services Administration, Office of Applied Studies. *www.samhsa.gov*.

"Similarity of Outcome Predictors Across Opiate, Cocaine, and Alcohol Treatments: Role of Treatment Services." A. Thomas McLellan et al. In G. Alan Marlatt and G. VandenBos, Eds. *Addictive Behaviors: Readings on Etiology, Prevention, and Treatment*. American Psychological Association. 1997. (technical)

Substance Abuse: A Comprehensive Textbook. Joyce Lowinson, Pedro Ruiz, Robert Millman, and John Langrod, Eds. Williams & Wilkins. 1997.

Toward a Psychology of Being. Abraham Maslow. VanNostrand. 1962.

Trauma and Recovery. Judith Herman. Basic Books. 1997.

Traumatic Stress: The Effects of Overwhelming Experience on Mind, Body, and Society. Bessel van der Kolk, Alexander C. McFarlane, and Lars Weisaeth, Eds. Guilford Press. 1996.

Critiques of the Disease Model, U.S. Drug Policy, and Treatment

(These are all great.)

Alcoholics Anonymous: Cult or Cure? Charles Bufe. SeeSharp Press. 1991.

The American Disease: Origins of Narcotic Control. David Musto. Oxford University Press. 1987.

The Awareness Trap: Self Absorption Instead of Social Change. Edwin Schur. McGraw-Hill. 1976.

Becoming Alcoholic: Alcoholics Anonymous and the Reality of Alcoholism. Rudy David. Southern Illinois University Press. 1986.

"The Disease and Adaptive Models of Addiction: A Framework Evaluation." Bruce Alexander. *Journal of Drug Issues, 17*(1), 47–66. 1987. (technical)

"The Disease Controversy: Of Myths, Maps, and Metaphors." Howard Shaffer. *Journal of Psychoactive Drugs, 17*(2), 65–76. 1985. (technical)

The Diseasing of America: Drug Treatment Out of Control. Stanton Peele. Lexington Books. 1989.

Drug Crazy: How We Got into This Mess and How We Can Get Out. Mike Gray. Routledge. 1998.

Drug Policy and the Criminal Justice System. The Sentencing Project. 2001. All sentencing policy publications can be obtained on their website: *www. sentencingproject.org*.

General Accounting Office. For a government report on the effectiveness of the DARE program of youth drug prevention, see their website: *www.gao.gov/new.items/ d03172r.pdf.*

Heavy Drinking: The Myth of Alcoholism as a Disease. Herbert Fingarette. University of California Press. 1988.

Hooked: Five Addicts Challenge Our Misguided Drug Rehab System. Lonny Shavelson. New Press. 2001.

I'm Dysfunctional, You're Dysfunctional: The Recovery Movement and Other Self-Help Fashions. Wendy Kaminer. Addison-Wesley. 1992.

INDEX

ABOUT THE AUTHORS

Patt Denning, PhD, Director of Clinical Services and Training of the Harm Reduction Therapy Center (San Francisco), is a licensed clinical psychologist. Beginning in 1972, she worked first in special education and then with mentally ill and substance-abusing people. In San Francisco she was a program director in residential treatment for people with schizophrenia and then worked with multiply diagnosed people as the director of a mental health outpatient team in a public health clinic serving a heavily HIV-affected community. Since 1993 she has been in private practice, working with people with a variety of emotional problems and those who need specialized help with their drug and alcohol problems. Dr. Denning has served on the faculty of two schools of psychology and is a Diplomate-Fellow in psychopharmacology. She holds a specialist certificate from the American Psychological Association's College of Professional Psychology in the treatment of substance use disorders and is widely recognized as an expert in both drug treatment and dual diagnosis. She is one of the main developers of harm reduction psychotherapy in the United States, trains professionals around the country, and has been named a media expert on dual diagnosis by the Partnership for Responsible Drug Information. Dr. Denning is the author of *Practicing Harm Reduction Psychotherapy: An Alternative Approach to Addictions*, as well as other publications on multiply diagnosed people.

Jeannie Little, LCSW, Executive Director of the Harm Reduction Therapy Center, is a licensed clinical social worker and certified group psychotherapist with 25 years' experience working in domestic violence, with families and children, with mentally ill adults, with drug users, and with homeless persons. As a therapist and in program management, she specializes in group therapy: she has developed a group program for homeless mentally ill substance users as well as long-term therapy groups for people with emotional and drug and alcohol issues. She trains other professionals on the topics of chemical dependency, dual diagnosis, harm reduction, and group treatment of substance abuse. She also provides ongoing consultation to numerous staff groups in outpatient clinics, outreach and drop-in centers, case-management programs, and housing facilities for multiply diagnosed clients. Ms. Little is the author of a book chapter and papers about therapeutic groups and harm reduction for dually diagnosed people.

Adina Glickman, LCSW, is a licensed clinical social worker with 15 years' experience working with adults with emotional as well as drug and alcohol problems. She is the Assistant Director for Peer and Academic Support at Stanford University, where she teaches courses in critical thinking and learning skills. While she is relatively new to harm reduction as a formal model, its basic principles have guided her since the beginning of her work as a therapist. She maintains a small private therapy practice in the San Francisco Bay area. In addition to her academic affiliation, she is also a writer, with several completed screenplays and three novels in progress.